AN UNGOVERNABLE FOE

AN UNGOVERNABLE FOE

*Science and Policy Innovation in
the U.S. National Cancer Institute*

NATALIE B. AVILES

Columbia University Press
New York

Columbia University Press
Publishers Since 1893
New York   Chichester, West Sussex
cup.columbia.edu

Copyright © 2024 Columbia University Press

Library of Congress Cataloging-in-Publication Data
Names: Aviles, Natalie B., author.
Title: An ungovernable foe : science and policy innovation in the
   U.S. National Cancer Institute / Natalie B. Aviles.
Description: New York : Columbia University Press, [2023] |
   Includes bibliographical references and index.
Identifiers: LCCN 2023040158 | ISBN 9780231196680 (hardback) |
   ISBN 9780231196697 (trade paperback) | ISBN 9780231551779 (ebook)
Subjects: MESH: National Cancer Institute (U.S.) | Neoplasms—prevention & control |
   Biomedical Research—history | United States Government Agencies—history |
   Health Policy—history | United States
Classification: LCC RC262 | NLM QZ 24 | DDC 362.19699/4—dc23/eng/20231002
LC record available at https://lccn.loc.gov/2023040158

Cover design: Elliott S. Cairns

CONTENTS

ACKNOWLEDGMENTS

An *Ungovernable Foe* has benefited tremendously from the contributions and support of a great and generous community of scholars. I have gained so much from so many relationships I developed over the many years it took to complete this project and regret that they are too numerous to acknowledge individually. Yet my success in completing this manuscript would not have been possible without the effort and input of those individuals. I acknowledge any errors or omissions herein as entirely my own.

The book before you began as an ambitious and wrong-headed dissertation that was tempered and put right by the efforts of an expansive and indefatigable community of scholars. Foremost, I thank my dissertation committee: Rick Biernacki, Cathy Gere, Tal Golan, Jeff Haydu, Martha Lampland, and Charlie Thorpe. They helped birth this project many years ago, and I hope they are pleased by how it has grown. The support I received from them and many others among the faculty and graduate students in the Department of Sociology and Science Studies Program at the University of California–San Diego (UCSD) made data collection for this project possible. I also thank Neil Gross and my colleagues in the Department of Sociology at Colby College, as well as colleagues in the Department of Sociology at Yale University and the University of Virginia, for supporting the subsequent development of this work intellectually and financially. Special thanks are due to the staff of these departments, including Nadine Amalfi, Beverly Bernhardt, Manny de la Paz, Joyce Holleran, Leslie Lima, Katrina Richards, Katherine Shiflett, and Susan Taniguchi.

I thank various interlocutors for their feedback on early drafts of the work that has matured into what you see in this book. Robin Scheffler has been an enthusiastic and supportive colleague and coauthor, and our collaboration was indispensable in allowing me to develop the theoretical framing of this book. Isaac Reed first sparked my interest in principal-agent models at the Radcliffe pragmatism conference in 2017, and Shan Aman Rana helped me develop this interest by engaging it from an economist's perspective. I am grateful for the special attention shown to early work by audiences at the 2015 Junior Theorists Symposium; 2015 UC San Francisco Biomedical Knowledge Working Group; 2017 Radcliffe Conference on Sociology and Pragmatism; 2017 Harvard Science and Democracy Network Conference; 2018 Yale Conference on Policy, Politics and Law of Cancer's History of Cancer Workshop; 2018 Initiative for Historical Social Science workshop at SUNY Stony Brook; 2019 Yale Comparative Research and Center for Cultural Sociology Workshops; 2021 TEMPO workshop at UVA; and 2022 SWAMP workshop at UVA. Attendees of several annual meetings of the American Sociological Association and the Society for Social Studies of Science also helped shape this project over the years.

I owe a great debt to the countless individual scholars who helped me think through this project over the years. In alphabetical order, I wish to thank: Jeff Alexander; Wisam Alshaibi; Jenn Bair; Michael Barany; Kevin Beck; Amy Binder; Vicki Bonnell; Rose Buckelew; Stan Chodorow; Nicole Denier; Monica Do; Steve Epstein; Nikolle Esteban; Jill Fisher; Brian Foster; Joan Fujimura; Danielle Giffort; Fiona Greenland; Harvey Goldman; Dan Hirschman; Carly Knight; Anurika Kumar; Gary Lee; Moran Levy; Kevin Lewis; Mary Lunn; Leigh Mante; Isaac Martin; Damon Mayrl; Megan McKenna; Chandra Mukerji; Dan Navon; Kwai Ng; Kelly Nielsen; J. P. Pardo-Guerra; Marcos and Lindsey Perez; Andy Perrin; Simone Polillo; Danielle Raudenbush; Josipa Roksa; Akos Rona-Tas; Joseph Rouse; Lauren Ruddy; Tad Skotnicki; Adam Slez; Iddo Tavory; Christena Turner; Janet Vertesi; Yingyao Wang; Josh Whitford; Nick Wilson; Chris Winship; and Patrice Wright. I deeply regret if I have neglected to include the names of anyone who aided or supported this project over the years and hope they see their contributions reflected in the text.

I was privileged to dig deeply into the archives thanks to the generous funding provided by the UCSD Department of Sociology and Science Studies Program. Mop-up work was also supported by funding from the Departments of Sociology at Colby College and Yale University. Other funding and support for the research and writing of this manuscript was provided by the Dean of Social Sciences and Center for the Humanities at UCSD; the University of California President's Dissertation-Year Fellowship; the Yale University Presidential Visiting Fellowship;

and the Department of Sociology at the University of Virginia. I am also grateful to the networks of graduate students and friends who provided company and hospitality during my time in the archives, especially Brandi Bernoskie, Cathy Collins, Pat Nighswander, Brenda Nishimura, and Eric van Rite. I give deep personal thanks to Doug Lowy and John Schiller for their oral history interviews and thank the historians and archivists who conducted the archived oral histories and preserved the documents that made this labor possible. Heartfelt thanks go to Barbara Harkins at the Office of NIH History; Judy Grosberg and Bridget Launi at the National Cancer Institute; Stephen Greenberg at the History of Medicine Division of the National Library of Medicine; Vanessa Mitchell and Sara Striner at the Library of Congress; and Tab Lewis at the National Archives and Records Administration at College Park. I am also incredibly grateful for the work of the many librarians, archivists, and staff members at these institutions. While too numerous to name individually, they each provided invaluable aid over the year and a half that I spent collecting the data referenced in this book.

I also thank Eric Schwartz and his team at Columbia University Press. Eric has been enormously supportive of this project and particularly gracious as I struggled to bring this book to fruition throughout the COVID-19 pandemic. Three anonymous reviewers offered invaluable advice on the manuscript for the Press, and I credit them with its improvement. Two chapters in this book appeared in print in modified form; I thank Sergio Sismondo and the anonymous reviewers at *Social Studies of Science* as well as Ed Hackett and the anonymous reviewers at *Science, Technology, & Human Values* for their feedback on these earlier versions.

Finally, I acknowledge and honor the family without whom I could not have accomplished this task. I am grateful for the limitless support of my husband, Ian, who took on so much labor to clear the space I needed to succeed in this and so many other things. A talented political sociologist in his own right, he also spurred this book in new theoretical directions, and it would not be the work that it is without his intellectual engagement and encouragement. I dedicate this book to him, and to our daughter, Lucrecia, who has given me something to strive for always. I also honor my father, Ernesto, and grandmother, Guadalupe, whose sacrifices in raising me made my future possible. Much love goes out to my brother, Alex, and Uncle Dan and Aunt Christina who have always been there to celebrate my accomplishments. I have also benefited from the support of my four-legged family members. My cats, Nimbus and Shale, by turns offered the enthusiastic embraces and judgmental indifference that kept reviewers' comments at the forefront of revisions. Shortly before completing this manuscript, my most stalwart companion in its production, Peanut, was diagnosed with a terminal hemangiosarcoma and died at the age of eleven. This book is also dedicated to her constant canine companionship, the loss of which brought home the ubiquitous tragedy of cancer in new and unexpected ways.

Some of the analysis included in chapter 3 was published in 2022 as "State Planning, Cancer Vaccine Infrastructure, and the Origins of the Oncogene Hypothesis," coauthored with Robin W. Scheffler, in *Social Studies of Science* 52 (2). A version of chapter 6 was published in 2018 as "Situated Practice and the Emergence of Ethical Research: HPV Vaccine Development and Organizational Cultures of Translation at the National Cancer Institute" in *Science, Technology, & Human Values* 43 (5).

AN UNGOVERNABLE FOE

INTRODUCTION

I n the first decades of the twenty-first century, cancer still reigns as the "emperor of all maladies."[1] In the United States, the average risk of being diagnosed with cancer at some point in one's life is 40 percent, and the average risk of dying from cancer is nearly 20 percent.[2] Although many Americans continue to navigate the cancer experience as an individualized medical drama, they do so in a cultural, political, and economic landscape that has come to view cancer as a *social* problem as well.[3] Almost a century ago, cancer became subject to some of the same collective interventions as many other vexing social problems of the era. Politicians began to worry over how cancer was affecting their constituents. Wealthy elites prioritized cancer as a target for philanthropic funding. Citizens affected by cancer mobilized to raise awareness and seed the scientific efforts that might one day eradicate the scourge. As the Great Depression eased, politicians emboldened by the New Deal's successes in improving social welfare created a federal agency that could bring the strength and will of the American government to bear on this terrible disease.

What does it mean to say cancer is a social problem today? There are different possible versions of the answer. For many, this has meant that environmental or industrial regulation is needed and that legal recourse should be made available to those who suffer from cancers brought on by deliberate exposure or malign neglect of state and private actors. Yet since the twentieth century, cancer has also been framed as a problem of scientific stewardship requiring national coordination and state governance. Though specific policy solutions to this problem have subsequently varied, their origins in the political environment of the 1940s continue to shape the general approach to scientific and policy problem solving still in use today. In this work of historical sociology,

I chronicle how agents employed in the intramural research program of the U.S. National Cancer Institute (NCI) developed distinctive approaches to solving the problem of cancer governance by innovating in the public interest. I aim to show how the institute's dual mission to fund cutting-edge science and improve the nation's health influenced these government researchers' scientific and bureaucratic practices in ways that shaped some of the most significant innovations in both cancer research policy and public health–oriented breakthroughs of the past seventy years. Focusing particularly on the unexpected case of cancer virus and vaccine research, I show how NCI agents' attempts to govern the nation's cancer effort under the watchful eye of Congress and advisors from the broader scientific community shaped how they conceptualized their own research agendas. In their mutual influence, NCI actors' scientific and bureaucratic tasks helped make the institute a leader in both science and policy, and their success serves as an important exemplar of how state bureaucracies help shape the social, political, and economic ecologies in which they perform their administrative functions.

THE NATIONAL CANCER INSTITUTE

The National Cancer Institute is the largest single patron of cancer research in the United States and around the globe.[4] When it was first established by the National Cancer Act of 1937, the NCI was chartered "for the purposes of conducting researches, investigations, experiments, and studies relating to the cause, diagnosis, and treatment of cancer; assisting and fostering similar research activities by other agencies, public and private; and promoting the coordination of all such researches and activities and the useful application of their results, with a view to the development and prompt widespread use of the most effective methods of prevention, diagnosis, and treatment of cancer."[5]

In 1944, the NCI was the first agency to branch off from the federal National Institute of Health, and its birth transformed that young bureau into the plural National Institutes of Health (NIH) as we know it today. As a component of the Public Health Service (PHS), the NCI was designed as a categorical, or single-disease-oriented, organization within the NIH and given a dual mission: first, "to seek fundamental knowledge about the nature and behavior of living systems" and, second, to ensure "the application of that knowledge to enhance health, lengthen life, and reduce illness and disability."[6] The need to realize this dual mission in scientific policy and practice motivated the NCI's approach to governance across several permutations throughout the twentieth century and continues to motivate the institute's approach in the twenty-first century.

Though its dual mission remains consistent, much has changed in the NCI since the time of its founding. In its youth the majority of the institute's research budget was allocated to intramural, or in-house, research conducted in a small confederation of federal laboratories and hospitals. But beginning in the late 1940s, the NCI benefited from an influx of funds that exponentially expanded its ability to fund extramural, or external, scientists in academic and nonprofit organizations. By the 1960s, the institute had come to resemble what we recognize as the modern NCI. The institute is now characterized by a diversity of intramural scientific efforts, ranging from laboratory inquiry to clinical research and epidemiology, conducted in laboratories and clinics spanning the Bethesda campus of the NIH and beyond; extramural grants supporting thousands of cancer researchers, teams, and centers in universities, hospitals, research institutes, and even small businesses across the United States and around the globe; both intramural and extramural support for studies that traverse the research spectrum from curiosity-driven research to clinical application; and approaches to organizing the national cancer research effort that range from undirected inquiry to directed research. In 2019, the NCI's budget totaled just over US$6 billion, of which more than US$4.5 billion was allocated to sponsor extramural cancer research in independent universities and nonprofits and just under US$1 billion allocated to intramural laboratories and clinics.

Though today the NCI is best known for its role in providing grants to academic researchers studying fundamental biological mechanisms and testing clinical treatments for cancer, one of the most fascinating and theoretically fruitful dimensions of the National Cancer Institute's innovation history can be found in the development of expertise in cancer virus research and vaccine development among the institute's own intramural researchers. From a technical perspective, it hardly seems natural or necessary that the NCI—as opposed, for instance, to its sibling National Institute of Allergy and Infectious Diseases (NIAID)—would have been a pioneering institute in virology and vaccinology. Cancer continues to be understood primarily as a degenerative disease necessitating personalized therapy, the kind of condition traditionally characterized *in opposition* to infectious disease and broad-based public health initiatives.[7] Yet there were numerous historical contingencies that led NCI scientists to develop expertise in virus research and vaccine development in response to the agency's mission to understand and eradicate cancer. It is thus instructive to analyze the development of virus and vaccine research competencies in the NCI as an unexpected and theoretically illuminating case of organizational innovation in an expert federal bureaucracy.

It may also be surprising that a federal bureaucracy can serve as a source of scientific and organizational innovation. If the NCI and other preeminent national institutes are any indication, career scientists in the federal government hardly deserve the reputation of federal bureaucrats as being stodgy and intellectually flaccid deadwood. Popular antipathy toward bureaucracy and antistatist suspicion about federal officials are common in American culture, but they are also mirrored in economic models that presuppose monetary incentives are the driving force behind labor-market distribution of scientists in academia, industry, and government. These models assume that the low possibility of monetary reward for experimental excellence in government laboratories would drive all but the most mediocre of scientists to prefer more lucrative alternatives in academia or the private sector over government toil.[8] Government scientists do have lower median salaries than those available at universities or firms and few opportunities for variable pay, so there appears to be little to motivate them to push the envelope in their research. Yet time and again, career NCI scientists can be found among the vanguard of the most innovative biomedical research subjects.

The apparent paradox that boundary-pushing and high-impact research emanates from the laboratories of government scientists illustrates the importance of considering the role *nonmonetary* incentives play in encouraging scientific innovation. Career public servants who find the social value of their work rewarding in and of itself may willingly forego opportunities to earn higher incomes in order to continue working in organizations that prioritize the public interest. Purposeful, driven, and invested in the public good, career NCI scientists seem to defy popular models of entrepreneurialism in biomedicine. The success of the NCI in virus and vaccine innovation thus invites us to reconsider some of our common assumptions about the role the state plays in the development of biomedical breakthroughs.

STATE BUREAUCRACY AND SCIENTIFIC INNOVATION

The first step toward appreciating the innovativeness of NCI scientists involves acknowledging the diversity of state bureaucracies in the United States and the NCI's distinctiveness among them. Contemporary sociologists now take it as a truism that the state is a fragmented rather than unitary agent.[9] Theorizing the distributed nature of governance in the contemporary United States shifts explanations of power closer to the characteristic structure of political organization as it is dispersed among the federal judicial, legislative, and executive branches and the machineries of state and local government. Alongside this injunction to reimagine the fragmented state is a similar reconsideration of state capacity. Once treated as a coercive tax-and-spend apparatus emerging from considerations of war and domestic regulation, the productive capacities of the state are now conceptualized by contemporary thinkers as seats of power and prosperity.[10] Thus, alongside foundational studies that addressed the role science and technology played in the emergence of the early modern state,[11] scholars now note that the contemporary state continues to play a prominent role in producing both scientific knowledge and the infrastructures necessary to disseminate innovations to the public.[12] Though quiescent, administrative agencies retain a central role in the political economy of science and technology in the United States.

A growing number of social scientists now endeavor to show how the state has managed to remain largely out of sight while playing such a significant role in innovation and economic growth.[13] In light of the centrality of state agencies such as the NIH to university research and the commercial pharmaceutical and biotechnology sectors, these agencies remain surprisingly undertheorized.[14] In the absence of a coherent national research policy that would make the state's productive role in innovation explicit, the structural configurations of the fragmented state operate to conceal the levers of agency-level policy making from observers more focused on market activity. As Suzanne Mettler has shown, contemporary modes of policy making that channel federal funds through nongovernmental third parties—such as grant funding for nonprofits—"obscure the role of the government and exaggerate that of the market."[15] The invisibility of government policy has perhaps encouraged a tendency to read the history of biomedical policy since the 1980s as the triumph of neoliberalism, where the state has shrunk in importance proportional to the rise of market forces driving innovation in the name of profit.[16]

This is not to suggest that the role of the state has been entirely ignored; work on science and the state has a long legacy in science and technology studies (STS).[17] STS scholars commonly deploy the concept of "coproduction" to analyze how scientific innovation interacts with and often plays a central role in projects of state building in countries such as the United States. Nevertheless, traditional STS approaches to analyzing the role of the state in scientific innovation have taken for granted that Congress, as the seat of lawmaking in the United States, is the primary driver of biomedical research policy. This legislative approach to analyzing policy has recently been challenged by studies that show it is not the congressional lawmaking process but instead the rules, procedures, and practices of agencies housed in the executive branch's expansive bureaucracy that give policies the force needed to shape the nation. The modern NCI was consolidated in precisely the historical moment when political scientists Karen Orren and Stephen Skowronek note the postwar American policy state crystalized around such semiautonomous administrative agencies, "endowing each with new resources for registering preferences in administrative operations [that] recast all of them as policy entrepreneurs." While scholars of the policy state have primarily focused on how and why Congress defers to expert bureaucrats in determining how legislation will be enacted, analysts urge us not to neglect the central significance of "other administrative instruments with important policy implications," including the minutiae of "priority allocation of resources, licensing, permitting, and planning," to the crafting of successful policies.[18] Together, these trends in policy craft and implementation within the federal government help us account for how agencies such as the National Institutes of Health can simultaneously be home to some of the largest and most innovative biomedical institutions in the United States yet be largely overlooked in a social science literature preoccupied with explaining how formal lawmaking affects market and private actors.

Thus, while coproduction has been effectively used by STS scholars to examine how institutional-level political environments for science policy help shape organizational dynamics in academia and industry, the tendency to reduce the role of government to legislative action elides the ordinary bureaucratic functions of the policy state.[19] Of notable exception is the work of Steven Epstein, whose analysis of bureaucratic procedure around the early HIV/AIDS epidemic and clinical-trial reform in the late twentieth century vividly illustrates the importance of agency-level innovations in the NIH to the development of policies that would only later be codified by Congress.[20] Epstein's empirical expositions of how agents in the NIH develop policies in response to the often competing demands of patient activists and congressional overseers and how these policies subsequently launch new "biomedical paradigms" that spread throughout the scientific community represent forebears of the current study. In analyzing the history of institutional transformations to the NCI, this study too contributes to the "new political sociology of science" that seeks to understand how the everyday practices of bureaucratic governance influence the production of science and policy alike.[21]

Reconsidering the Scientist-Bureaucrat

To better grasp how innovative science and policy emerges in the NCI, I first conceptualize the institutional dynamics structuring this bureaucracy. Though this study is firmly oriented toward sociology and STS, I find that framings of administrative policy craft from political science and economics effectively summarize the structural problematic faced by expert bureaucrats in agencies such as the NCI. These allied disciplines have conceptualized policy making in federal agencies—which are beholden to stakeholders in Congress who authorize and fund them—through the lens of principal-agent models.[22] Principal-agent models offer a stylized rendering of one of the central conundrums of accountability in democratic governance: principals (such as members of Congress) depend on more knowledgeable agents (such as bureaucrats) to enact policies, but relying on agents entails balancing the benefits of delegation against the costs of oversight. Too much oversight over agent activities consumes time and energy the principal wishes to allocate elsewhere, yet giving agents more discretion risks those agents developing policies that do not reflect the principal's best interests. When the matter at hand involves scientific policy, the distribution of expertise creates additional concerns because principals often lack the expertise to independently evaluate or hold accountable the technical products of scientists.[23] Agents possess more relevant technical knowledge necessary for making informed policies, so principals must necessarily allow far greater deference to their expertise.[24] The principal's objective, then, is to offer incentives that will motivate agents to work in optimal alignment with the principal's interests and minimize the effort they must expend monitoring said agents.

Political scientists have applied principal-agent models to federal bureaucracies to analyze how the policy state emerges from the conditions that enable bureaucrats to learn the requisite skills for designing informed policies within these agencies. As Sean Gailmard and John Patty argue, the "incentives for administrative actors to acquire policy expertise result from the organizational structure and political position they occupy as created by political principals, in particular Congress."[25] The expertise necessary to create effective policies is endogenous to bureaucracies; that is, it is the outcome of bureaucrats acquiring expertise and learning how to craft it into effective policies and procedures over time in accordance with the mission bestowed upon their agency. Based on the assumption that "policy rents," or the ability to extract more of their own policy preferences from agency rulemaking, incentivize bureaucrats to continue acquiring expertise, structuring agencies so they have greater autonomy from oversight by political principals allows bureaucrats to apply their distinct expertise to develop more innovative and effective policies than Congress would ever be capable of designing. Under this model, policy drift—where the direction of an agency's policies leans toward bureaucrats' expert preferences, possibly in departure from the preferences of their principals—is an inevitable but tolerable trade-off for agency effectiveness.[26]

In agencies such as the NCI or the other national institutes with dual missions to fund meritorious science and improve national health outcomes, policies are crafted and executed by expert scientists who are simultaneously doing science and acquiring the kind of bureaucratic expertise Gailmard and Patty identify as the basis of learning to govern in the policy state. This overlapping scientific and policy expertise can elude standard applications of the principal-agent approach. For instance, when the STS scholar David Guston applied the principal-agent perspective to analyze the NIH Office of Technology Transfer, he identified this unit as a "boundary organization" whose bureaucratic mission means that "negotiating . . . contingencies [between science and politics] becomes the organization's daily work, involving . . . a collaboration between the interests of the principals and those of the agents."[27] But working alongside the technology transfer specialists whom Guston studies, whose work is primarily bureaucratic and based on a "division of labor" that separates their "paper work" from intramural scientists' "laboratory work,"[28] is a special class of intramural scientists who are simultaneously productive biomedical researchers *and* civil servants working to manage a federal bureaucracy. To better capture the central role that these NCI intramural researchers play in shaping scientific and policy innovation, it is necessary to conceptualize how these actors come to embody both kinds of expertise. I distinguish such NCI intramural researchers from primarily bureaucratic personnel by their dual role as "scientist-bureaucrats," a construct that captures how their day-to-day lives are organized around *both* scientific and bureaucratic activities. Scientist-bureaucrats are researchers who obtain administrative positions in the institute and thus occupy organizational roles that tack back and forth between the bench and the boardroom. The concept of the scientist-bureaucrat highlights the hybridity of roles held by government-salaried scientists who participate in state policy and scientific governance in tandem with their active research agendas.

The work of scientist-bureaucrats encapsulates an approach to science and policy that reflects the dual nature of the NCI's mission and is complemented by a distinct governance structure. Unlike regulatory agencies tasked with monitoring private industry, the NCI is a policy organization and a patron of scientific research conducted partly in-house but overwhelmingly in the nonprofit sector by extramural scientists. Since its inception, the NCI has maintained an advisory apparatus inclusive of members from the broader scientific community to help fulfill its organizational mandate. While some of their functions relate to decisions around grant allocation,[29] these advisory bodies also maintain a role in governance where they help ensure the NCI's policies are technically sound and consistent with scientific judgments of quality. In their broader governance capacity, the members of the scientific public who sit on these advisory committees can more accurately be regarded as additional principals who entrust the NCI to formulate policies in accordance with their own standards of good science. Given this aspect of agency design and the fact that the degree of agency autonomy from congressional control means most policies emanating from the NCI are authored by scientist-bureaucrats in consultation with and deference to advisory boards, I argue that governance of cancer research policy is more appropriately characterized by multiple-principal models that envision the NCI as serving two masters—the broader American public as represented by principals they elect to Congress and a scientific public as represented by principals appointed to expert bodies that advise the institute.[30]

The need for NCI policies to serve the interests of both principals complexifies the problematic of agency accountability because it raises concerns that the needs of one principal may be prioritized over those of the other. Political scientist Daniel Carpenter has compellingly demonstrated through historical case studies that similar scientific bureaucracies tend to enjoy greater autonomy from congressional oversight in part because of the technical complexity of the information that substantiates their policies.[31] Though there are numerous possible solutions to the accountability problems generated by multiple principals in conflict, one common governance solution is of particular relevance to the NCI. This solution involves delegation of oversight to a mediating entity that represents the interests of the multiple principals while mitigating their potential conflict. An intermediary of this sort interfaces with the NCI in the form of the National Cancer Advisory Board (NCAB), which since the 1970s has been staffed by both political appointees and preeminent scientists who together represent the concerns of both public interests. While the NCAB may appear similar to other scientific advisory committees composing what STS scholar Sheila Jasanoff calls the "fifth branch" of U.S. government, it lacks the kind of adversarial stance that scientific advisory boards often take toward regulatory agencies.[32] Whereas those advisory boards are often at pains to separate their scientific advice from the policies and rules the agencies they advise may produce, the NCAB has by statute been granted a more direct and participatory role in rule making and grant allocation at the NCI, where it authorizes everything from grant approvals to intramural program reviews and new national initiatives or consortia.

The close integration of the NCAB into procedural routines of governance at the NCI, coupled with the accord between NCI scientist-bureaucrats and their colleagues qua scientists, suggests that the NCI's scientific principal will hold greater sway in monitoring and oversight of its policies than its congressional principal.[33] Representation of more informed members of the scientific community so proximate to agency deliberations enables advisory boards to have greater substantive input on NCI policies than members of the general public. While their expertise may disadvantage the interests of more distant congressional principals, it also provides a formal channel through which policies can be informed by extramural scientific perspectives that will enhance their technical adequacy and innovativeness.[34] The advisory board structure also indicates a distinct advantage to involving the NCI's scientist-bureaucrats in agency policy. Oversight from scientific advisory boards holds NCI scientist-bureaucrats accountable to congressional and scientific principals in the same venue, recapitulating the agency's dual mission in the organizational practices through which scientist-bureaucrats learn how to govern. But the very fact that they learn how to govern at the same time they learn how to advance their own research suggests an important modification to traditional principal-agent analyses of federal funding agencies that assume the requisite scientific expertise needed to meet agency missions does not exist in those agencies and must be delegated to outside scientists via extramural grants.[35] The existence of robust scientific expertise in its intramural research programs makes the NCI more than an intermediary—it is in itself capable of producing mission-critical science at the same time it creates the rules and procedures that help it enforce policies through the organizational work of scientist-bureaucrats who come to embody both capacities at once.

The multiple-principal framework thus gives shape to the structural systems of accountability that apply to NCI scientist-bureaucrats as they formulate policies meant to address the institute's dual mission. However, social scientists caution that principal-agent models, when extended to empirical case studies, should not be assumed as descriptions of design or intent that can be straightforwardly attributed to agencies or actors.[36] Instead, these models help elucidate the generic opportunity structures and power dynamics that obtain in particular problem situations confronted by federal bureaucrats. In the case of the NCI, describing problems of accountability to the agency's congressional and scientific principals using this model is an opening salvo in the effort to theorize precisely how the dual mission of the NCI remains salient as a foundation for scientific and policy innovation in the institute. On the other hand, the emphasis principal-agent theories place on monitoring and incentives fails to adequately specify how scientific conduct in particular comes to inform NCI agents' approaches to their expert bureaucratic practices.[37] To better capture the complexity of problem solving that unfolds as NCI scientist-bureaucrats iteratively learn how to innovate and govern in the same organization, I ground my theoretical approach to scientific and bureaucratic action in the tradition of philosophical pragmatism.

Prominent in both sociology and STS as an approach to analyzing scientific practice and organizational life, pragmatism offers an alternative theoretical grounding to the rational actor theory used by advocates of the principal-agent approach.[38] As the pragmatist sociological theorist Josh Whitford notes, actors in real-world situations typically do not confront a well-delineated menu of decisions that they can weigh against their own well-worked-out preferences to select the course of action that maximizes a given utility function.[39] Rather, actors' goals are emergent from situated conduct in an environment against which actors formulate the means and ends of problem solving in parallel. The classical pragmatist philosopher John Dewey theorized that actors formulate courses of action by sussing out "ends-in-view" to act toward and use the outcomes of those actions to reshape their environments to better enable subsequent action. These lines of action can be analyzed as trajectories wherein the ways actors evaluate different strategies and aims are emergent from the practices they develop to transform their material and symbolic environments to make them more amenable to future problem solving. To a great extent, these lines of action track habits that actors have already developed, which condition not only how they respond to the material dimensions of an environment but also how they (often creatively) acquire new expertise and learn to interpret their own desires for particular outcomes in light of the situation they confront. As a historical analysis of the NCI shows, this pragmatist approach is more adequate than the rational actor theory of principal-agent models in accounting for how scientist-bureaucrats both learn to govern *and* develop novel scientific innovations as part of their everyday organizational tasks in the NCI.[40] As scientist-bureaucrats attempt to define and solve problems against the dual mission and accountability structures of their environment, they learn to act in ways that are productive of both bureaucratic and scientific innovations. These innovations in turn alter the environment for defining problems and acting toward their solution in the future.

One crucial adjustment that follows from grounding innovation in a pragmatist microfoundation is a de-emphasis on stylized models of information development and transmission as the primary source of expertise commonly found in political science. As a historical sociologist and STS scholar, I instead ground my analysis in contextualized empirical accounts with an eye toward unpacking the practical activities around which scientist-bureaucrats organized their everyday lives in the NCI. To be sure, information, particularly from external sources, remains relevant to the environment in which both scientific and bureaucratic routines in the NCI unfolded, but this information becomes salient to the extent scientist-bureaucrats can incorporate it into their practices. The shift from emphasizing information to emphasizing practice not only is more faithful to the general theoretical disposition in STS to view scientific expertise less as a body of knowledge and more as a set of practical competencies but also aligns with recent shifts toward analyzing practice in organization studies.[41] Practice theories of organization reject the reduction of bureaucratic agencies to formalized information flows and instead conceptualize them as localized routines and performances unfolding in material and temporal arrangements buttressed by formal rules, collective memories, and actors' embodied skills.[42]

Emphasizing the significance of environed bureaucratic and scientific practice to the organizational lives of NCI researchers also exposes the need to modify one final assumption most principal-agent models make about the incentives that keep civil servants in the federal government despite the greater potential for monetary reward in the academy or private industry. NCI career scientists are quintessential "motivated agents," or "agents who pursue goals because they perceive intrinsic benefits from doing so" that outweigh the extrinsic benefits of higher compensation in organizations whose missions do not align as closely with their values.[43] Though NCI scientist-bureaucrats are undeniably motivated by nonmonetary incentives, they may not straightforwardly conceptualize these incentives in relation to policy rents as principal-agent models of policy learning assume.[44] As we will see, NCI scientist-bureaucrats consistently cite their ability to do innovative research with a public health impact as the primary incentive keeping them in the federal government. Other STS scholars have suggested that academic scientists often perceive bureaucratic tasks as unwanted impositions upon their research practices[45]; however, scientist-bureaucrats working in the federal government offer a distinct counterexample where fulfilling the mission of the bureaucracy motivates both their scientific and career aspirations. It is only in applying a pragmatist perspective to study how means and ends emerge in both scientific practice *and* bureaucratic tasks that we can account for the process whereby NCI scientist-bureaucrats transform their dual expertise into both scientific and policy innovation. Embedding their actions in the organizational life of a scientist-bureaucrat is precisely what will allow us to explain how the research of NCI scientists is so unexpectedly innovative and effective.[46]

A THEORY OF INNOVATION AS ENVIRONED SOCIAL LEARNING

In addition to the distinctive structures of governance that shape organizational life, the NCI provides characteristic *cultural* resources scientist-bureaucrats often draw upon in developing innovative approaches to scientific and bureaucratic problems. As Erin Metz McDonnell observed of pockets of government bureaucratic competence that nurtured administrative capacity in otherwise weak developing states, "iterative and endogenous change process[es] of organizational culture" can enable the emergence of distinctively efficacious bureaucratic niches around particular work subcultures.[47] Where McDonnell attributes the efficacy of these bureaucratic units to the "dual habitus" bureaucrats cultivate in response to their structurally marginal positions vis-à-vis local cultural systems of patrimonialism and corruption, the tension confronting NCI scientist-bureaucrats results from their dual commitments to the cultures of science and public service as enshrined in their practical enactments of the institute's mission.[48] Career scientist-bureaucrats at the NCI learn how to participate in administrative governance and policy craft alongside their day-to-day scientific conduct. The NCI thus provides another crucial elaboration of how the "bureaucratic ethos" McDonnell shows is necessary to developing local competence gains coherence through the routine *practices* composing organizational life. In the case of scientist-bureaucrats, the publicity and materiality of scientific practices provide a theoretical legibility to the concept of practice that is often missing in bureaucratic roles constructed around activities that leave behind few permanent traces beyond paperwork.

The case of scientific and bureaucratic innovation in the NCI is thus an illuminating one for both sociological studies of state bureaucracy and STS approaches to situated scientific innovation. Scholars of STS have sometimes remarked upon the need to more carefully specify the role formal organizations play in shaping scientific innovation, a problem some have recently taken up in earnest.[49] This study further develops the growing STS emphasis on formal organizations with attention to how organizational structure and culture create durable mechanisms whereby the broader institutional environment as well as the grounded activities of organizational actors mutually constitute one another. A similar ecological perspective on scientific environments has been carefully developed by social worlds scholars in STS who are similarly inspired by sociological interpretations of pragmatism.[50] Developing the pragmatist social worlds perspective one step further, I analyze how organizational culture influences scientific practices using the insights of the philosopher of science Joseph Rouse, who combines STS scholars such as Hans-Jörg Rheinberger with neopragmatist thinkers such as Robert Brandom to conceptualize scientific innovation as lineages of linguistic and material niche construction.[51] I use this approach to study innovation in the NCI as emerging in relation to the ongoing practices that organize scientist-bureaucrats' everyday lives within the organization that employs them. Scientist-bureaucrats' research practices are beholden not only to the material configurations of their laboratories or clinics but also to the performances of managerial and scientific competence they must enact to maintain them as functioning components of formal organizations. Yet their scientific practices are not neatly separable from their organizational performances. Social worlds analysis suggests that these performances are sustained by the material and institutional infrastructures that enable them to produce and interpret scientific results. Rouse's concept of the dual normativity of scientific practice offers a reinterpretation of Dewey's conception of the dual emergence of means and ends by showing how scientist-bureaucrats act toward the material and institutional dimensions of their environment in formulating actionable and meaningful definitions of what is "at issue" (i.e., how to interpret what phenomena are being generated) and "at stake" (i.e., how to interpret the broader meanings and implications of these phenomena) in a given scientific or bureaucratic performance. Together, these ecological and pragmatist theories offer the means to conceptualize the dynamic interplay between organizational routines and their broader environments and to analyze how organizational and institutional phenomena interpolate into systems of scientific innovation and vice versa.

I proceed from this ecological approach to scientific innovation by analyzing innovation as a process of *environed social learning*. This learning process is collective and involves groups iteratively defining problems and their solutions in light of the structural, cultural, and material environments in which they act.[52] In this model, innovation is the outcome of durable transformations to a collective's environment that emanate from alterations to scientific and organizational practices. In relation to the specific case at hand, this theory allows me to show how scientists studying cancer viruses and vaccines in the NCI defined the issues and stakes of their research in ways that instantiated different interpretations of the institute's dual mission in the scientific and bureaucratic routines they enacted. By shaping how they interpreted the issues and stakes of science and policy together, the dual mission often motivated scientist-bureaucrats to change their circumstances for acting into ones more amenable to public health–relevant science.

By analyzing scientific and bureaucratic innovation over time, I am able to identify some common elements of the collective and temporal dynamics of environed social learning. I capture these elements in a tripartite heuristic that proceeds from the emergence of new issues and stakes in *episodes of colligation* to their serial instantiation in routine practices that *iteratively encode* these issues and stakes in the environment, culminating in the development of new *innovative competencies* that did not exist before in the organization. While this heuristic is communicated in phasic form, the dynamics driving the overall learning process involve complex feedback loops that can terminate or repeat in ways that sometimes disrupt neat transitions between phases. Nevertheless, labeling different stages of the environed social learning process provides a means to highlight their operation throughout the case studies examined in the chapters that follow.

Phase 1: Episodes of Colligation

Environed social learning often begins in an episodic fashion, as a researcher confronts a problematic situation that the researcher comes to define as relevant to their scientific and bureaucratic practices. These problem situations are often produced by the distinct ecological dynamics of the organization, which make new infrastructural configurations, novel experimental findings, shifts in resources or materials, urgent public health crises, or institutional reconfigurations salient to the scientist's conduct. Here the organization's congressional and scientific principals may play an instrumental role, as they can alter the material or symbolic presentation of problem situations to make them relevant to the mandates of the bureaucracy or the researcher's scientific conduct.

In rare instances (innovation is, after all, a rare occurrence), the problem situation confronting the scientist precipitates a moment of colligation. Colligation describes the process whereby a novel element becomes activated as part of the scientific and organizational practices of a collective. I borrow this concept from its formulation by sociologist Richard Swedberg as "the idea that scientific phenomena consist of facts that are bound together in an analytically useful manner through an idea."[53] However, colligation in my formulation demands that the newly minted understanding be articulated through performances that enact it as a meaningful scientific or bureaucratic construct. These performances, when committed into ongoing practice, initiate the next phase of environed social learning.

Phase 2: Iterative Encoding

In order for a newly colligated understanding to persevere, it must be enacted across several subsequent iterations. However, iteration does not merely function to justify or clarify a new understanding; in experimental and organizational routines, iterations are often *generative* of the material and cultural conditions that enable performances to successfully articulate new practices.[54] In the context of experiments, material apparatus must be tinkered with over several repetitions to produce the desired phenomenon. In the context of bureaucratic routines, several attempts may be made across a variety of interactive media such as reports or meetings before organizational changes can be performed into existence. Given the structural configuration of the scientific and bureaucratic environment, these successive attempts to articulate the newly colligated understanding will inform one another as researchers use them to develop scientific and bureaucratic expertise.

The newly colligated understanding will endure to the extent it is successfully encoded into scientific and organizational routines. Here I use the concept of encoding developed by the sociologist Andrew Abbott to describe how the historicity of events is preserved such that those events can influence subsequent action "across the succession of contingent presents to the one present of now."[55] Rouse helps us understand how the dual normativity of scientific practice, which always involves consideration of what is at issue and what is at stake, allows for the simultaneous encoding of scientific and bureaucratic concerns in iterative experimental performances. To the extent that scientists also interpret their bureaucratic roles in light of their scientific experiences, encoding creates a feedback dynamic spanning these two varieties of organizational tasks. Once again, it is worth remembering that encoding can fail, either because any of the scientific or bureaucratic performances are unsuccessful or unpersuasive or because other understandings or routines crowd out the novel ones proposed.

Phase 3: Innovative Competencies

In those uncommon instances where innovations are successful, the environment for conducting research or enacting policy will have been transformed to enable new scientific and bureaucratic practices. Consistent with Keith Sawyer, I "distinguish between 'creativity' as the ideas or products generated by individuals, and 'innovation' as the successful execution of a new product or service by an entire organization."[56] This definition foregrounds how successful innovation requires successive collective performances across extended temporal periods. The environed social learning process provisionally concludes with the formation of new competencies, a concept that refers to the acquisition of conceptual schemas, practical skills, and material transformations to the environment that increases organizational actors' capacity to act effectively in pursuing their goals. In the case of scientific bureaucracies such as the NCI, these competencies may be instantiated in new policies, infrastructures, or scientific products—and are often applied across these settings all at once. As opposed to informational models of policy making, the concept of capacities allows us to emphasize how knowledge and expertise are often embedded in new collective practices or changes to the material configuration of the environment and in new formal policies, rules, or procedures.

—————•◦•—————

Studying environed social learning involves not only tacking back and forth between macro-level institutional interactions and meso-level organizational learning but also following the periodic resurgence of common problems over time. As the endogenous production of mission-relevant policies emerges from the scientific and bureaucratic lives of NCI employees, the learning process facilitates both policy and scientific drift. The process of environed social learning shows how drift emerges from the co-construction of scientific and policy innovations on the basis of how inquiry iteratively unfolds in the distinctive environment of the NCI. Yet the structural configuration of the NCI within its institutional ecology leads tensions that inhere in the dual mission of the institute to boil over in crucial historical moments that bring increased scrutiny from congressional or scientific principals. We can derive broader lessons about how these tensions are reconciled from comparisons across innovations at the NCI throughout its history by drawing upon the method of "reiterated problem solving"[57] to analyze regularities attributable to the institute's distinctive environment. As a comparative-historical method, reiterated problem solving focuses on sequences of events that repeat across different time periods and revolve around attempts by historical actors to address similar structural problems while integrating insights from past attempts at their solution. More important, reiterated problem solving provides a method for analyzing how solutions to antecedent problems shape the environments to which subsequent iterations respond. When it comes to analyzing evolving approaches to biomedical stewardship in the NCI, reiterated problem solving provides a rich approach to using single-case temporal comparison to develop theories about the relationship between cancer research, bureaucratic practices, and long-term policy changes. The careful attention this approach demands to structural conditions, practical legacies of problem solving, and actors' cultural understandings of the aims they pursue contributes to my ultimate objective of offering an ecological account of scientific and policy innovation at the NCI.

STUDY DESIGN AND METHODOLOGY

The arguments made in this book are based on analysis of historical sources that chronicle the scientific and bureaucratic activities of select intramural researchers employed in the National Cancer Institute from 1948 to 2018, as detailed in the appendix of this book. The most significant source of documentary evidence is derived from the NCI's annual reports, which describe the scientific and programmatic operations conducted by researchers in the intramural program each fiscal year. These annual reports were supplemented and verified with additional archival documents related to administration and governance at the NCI. Of particular relevance were meeting minutes and videocast recordings of the NCI's National Cancer Advisory Board and Board of Scientific Advisors. Other evidence I draw upon in formulating my argument comprises primarily administrative and scientific documents produced by the NCI or its principals, such as fact books, technical reports, external reviews, congressional budget reports, and congressional testimony. I also draw upon published and unpublished memoirs detailing the efforts of NCI scientist-bureaucrats involved in the institute's virus and vaccine programs, as well as oral histories collected by the Office of NIH History and myself. Periodicals, such as *Science* and the *Cancer Letter*, routinely form important historical context for my analysis.

My claims about how the dual mission of the NCI affected scientific innovation are based on analysis of a theoretical sample of thirty-six principal investigators (PIs) in the NCI's Intramural Research Program whose projects addressed cancer viruses or vaccines (see table A.2 in the appendix). This sample was strategically selected to capture scientists employed in performance of virus and vaccine research throughout the major periods of study and who represent a diversity of career trajectories, from those with brief tenure in the institute to those with decades-long careers, and scientists who selected into administrative leadership positions as well as those who did not. Temporal comparisons across these groups highlight important variations in organizational environments and innovative outputs, which led to the development and refinement of the model of environed social learning described in this study. Though historical analysis of each of these projects was crucial to the development of the explanation offered in this study, I forego analysis of each individual project in the text in favor of a narrative approach that better captures the complexity of interrelationships between scientific and policy work among career scientist-bureaucrats. Though this narrative accounts for notable scientific and bureaucratic failures, my concern with highlighting the processes resulting in innovation outcomes leads me to emphasize successful instances of innovation.[58] The reader should bear in mind that successful innovation, though an outcome of great theoretical interest, is by no means the most representative outcome of the average research project at the NCI or elsewhere.

In addition, I present the results of within-case temporal comparisons of environed social learning episodes in the NCI as of theoretical value rather than expansive scope or generality. In this study, I do not systematically compare cancer virus and vaccine research in the NCI to research in academia or the private sphere.[59] While this limits my ability to generalize arguments about research at the NCI to virus and vaccine research generally, the purpose of this study is more to mine theoretical insights from overlooked federal research than it is to offer a generic model of innovation in cancer research as a whole. The NCI's apparent uniqueness relative to other research organizations and federal bureaucracies often proves a theoretical strength, in that many of the factors other analysts use to explain scientific and policy innovations (like monetary incentives) are absent in this context, while others (like mission-oriented projects) are enhanced. Readers should bear in mind that this study is more an abductive theory-generating exercise than a deductive experimental one—though there is certainly space enough for both approaches in the amply provisioned yet relatively unexplored territory of federal cancer research.

Why Virus and Vaccine Innovation at the NCI?

Although virus research and vaccine development are less commonly associated with cancer prevention and treatment than are genetic research or chemotherapy in the public imagination, they nevertheless have occupied a significant place in the NCI's scientific portfolio almost since the agency's inception. In fact, cancer virus and vaccine research has been an unusual strength of the NCI's intramural program since the late 1940s. At that time, though evidence that viruses could cause cancers in mice, chickens, and rabbits had been established, the hypothesis that human cancers may be caused by viruses remained controversial among most medical researchers.[60] By the 1950s, the NCI had become a central hub for producing research on cancer viruses and vaccine candidates, training cancer researchers and virologists in emerging methods, and producing the materials and techniques (including tissue cultures, viral reagents, and animal models) that would enable virus cancer research to spread throughout the United States. Over the ensuing decades, these competencies in virology and vaccinology would continue to be nurtured in the NCI, where a succession of scientists, often kept on after training under more senior NCI scientist-bureaucrats, would establish their own laboratories and forge new experimental paths in the institute. In addition to research of direct relevance to oncogenic, or cancer-causing, viruses, these NCI scientists would conduct research that informed developments in basic theories of cancer causation, such as the oncogene hypothesis discussed in chapters 2 and 3, and therapies for non-oncogenic viruses and sequalae, such as HIV/AIDS as discussed in chapters 4 and 5.

Beyond these clinical and laboratory innovations, many policy developments must be contextualized in light of cancer virus and vaccine research in the NCI. In the current academic atmosphere, critiques of innovation tend to take for granted that the infiltration of corporate profit-seeking logic into all facets of research (including academic life) presents the greatest barrier to using biomedical breakthroughs to enhance the public good.[61] While the for-profit nature of American medical care justly elicits such critiques, the history of virus vaccine innovation is less straightforward. Alongside some famously innovative private pharmaceutical firms such as Merck, government researchers at the Walter Reed Army Institute of Research and the National Institutes of Health have historically played a vital role in vaccine innovation.[62] Of course, the absence of public infrastructure for scalable vaccine manufacture and distribution ensures that the commercial pharmaceutical industry will continue to play a publicly prominent and technologically essential role in vaccine research and development. But as private pharmaceutical entities have largely disinvested from in-house virus and vaccine discovery research, and biotechnology remains a high-turnover sector, government and academic researchers continue to conduct much of the early-stage research that contributes to successful vaccine innovation.[63] It thus remains essential to study the processes that lead these scientists to identify and test promising vaccine compounds in their own institutional environments, where the logic of commercial capitalism does not heavily incentivize their day-to-day decision making.

Another characteristic of intramural science at the NCI that makes it distinct from other research units in academia or commercial industry also presents one of its major theoretical strengths as a case study. In the NCI, non-monetary incentives predominate because monetary incentives are statutorily limited for civil servants. As federal employees, NCI scientists who invent even blockbuster innovations must surrender their intellectual property rights to the U.S. government. While they are permitted to collect royalties on any innovations licensed for commercial development, these royalties have historically been capped at $100,000–$150,000 per annum.[64] The financial opportunities available to NCI scientists are thus distinctly disadvantaged compared with those available to either academic scientists, who can profit handsomely by spinning off promising innovations into multi-million-dollar start-ups, or industry scientists, who can reap additional rewards from stock options and corporate bonuses. Furthermore, "according to scientists, technology transfer specialists, and the General Accounting Office, the monetary incentives provided by royalty-sharing are not effective in changing behavior" of intramural scientists at all.[65] By studying scientists for whom major financial incentives cannot reasonably be said to motivate the additional risks of pursuing novel innovative research, this study can isolate more general social factors that affect innovation in scientific research.

Yet scientist-bureaucrats studying cancer viruses and vaccines are also distinctive compared with many of their intramural colleagues. With the majority of studies in the intramural program addressing either the fundamental biological causes of cancer, development or testing of clinical diagnostics or treatments, or epidemiological trends, virus and vaccine research constitutes only a small percentage of scientific effort at the institute. Nevertheless, scientific leaders in the virus and vaccine programs have come to occupy some of the most prominent positions in the institute, with a disproportionate number of these personnel occupying assistant directorships or directorships relative to the number of NCI personnel conducting other forms of cancer research. The presence of unusually successful cancer virus and vaccine researchers in NCI leadership thus raises interesting questions about how novel areas of expertise emerge and are nurtured in organizations.

Virus and vaccine innovation is also a strategic site for examining the bureaucratic and scientific prerequisites for successful translation of "basic" science discoveries into "applied" public health technologies.[66] Scientifically, virus and vaccine studies have the potential to span the boundaries of fundamental, clinical, epidemiological, and public health research. This makes them distinct from more common cancer innovations that typically entail the development of combination chemotherapies or chemical entities, which tend to move slowly from laboratory study into small-scale human trials and only rarely into epidemiological analysis or public health policy, as successful cancer drugs tend to be licensed for individual medical use rather than as large-scale public health interventions. Additionally, because they are relatively underrepresented in the institute's armamentarium, vaccines lack the established organizational channels that other experimental new drugs pass through in the NCI. This becomes evident in the case of HPV vaccine development and testing discussed in chapter 6, where the need for NCI scientists inexperienced in vaccine development to navigate uncharted bureaucratic waters demanded they engage creatively with available organizational resources. Finally, unlike cancer drugs, vaccines rarely reach blockbuster status for private pharmaceutical companies—one of the major reasons they have been minimized in most of these companies' portfolios since the 1970s.[67] This tips the risk-reward balance for scientists motivated by monetary rewards against entering into this line of research, lending additional support to NCI researchers' declared public health motivations for doing vaccine research over assumptions of profit motive.

Finally, studying cancer virus and vaccine projects at the NCI offers a sustained glimpse into how scientists' interpretations of the NCI's dual mission to both produce innovative science and improve cancer outcomes for Americans has evolved. Since the mid-twentieth century, as the landscape for medical delivery has undergone major shifts that fundamentally altered the ways Americans accessed and paid for care, vaccines have remained comparatively stable as public health technologies. Holding the public health strategy of vaccination constant highlights how changes in the material and social environments for research nevertheless drew upon cultural understandings of how investment in biomedical innovation could ameliorate health inequalities in postwar American society. Throughout various periods of its existence, the institute has developed different strategies for articulating its dual mission alongside the cancer research its constitutive scientists conduct. As a result, there are periods where the NCI articulates distinct organizational solutions to reconciling the sometimes competing ideals of scientific innovation and public service. Comparing the processes whereby these organizational solutions emerge, are stabilized, and decline is instructive for understanding how scientific and bureaucratic decisions interact to shape how the tensions between the two missions are negotiated in and through NCI scientist-bureaucrats' practices. Over time, processes of environed social learning allow NCI scientist-bureaucrats to refine otherwise ambiguous policy regimes into meaningful performative guides for further action. In part, I argue, they do this by elaborating what is at issue and what is at stake for scientific and bureaucratic practices—an elaboration that leads NCI scientists to articulate ongoing practices in both spheres of action in ways that belie any attempt to draw firm boundaries between them.

OVERVIEW OF THE BOOK

This book proceeds chronologically in roughly decadal fashion, narrating interrelated scientific and bureaucratic innovations that emerged from the efforts of intramural researchers to realize the NCI's dual mission in policy and scientific practice. Throughout these chapters, the focus is on illustrating how NCI agents interpreted not only the issues and stakes of their ongoing research but also the organizational problems of realizing the institute's dual mission in bureaucratically plausible procedure and policy. As scientist-bureaucrats specializing in virus and vaccine research attain leadership positions in the agency, their approaches to addressing policy problems continue to be informed by lessons they took away from prior episodes of social learning in the laboratory or clinic. At the same time, successful policies alter the broader scientific ecology in ways that feed back into both scientific and policy problems that confront these scientist-bureaucrats, particularly in the form of congressional and scientific principals' sometimes competing demands that the institute demonstrate it has been accountable to its dual mission of supporting biomedical science and improving health.

Chapter 1 introduces the structural and institutional environment confronting the modern NCI through an analysis of organizational changes that took place throughout the 1940s and 1950s. These changes added a distinct role for scientific principals in institute governance through the NCI's advisory boards, which imposed standards and concerns for good policy making that were different from those of congressional principals. Notably, influential disease lobbyists and their congressional supporters pushed for an interpretation of biomedical research funding as an instrument for ameliorating cancer-related morbidity and mortality in a country that had definitively rejected the possibility of universal health care reform. In addressing the policy demands of these principals, NCI leadership reconstituted the organization's mission around emerging ideas about the relationship between science and policy that set the stage for the scientific and bureaucratic innovations detailed in later chapters. In the process, the NCI's principals modernized the organization around an interpretation of its dual mission as an agency that funded cancer research in order to improve the nation's health. The 1950s closed with Congress and the public increasingly calling for accountability from the NCI in the spending of its now generous appropriations.

In chapter 2, I analyze how an emerging emphasis on viruses as possible causes of leukemia and other cancers in the NCI's intramural program offered a compelling policy solution to the institute's dual mission: a cancer vaccine. Throughout the 1960s, NCI scientists applied their interpretation of the scientific urgency around cancer virus studies to the construction of a targeted cancer vaccine initiative called the Special Virus Leukemia Program. Inspired by Cold War systems planning used in weapons and aerospace development, NCI scientist-bureaucrats designed the "convergence technique" to manage discovery-oriented cancer research in service of the ultimate goal of innovating vaccines to prevent human leukemia. As the Special Virus Leukemia Program's own cadre of "scientist-managers" iteratively enshrined their scientific interpretations of the issues and stakes of ongoing research into this bureaucratic planning apparatus, the program came to increasingly focus on RNA virus studies, which it supported through the work of expansive networks of contracted scientists stationed throughout academia and industry.

Chapter 3 explores how optimism around the NCI's novel scientific-bureaucratic approach to virus and vaccine innovation helped spur the declaration of a "War on Cancer" in 1971. Despite congressional support for the NCI's targeted planning enterprise, emerging scientific problems within the virus cancer programs led to redefinitions of the programs' stakes away from vaccines and toward a novel explanation of cancer causation called the "oncogene hypothesis." Concurrently, changes in rules governing bureaucratic advisory boards empowered scientific principals in institute planning, many of whom called on the NCI to abandon targeted research in favor of grant funding for independent academic scientists. The combination of shifting research goals and the rebalancing of power among congressional and scientific principals led to the dissolution of the institute's targeted virus programs—ironically, on the very eve of the discovery of the first human cancer retrovirus.

The NCI's once-maligned targeted retrovirus studies would soon prove fortuitous as the nation faced an exploding HIV/AIDS epidemic in the early 1980s. Chapter 4 explores how a new NCI director, rehabilitating the institute in the eyes of scientific principals who criticized its past attempts to target health-relevant virus research, took a different tack toward confirmatory evidence that viruses caused cancer and related diseases in humans. As reports of the syndrome that would come to be known as AIDS surged in the United States and around the globe, NCI cancer virus researchers such as Robert Gallo applied knowledge and resources accumulated in part from the now-defunct targeted programs to fuel collaborations that identified the viral cause of AIDS and led to the innovation of a screening assay for detecting HIV in the nation's blood supply.

Chapter 5 illustrates how informal collaborations between Gallo's laboratory and clinicians in the NCI's Clinical Oncology Program led to the development of the first generation of effective HIV/AIDS therapeutics, including the drug AZT. With the NCI's previous contracting capacities for virus cancer studies now gone, NCI clinicians such as Samuel Broder relied on collaborations with commercial pharmaceutical companies to scale up anti-AIDS drugs for public use. However, loss of scientific credit for AZT research, combined with its high price tag, undermined NCI scientist-bureaucrats' interpretations of the issues and stakes of their research efforts. Learning from these outcomes, NCI scientist-bureaucrats changed the institute's intellectual property policies in an attempt to ensure future drug development would better serve the institute's public health mission.

In chapter 6, I show how scientific and bureaucratic lessons from HIV/AIDS research and drug development informed the creation of the NCI's first policies designed to foster "translational research," an emerging concept referring to policies that would help move innovations from the laboratory to the patient. Though initially oriented toward extramural granting practices out of a need to balance scientific principals' demands for basic research funding with congressional principals' challenges around realizing disease reduction, initiatives soon turned inward to the organization's intramural research capacities as well. Research into vaccines against human papillomaviruses provided compelling models for translation in the institute, and intramural scientist-bureaucrats soon learned how to define the issues and stakes of HPV vaccine innovation in concert with evolving concerns about how the NCI could best realize its health mission. From these learning episodes, NCI scientist-bureaucrats came to consider the institute as occupying a distinct role in research and development vis-à-vis industry, a perspective that continued to inform subsequent attempts to refine translational research policies into the new millennium.

Chapter 7 details how translational research policy continued to develop in the midst of political shifts that aimed to advantage private commercial entities in NCI policy. Despite the presidential appointment of a decidedly pro-market NCI director in 2001, scientific principals and NCI scientist-bureaucrats resisted attempts to redefine their mission around a model informed by commercial business management. Instead, scientist-bureaucrats and their advisors continued to shape translational research policies toward alternative definitions of the issues and stakes emergent from their ongoing research and governance practices. The statutory exclusion of commercial interests from policy making was combined with NCI scientists' commitment to their dual mission to largely insulate many important programs in the institute, such as the extramural Rapid Access to Intervention Development (RAID) drug development program, from industry preferences. The enduring approach to translational research policy that became integrated into the institute instead reflected scientist-bureaucrats' understanding of the NCI as a complementary and even countervailing influence on the innovation environment. This understanding continued to shape institute policy under subsequent directors throughout the 2010s, culminating in the NCI's approach to forming scientific priorities under the "Beau Biden Cancer Moonshot" legislation.

I conclude the book by revisiting the lessons about innovation as environed social learning communicated across within-case comparisons in this study. I reflect upon the broader trajectory of environed social learning across seventy years of intramural cancer virus and vaccine research and consider the lessons this case may hold for sociologists, STS scholars, and analysts of biomedical research policy in the United States.

CONCLUSION

Despite the centrality of cancer to Americans' cultural and medical lives, few sociologists have made cancer research itself an object of sustained study. This book contributes to a small but growing literature in sociology and STS that examines the production of scientific knowledge and innovation around cancer,[68] exploring the curious case of viral cancers and cancer vaccines. It shows how organizational structure and culture shape scientific innovation and offers an unexpected case illustrating how the fragmented American state has functioned to produce the goods, services, knowledge, and infrastructure driving economic growth in significant sectors of the biomedical economy since the postwar period. In the process, it advances theories of innovation that show how the close interconnection between scientific and bureaucratic practices allows NCI actors to develop distinct policy expertise that simultaneously shapes the trajectory of biomedical research innovation and governance in the United States.

CHAPTER 1

MEDICINE, MELIORISM, AND THE MAKING OF A MODERN NCI

The National Institutes of Health (NIH) emerged in 1930 out of humble beginnings in the Hygienic Laboratory, a Progressive Era institution that aimed to improve public health in the United States through the advancement of scientific research relevant to human thriving.[1] Buttressed by popular support for scientific medicine and the conviction of policy makers that the government had a role to play in coordinating and supplementing research funded by universities, philanthropies, and commercial enterprise, the NIH was envisioned as a place where government scientists applied cutting-edge knowledge to problems of concern to the nation. In the 1940s and 1950s, the NIH and its constituent institutes would become central to attempts by the federal government to achieve "the ultimate goal . . . to control and if possible 'conquer' disease, thereby improving the people's health. To attain that goal, an intermediary goal was understood: the biomedical research enterprise must be built up, and institutions and individual researchers supported. That, in turn, would require great amounts of money, and Congress thought the government should be willing to spend it."[2] With support from principals in Congress, the National Cancer Institute (NCI) would become a pioneer in the formulation and execution of this goal.

When the NCI was first established in 1937, it was independent of the NIH within the U.S. Public Health Service and was not formally subsumed under the NIH until the Public Health Service Act of 1944.[3] As the historian Richard Mandel points out, the institutes' focus on providing grants-in-aid to extramural scientists was a distinctive holdover of New Deal–era policy that would become a hallmark of funding at the NIH.[4] The basic bureaucratic structure of review and approval for research grants to university investigators was developed at the NCI during its first few years of existence. Under this structure, "study sections" of intramural NCI scientists (and, later, extramural scientists) provided a first layer of review that passed on meritorious applications for approval by the National Advisory Cancer Council (NACC), a committee staffed by extramural scientists and clinicians.

In designing the National Cancer Institute, Congress built into the organization's governance structure a means to represent the expertise of nongovernment scientists in federal policy making. The National Advisory Cancer Council originally comprised six experts in science and medicine, with the surgeon general serving as chair ex officio. The NACC was from its inception constituted

> to make recommendations to the Surgeon General with respect to carrying out the provisions of the [National Cancer Act of 1937]. Specifically, the Council is authorized to make recommendations in regard to cancer research projects submitted to it or initiated by it; to spread information about cancer studies "for the benefit of health agencies and organizations, physicians, or any other scientists, and for the information of the general public;" and "to review applications from any university, hospital, laboratory, or other institution, whether public or private, or from individuals, for grants-in-aid for research projects relating to cancer, and certify approval of projects deemed worthy of support."[5]

The NACC thus provided oversight in executing the new institute's charter as well as a layer of scientific peer review that guaranteed the quality of sponsored projects. Unlike advisory boards in regulatory agencies whose charters extend only to providing advice for policy formation that takes place further along bureaucratic or legislative channels,[6] the NACC from its inception played a direct role in shaping policies in concert with bureaucratic leadership at the NCI.

This distinctive composition of the NACC and its relation to the NCI provided a means to incorporate the interests of the scientific public distinct from Congress. Recognition of how the agency's design integrated scientific principals into governance and administration clarifies that the scientific community has always had a mechanism for influencing policy in the NCI. This creates an important analytical distinction between how NCI scientist-bureaucrats must be responsive to the scientific community, routinely conceptualized as those working in public or nonprofit academic, medical, and research institutions, and how they might be responsive to tertiary special interests. The structure of the NCI makes the agency accountable to advisory board scientists in a way that is similar to its accountability to Congress as an important participant in the mechanisms of agency governance. Special interests, on the other hand, remain external to the statutory governance structure of the institute, and those wishing to sway or capture institute decision making would have to seek indirect means of communicating preferences and influencing policy at the NCI.

In the 1940s, congressional lobbying emerged as the dominant means whereby tertiary special interests could influence the nation's biomedical research agenda. Since that time, disease lobbyists in particular have played a prominent role in spurring Congress to invest in research in the NIH, up to and including the establishment of new categorical disease institutes.[7] Yet public policy scholars who have measured the influence lobbyists have over the appropriations and allocations process at NIH have found a complex relationship between lobbyists' agendas and research policy emanating from the institutes. Starting with the premise that the institutes' scientific and health missions can stand in tension as scientific principals emphasize research investment and congressional principals and disease lobbyists emphasize health gains, Bhaven Sampat notes that NIH administrators have cultivated political "savvy" in generating broad bipartisan support for the institutes throughout the postwar period.[8] While the overwhelming majority of the NIH budget is reserved for funding investigator-initiated extramural science, the NIH has been adept at using its remaining funds to create targeted programs that provide "safety valves" for meeting disease lobbyists' interests while largely avoiding "hard" congressional earmarks that reserve significant funds for specific initiatives demanded by lobbyists.[9] In this manner, the NIH has maintained autonomy in policy making and avoided the kind of special-interest penetration that would allow forces outside the agency to drastically shape its policies. As Hegde and Sampat demonstrate, even those lobbyists who are successful at inserting their agenda into institute appropriations secure only "soft" earmarks (i.e., nonbinding congressional recommendations to invest more funding in diseases of interest).[10] This means that lobbying from disease advocates, businesses, and other special interests has limited effect on shaping the research agendas of the institutes.[11] Overwhelmingly, these decisions are made according to standards of peer review and portfolio management internal to the statutory governance procedures of the National Institutes of Health.

Ironically, the relative autonomy the NIH now enjoys in scientific policy making resulted in part from early efforts by lobbyists to make the NIH—but especially the NCI—a strategic mechanism for improving Americans' health. As the prospect of founding a national health care system in the United States faded in the immediate postwar period, a coalition of lobbyists led by notables such as Mary Woodward Lasker turned toward medical research funding as an alternative to direct health care reform. Their ambition was to increase investments in basic medical science, on the assumption that such discoveries would beget improvements in medicine and public health. In the process of lobbying Congress for increased public investment in medical research, they helped spur a period of extraordinary growth in funding for the NCI that enabled the institute to fundamentally transform the nation's biomedical research infrastructure.

We can understand the policy environment that developed between disease lobbyists, Congress, scientists, and the NCI in this period through the concept of meliorism. In this scheme, the problem of governing cancer has been approached with what the pragmatist philosopher Colin Koopman calls a "melioristic sensibility," defined by an orientation toward "the improvement of political realities on the basis of resources already available within the very realities" of a given situation.[12] In this context, biomedical innovation was understood as a readily deployable tool to eliminate disease in the absence of political will for health care reform. Meliorism offers a perspective for analyzing what the historian of science Robin W. Scheffler has called the "biomedical settlement" in cancer research funding. The biomedical settlement entailed "the tacit promise that in lieu of providing health care to its citizens directly, the government could foster public welfare through biological investigations of disease."[13]

Yet the lobbyists and members of Congress whose biomedical settlement would funnel through the meliorative programs of the NIH left open-ended the answer to the question of how best to steward the nation's cancer research effort and depended on agencies such as the NCI to develop the policies and scientific products that would make their aspirations a reality. The open-endedness of melioristic politics allowed for the growth of biomedical investment in cancer research in the absence of well-specified congressional policies or presidential agendas. This led to the situation that the historian Stephen Strickland described in 1972 as one where "there has been no centrally issued, widely promulgated summary statement of what nonetheless has developed into an unmistakable government commitment" to biomedical research.[14] Strong congressional support for a growing biomedical budget, driven in part by enthusiastic disease lobbyists, created an environment where the NCI was given remarkable autonomy to mobilize the scientific expertise of its bureaucratic corps toward creating the policies that would transform such an investment into health gains.

CARVING OUT A NICHE FOR
FEDERAL MEDICAL RESEARCH POLICY

The technological optimism of postwar America, boosted by the memory of wartime innovations in antibiotics and peacetime developments in vaccinology and chemotherapy, sets the stage for the legislative and organizational changes that modernized the National Cancer Institute. A truly national medical research policy landscape first emerged from defense-related demands during World War II.[15] Under the leadership of Vannevar Bush of the Office of Scientific Research and Development (OSRD), the Committee on Medical Research mobilized military, Public Health Service, and civilian scientists and medical personnel to address the needs of soldiers fighting in multiple combat theaters around the globe. Given "a direct presidential mandate . . . and what was tantamount to a blank check," the committee signed off on hundreds of contracts that led to path-breaking developments in antibiotics, sulfonamides, and many other medical technologies.[16] Bush's ambitions to continue support for research in peacetime converged with ongoing efforts to reorganize the Public Health Service (PHS). In 1944, the Public Health Service Act extended the mission and funding powers of the Committee on Medical Research to the PHS.[17] The prevailing policy climate in the executive branch assumed federal patronage of "medical research had become a vital prerequisite for developing the national health care system."[18]

The flowering concord between medical research and a prospective national health care system had its own advocates in Congress. Military health screenings of American civilians during World War II "uncovered shockingly bad health conditions among the nation's young men," 40 percent of whom were deemed medically unfit to serve.[19] National reporting on these conditions spurred congressional action, led by Senator Claude Pepper, to investigate how "the expenditure of more [public] funds in medical research would lead to a longer life and better health for the people of the country."[20] Yet the issue of how to ensure that research would realize these health improvements was politically fraught.

Pepper's own efforts were caught between the American Medical Association's (AMA) objections to anything smacking of health reform and Bush's ambition to found an independent agency dedicated to funding basic research. President Franklin Roosevelt's own physician, Ross McIntyre, asked Pepper "not to hold hearings on the question of a special medical research agency" until Bush's proposal could be heard (though he also personally advised Roosevelt against a health component to the Social Security bill).[21] The AMA had supported establishing a science agency under the condition that it respect the medical field's autonomy; under the Truman administration, however, federal support for medical research and investment in a national health program would be considered part and parcel of the same effort.[22] Both issues around science policy and health reform were deadlocked.

Scholars have noted that this political impasse created an opportunity for the extant Public Health Service to "[step] into the policy gap" left for medical research.[23] The crucial maneuver made on the part of PHS leadership involved claiming a large portfolio of orphaned wartime medical research contracts from the OSRD. While Bush had planned for these contracts to transfer to the new science agency he hoped to found in 1945, ongoing conflict stalled the proposed agency and left these active contracts in need of management.[24] Though initially resistant to efforts to modify the PHS's structure or charter and cautious about the pace of agency growth, PHS officials soon accepted an expansion of their mission through the transfer of active medical OSRD contracts to the fledgling National Institutes of Health. Once completed, the transfer of these contracts significantly increased the NIH budget—from $180,000 in 1945 to $4 million in 1947.[25] The influx of funding put muscle behind the NIH's push to make its explicit "objective the improvement of the nation's health through the acquisition of knowledge in all the sciences related to health."[26]

The historian Daniel Sledge points out that the track record the Public Health Service established with local offices in the South in combating endemic health issues and epidemic diseases helped it secure political cache and become central to health care debates in the first half of the twentieth century. The political clout the PHS garnered through these efforts enabled it to play a significant role in shaping federal health policy once it became a serious issue in the 1940s. Early in the Progressive Era, the PHS had laid the groundwork for the constitutional and policy legitimacy of a national health care system, going so far as to advocate for some form of insurance or federal subsidy to ensure Americans had access to necessary medical services. The stance the PHS developed in the 1910s, which "argued in favor of an intergovernmental system that would seek to collapse distinctions between public health and individual medicine," would go on to inform the "vision of health policy" the PHS proffered for decades to come.[27] Of particular importance to this vision was PHS official Thomas Parran, Jr., surgeon general from 1936 to 1948, who put the agency "often at the center of health policy making" throughout his tenure. Parran offered a distinct model for the federal government to assist in the funding and provision of medical services throughout the country. Under this model, sophisticated infrastructure in the form of local centers interconnected with state and federal initiatives would enable public health to work hand-in-hand with health care delivery.[28]

Parran's bureaucratic vision of the PHS and its constituent agencies ran counter to the agendas of influential special interests in the medical community. Throughout the twentieth century, the powerful AMA was reliably opposed to any legislation that threatened the total autonomy of the medical profession from external control. The 1937 founding of the National Cancer Institute was no exception. Here the AMA objected to the provision of advisory councils over the new institute as presenting a "danger of putting the government in the dominant position in relation to medical research."[29] Despite such principled objections, the AMA never came to exhibit the kind of hostility toward medical research policy as it did toward direct attempts to regulate medical practice or enact health care reform. By the mid-1940s, the AMA had assumed a "neutral" stance toward medical research policy, preoccupied as it was with efforts to combat Truman's proposed health plans and other sporadic attempts to legislate health care or advance programs of compulsory medical insurance.[30]

Indeed, medical research investment would become a viable avenue for federal policy expansion in part because of the timing of its introduction alongside health care reform proposals. It was increasingly clear to leadership at the AMA during Roosevelt's first administration that the physicians' lobby had acquired an obstructionist reputation. The AMA had no plans to back off from its objection to national health insurance but would have to make some concessions in the face of a mounting effort in the executive branch to enact some federal reform. So as not to erode the goodwill and hard-won cultural authority of allopathic medicine in the United States, the AMA gradually took a conciliatory approach to expanding public health efforts.[31] With controversy over national health insurance still raging, the National Conference on Economic Security's final report on health could only offer a consensus opinion on the expansion of existing public health infrastructure as a means of ensuring access to inexpensive preventative care.[32] For their part, officials in the Public Health Service regarded both public health and health insurance for individual medical care to be inseparable from the broader goal of ensuring the nation's health. Yet in the absence of clear consensus or strong presidential support for health insurance, they too were forced to default to a program of public health research and infrastructure only.[33]

Plans for a national health care program were again pursued in earnest under the Truman administration. Truman's 1949 National Health Plan offered a five-pronged approach to addressing the health needs of the postwar nation. Foremost among these was a controversial national health insurance package (sometimes called the Wagner-Murray-Dingle proposal after its perennial congressional sponsors), but also included was expansion for hospital construction; scholarships for medical school students; federal grants to medical schools; and expanded funding for medical research. Though each of these programs was in principle anathema to the tack the AMA had traditionally taken, medical research funding was the very least of its concerns. The remaining programs, aimed directly at the nation's health care delivery apparatus, attracted the full force of the AMA's formidable fury. Framing national health care as a slippery slope toward communism, the AMA's public relations machine quickly eroded support for Truman's policies.[34] Truman would eventually abandon his health care reform ambitions when the United States became once again embroiled in international conflict in Korea. Still lacking strong executive leadership, the fragmented field of health agencies at the federal level continued to pursue piecemeal and agency-centered approaches to health policy in the postwar period, conditions that encouraged the growth of myriad disease-specific lobbies like those that would soon emerge around cancer research.[35]

FEDERAL MEDICAL RESEARCH AS
SUBSTITUTE AND COMPROMISE

After the failure of Truman's health care reform efforts, prominent philanthropists sought a compromise to direct federal funding for medical care by sponsoring investment in disease research instead. This new strategy involved placing significant responsibility for improving chronic disease outcomes in the hands of medical researchers funded by taxpayer monies. As the sociologist Paul Starr argues, the extraordinary growth of scientific medicine in the postwar United States "offered the prospect of improved well-being without requiring any profound reorganization of society."[36] Working around opposition from the American Medical Association proved a major impetus toward this substitute strategy. "Public support for medical research, hospital construction and other forms of resource development . . . posed fewer problems for the AMA than did health insurance. These programs typically increased the capital resources of the system (scientific knowledge, physical infrastructure) without limiting physicians' income from it."[37] The success of medical research during and after wartime, notably in the form of polio vaccination, persuaded American politicians that "opponents of national health insurance could display their deep concern for health by voting generous appropriations for medical research."[38] Though the AMA continued to block direct support from the NIH for medical education throughout the 1950s, postwar proponents of science, technology, and innovation policy convincingly argued that investment in medical research would lead inexorably to job growth.[39]

The historian of science Angela Creager has demonstrated the significance of voluntary health organizations to mobilizing the federal investment in cancer research.[40] No history of the grand ascent of medical research lobbying in this period is complete without due attention to the efforts of Mary Woodward Lasker (figure 1.1). Already a successful entrepreneur when she married advertising magnate Albert Lasker, she soon became a fixture among the country's elites because of her tireless philanthropic and political activities. Lasker was more attentive perhaps than others of her stature to the fact that "most people could not afford proper medical care, and that a family's entire savings could be wiped out by a single prolonged illness."[41] Lasker was thus "strongly committed to national health insurance and federal support of medical education," though her pessimism about AMA opposition to these policies meant she "was never deeply involved in the legislative debate on either issue."[42] Yet as it became clearer to Lasker and her allies that "the AMA did not oppose federal support of medical research, but, in fact, tacitly supported it," she and her confidantes "were forcefully directed to medical research partly because other avenues of health policy were effectively closed."[43]

Lasker's lobby became known as the "noble conspirators" who, through Congress, appropriated millions for federal biomedical research toward the ultimate

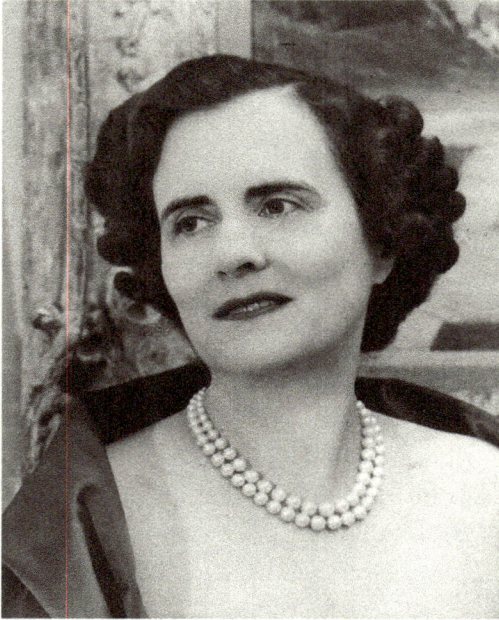

1.1 Mary Woodward Lasker, circa 1957.

Photo credit: Columbia University Rare Book and Manuscript Library, Mary Lasker Papers.

goal of eliminating the nation's greatest health threats.[44] Lasker was aided in her philanthropic efforts by Florence Mahoney, the wife of a southern newspaper magnate. Mahoney had once entertained aspirations to a career in medicine but surrendered these to the prevailing social norms that discouraged women of station from entering into this (or any) profession.[45] Lasker's extensive history with voluntarist health societies and medical professionals "had convinced her that the private sector, alone, could never make sufficient headway against disease."[46] Lasker and Mahoney thus joined forces in an ambitious plan to transform the landscape of American medical research by "getting government involved in medical research in a big way."[47] As elites, Lasker and Mahoney benefited from Rolodexes brimming with names of consequence, from politicians to philanthropists and public figures. Lasker in particular proved adept at mustering compelling witnesses for public congressional hearings in favor of increased medical research funding. This strategy she deployed throughout the postwar period to enviable political success.

Lasker and Mahoney's first major lobbying target was, fortuitously, Senator Claude Pepper. Both women were connected to Pepper socially and found in him a natural ally for the cause of advancing health through federal investment in medical research. In 1944, in exchange for their generous financial and editorial support of his reelection campaign, Lasker and Mahoney boosted Pepper's agenda to expand the Public Health Service's role in controlling the diseases that loomed largest in the public imaginary.[48] Chief among these was the terrifying specter of cancer.

Lasker's foray into government lobbying was only one part of her multi-pronged attack on cancer. Lasker had previously used her and her husband's philanthropic power to raise funds for the American Society for the Control of Cancer. After shortly becoming disillusioned with reluctance on the part of the society's surgeon leadership to invest in research, Lasker took over the organization and secured a commitment from its executives to devote one-quarter of the newly renamed American Cancer Society's (ACS) funds to cancer research. Her involvement in lobbying for increases to federal spending on biomedical research was similarly motivated by her frustration with medical professionals who insisted on shoring up professional autonomy over launching new efforts to improve cancer outcomes through innovation. By bringing federal science agencies into the mix, Lasker's hope was to develop a national infrastructure that would serve "as a supplier of research and training services, while the ACS would focus on public education and innovative science."[49]

The recent defeats of stand-alone health care and science-funding bills signaled to the enterprising Lasker that lobbying for increased annual appropriations could be a lower-risk, higher-reward strategy than attempts to back direct legislation.[50] Lasker thus recruited an army of sympathetic physicians, scientists, administrators, and activists who could serve as expert witnesses in routine congressional testimony or could otherwise persuade subcommittee members to increase appropriations for cancer research efforts.[51] In addition to controlling the country's largest voluntary association devoted to cancer, "by the mid-1950s Lasker exercised substantial influence over both the expert advice supplied to Congress about cancer and the machinery of appropriations for federal spending on biomedical research."[52] These circumstances, coupled with the AMA's "indifference toward cancer research" policy, concentrated tremendous power in the Lasker lobby.[53] Though public support for cancer research was mounting in this period due in part to the success of chemotherapy in treating childhood leukemia, Lasker's lobby played a far more influential role in these increases than did pressure from constituents. In securing congressional funding to advance chemotherapy in the early 1950s, Lasker and her lobby even surmounted a cool attitude toward chemotherapy among members of NCI's leadership.[54]

Congressional lobbying also gave Lasker and her allies the opportunity to circumvent opposition from members of the scientific community whose ideas about science policy ran counter to theirs. The medical research policy environment of the immediate postwar period was markedly different from the one Lasker and her allies envisioned. Vannevar Bush's inspired take on a National Science Foundation (NSF) was not universally shared, as other prominent voices (such as National Academy of Sciences president Frank Jewett) insisted that peacetime research and development could return to its idyllic prewar days without losing any integrity. For most physicians and scientists, this would entail a return to universities and hospitals that considered intensive research marginal to their missions. Scientists employed in private industry where the bulk of research and development monies were then spent would remain focused on research with potential commercial application. Voluntarist societies would remain fixed on improving the delivery and quality of medical care to the afflicted. For their part, the Rockefellers, Carnegies, and other research foundations could continue allocating their small millions to the handful of projects deemed worthy of private support.

But the status quo ante did not suit Lasker's ambitions, and she did not have to look far to find prominent physicians and researchers who agreed with her. She gathered these powerful allies to testify during Pepper's hearings in 1944, where they forcefully argued that the nation's patchwork system of private investment in medical research was woefully inadequate to fund the kind of cutting-edge inquiry that would finally rid the American people of common scourges such as cancer, arthritis, and heart disease. Lasker armed herself and her allies with a compelling new rhetoric: not only should the nation invest more money in medical research, but also its investments should equal the burden these diseases imposed upon society.[55] Assigning medical research value proportionate to that of lives lost or comparing the losses to disease with those due to military conflicts quickly became a theme in the debates over how to fund medical research in the immediate aftermath of World War II.[56] Its broad resonance with policy makers and the public helped propel medical research to national prominence alongside other notable discussions of how to ensure the general welfare and prosperity of the American people in peacetime. Lasker ensured her agents had the statistics to back up their claims as well. Behind the unflappable philanthropist was an army of hand-picked Madison Avenue marketing wonks whose efforts ensured the Laskerites' messaging was as convincing to members of Congress as it was to their constituents.

Learning Biomedical Research Policy at the NIH

Despite her personal charisma and singular significance, Lasker was far from the prime mover of medical research policy in the 1940s. Lasker's own position, and the strategies enjoined by fellow travelers, were of mutual influence. Indeed, throughout this period of sometimes chaotic legislative maneuvering can be found episodes of clear social learning where the NIH and NCI grew their bureaucratic capacity to plan and enact biomedical research policy. Lasker and Mahoney worked through sympathetic legislators such as Senator Matthew Neely, who had once scolded the NIH for its attempt to cap appropriations to an amount they deemed able to responsibly spend, to spur the institutes toward bureaucratic innovation.[57] As the NIH at this time "seemed only able to react—sometimes reluctantly, always slowly—to priorities urged by others," Lasker adopted a similar tack to Neely's in cajoling the NIH to action via constant appropriations increases.[58] Under the leadership of NCI director Leonard Scheele, the NIH acquired new bureaucratic competencies to accommodate the growing desire among lobbyists and their congressional allies to fill the nation's biomedical research coffers. Reasoning that the NIH could work on a long-term plan to find use for an increase in funding, institute leadership emboldened its budget requests by tripling NCI expenditures beginning in fiscal year 1947.[59] Scheele was elevated to the Surgeon General's Office in 1948 and in this position encouraged ongoing relationships between the lobbyists and the NCI. Lasker in turn warmed to the idea of the NCI leading the nation's cancer research enterprise. The resulting détente helped solidify the NIH's role as the preeminent federal funding body for biomedical research against all would-be usurpers, including the NSF.

But it was NIH scientist-bureaucrat James Shannon who would seize upon the strategy that helped change the national institutes into the modern research and policy centers they are today. Shannon rose quickly through the ranks of the NIH and was soon venerated for his skill as an administrator whose

> vision of the grand design [of the NIH] . . . enabled him to serve so effectively
> as director general of the medical research enterprise, sitting between those

on one side who fashioned a policy they believed and expected would bring the American people into a new age of good health and long life, of freedom from fear of disease; and on the other, those scientists who pursued truth, who pushed back the frontiers of knowledge bit by bit, who day to day engaged in the meticulous and fascinating effort to find new answers to old or new, particular or general, scientific problems. The two groups did not unreservedly trust each other, although their mutual dependence was crucial.[60]

In 1954, then Associate Director Shannon "sensed an opportunity" to elevate the NIH as the leading agency in sponsoring biomedical research (a role that lately seemed threatened by the Eisenhower administration's efforts to better define a funding jurisdiction for the fledgling NSF).[61] Under the advisement of NIH Office of Research Planning chief Charles Kidd, Shannon strategically positioned NIH grants as investments in inexpensive public health innovations such as the newly minted polio vaccine. By funding investigators such as Jonas Salk, the NIH's modest investments in prevention could eliminate the need for massive expenditures on health care. By indirectly funding clinicians in universities as scientific investigators, NIH grants could also circumvent AMA objections to direct support for medical training.

Under Shannon, the NIH's goal was to ultimately develop an infrastructure capable of coordinating the nation's biomedical research enterprise and integrating its fruits into health policy, if not medical practice. The NIH had an opportunity to vividly demonstrate its leadership when it intervened to standardize and screen polio vaccine lots after the devastating quality-control failures by Cutter Laboratories that led to a polio outbreak in 1955. Its success in rapidly scaling up vaccine production led to a reversal in the Eisenhower administration's attitude toward biomedical research funding. When James Shannon ascended to the NIH directorship in 1955, he took over an organization experiencing dramatic increases in funding and political favor.[62]

Between 1955 and 1960, the NIH budget grew from $81 million to $400 million.[63] In the first years of major influx, the brisk pace of funding expansion "unsettled every aspect of institutional life at NIH."[64] The NIH and its component institutes quickly grew in complexity in an attempt to adapt to this congressional largesse, particularly around programs that channeled funding into building research facilities and other infrastructure. Funding dispensed to these infrastructure projects was often accompanied by "informal program development" efforts that aimed to steer researchers and clinicians toward particular policies and practices.[65]

As Scheffler notes, the efforts of Lasker and her colleagues effected nothing short of a change in the political culture of biomedical research funding.[66] Yet critics of the Lasker-led medical research lobby feared that the lobby's single-minded focus on the diseases that most terrified Americans may have made the lobby's strategy a victim of its own success. "The aim was to make medical services more available, but there was little thought as to whether such an investment might actually make any difference in health."[67] As Strickland sharply observed in 1972: "Federal biomedical research and related programs have carried a heavy burden over the last 25 years. Unaccompanied by the real thing, medical research has *had* to serve as a 'national health insurance.' Lacking a comprehensive system for the delivery of existing health knowledge and health care techniques to all persons specifically in need, the country has seemed to expect that new results of medical research, and the expanding presence of a research enterprise in medical schools and university science departments and hospitals, would suffice, following a kind of 'trickle-down' theory, to produce better health for the American people generally.[68] The challenge of how to formulate policies that would meet such demands would fall on the scientists tasked with managing the growing bureaucracy of the NIH and its component institutes.

CONGRESSIONAL PRINCIPALS FIND BIOMEDICAL FUNDING A HOME

Significant transformations in the intramural laboratories of the NCI followed from attempts to position this federal research agency as a surrogate mechanism for expanding health care access through the legislative system and its interfaces with public and private interest groups. In the 1940s and 1950s, U.S. spending on medical research grew exponentially; most of this growth occurred in the context of distributed and investigator-driven research grants and in the absence of any unified philosophy of governance for the nation's investment.[69] Control over the evaluation and allocation of federal moneys was left to the directors of each categorical institute within the NIH, to whom policy making for the nation's biomedical research portfolio was also delegated by statute.[70] The sacred autonomy of funded investigators in dispensing with their grants in accordance with their professional judgment prevailed in the absence of explicit policy design. The combination of extramural granting overseen by dual layers of study section and advisory board peer review, and informal governance over the intramural program via advisory groups of institute and lab or clinic leaders, allowed the NCI to "become the prototype for other NIH institutes . . . [and] an integral part of NIH through a variety of policy and procedural means."[71] In its substance, NCI policy often reflected the opinions and dispositions of key intramural personnel, who advised NCI director John Heller (1948–1960) on most matters of scientific or bureaucratic importance.[72]

The NCI's growing reputation for research excellence was matched with "statutory obligations for disease control" distinctive among the institutes.[73] In 1937, the bulk of the NCI's first year of funding was allocated to a program providing radium for the treatment of medically indigent cancer patients across the country.[74] Yet the interpretation of the NCI's mission as involving immediate cancer care subsidy was short lived, and the institute's advisors quickly transitioned to a sustained emphasis on research and training support as the only politically viable budgetary position. By the 1950s, the NCI's most direct efforts to coordinate cancer control programs at the level of state and local health departments foundered in the fragmentation of services between government and private practice.[75]

At the same time the NCI was unloading direct-care programs elsewhere in the PHS, public enthusiasm for cancer chemotherapy was mounting, and the American Cancer Society was drumming up support for the new technique in congressional hearings. When Lasker and her ally, famed chemotherapist Sidney Farber, were appointed to the National Advisory Cancer Council in 1953, they obtained significant oversight over policy and planning in the NCI's fledgling chemotherapy program. Lasker leveraged her position in the institute's governance apparatus to ensure the program focused on developing new curatives.[76] Yet NCI scientist-bureaucrats defined the issues and stakes of chemotherapy research and development differently from Lasker and funneled the institute's investments toward projects that emphasized the still inchoate nature of these therapeutics above their potential for immediate clinical success. Thus, when Congress earmarked appropriations funding to establish the Cancer Chemotherapy National Service Center (CCNSC) in 1955, NCI administrators designed a "large-scale, broad-scope, nondirected chemotherapy program" that "reflect[ed] the NCI's misgivings about the intellectual worth of screening" over Lasker and her congressional allies' therapeutic optimism.[77]

In the first five years of its operation, the CCNSC's budget grew to more than $30 million, its galloping expansion "driven by powerful political forces."[78] Yet Lasker and her supporters' plans for ramping up the chemotherapy program met resistance from the NCI's Kenneth Endicott, who had been appointed chief of the CCNSC at the program's inception. Endicott cautioned that growing too aggressively jeopardized NCI scientist-bureaucrats' ability to manage "a smooth, efficient cooperative program."[79] At the same time that NCI personnel found ways to push back against lobbyists, "the NIH and the political forces that sustained it in the late 1950s and early 1960s achieved a remarkable degree of autonomy from external political control."[80] The growing disconnect between congressional support, spurred by the Lasker lobby, and the NCI's own operational routines would lead to more explosive conflicts over planning and contracting in later years.

Despite the lack of a coherent national cancer research policy and growing tensions between disease lobbyists, Congress, and the NCI, funding for the institute continued to grow. The NCI budget quintupled in the decade between 1952 and 1962 alone.[81] As Strickland argues, the NIH rose to prominence as the nation's leading medical research entity "from the aggregate condition that scientific talent, political interest, popular concern, [and] hence federal dollars had no place else to go."[82] Political stalemates and divided government prevented broader planning around the many bills in support of enhancing medical research that sailed through Congress on public and special interest support. These moneys defaulted to the NIH as the federal agency with standing authorization to dispense funds immediately and to their intended use. Yet "the key members of Congress, research lobby leaders, and biomedical science bureaucrats had never sat down together and drawn up a set of goals or even a strategic plan for attaining goals presumably shared, implicitly agreed upon."[83] And while Lasker had cozy relationships with powerful committee members in Congress, she lacked a similar closeness with most NCI scientist-bureaucrats. Indeed, NIH director Shannon was careful to shore up the institutes' autonomy to protect its internal policy processes from interference by lobbyists such as Lasker, whom he preferred to keep at arm's length.[84] Agency autonomy was important in preserving the policy initiative of the scientist-bureaucrats who in fact designed most biomedical research policies. Though they "appeared to be congressional directives to the agency," Shannon insisted these policies "were in fact directives that NIH had approved in advance if not originated."[85] The NCI's attempts to maintain control over research programs funded by Congress through pressure from

Lasker's lobby further spurred agency bureaucrats to wed scientific expertise and administrative procedure in an effort to preserve their autonomy.

CONCLUSION

By the end of the 1950s, funding for medical research had taken on a life of its own in Congress. Few on Capitol Hill dared openly object to funding biomedical research. Moreover, the impression of fervent public support for investment in disease cures (brought to life in part by the polling and publicity efforts of Lasker, Mahoney, and their lobbying apparatus) elevated medical research to a bipartisan policy agenda. Campaigning for the presidency in 1960, John F. Kennedy promised to accelerate the nation's investments in biomedical research and infrastructure so that "what has already been accomplished in polio and T.B. . . . might soon be accomplished for cancer."[86] Yet by this time, Congress had become "convinced that the executive did not intend to offer leadership" on biomedical research policy and "all but ignored the traditional executive policy-directing, pace-setting machinery" embodied in the office of the surgeon general.[87] Congress treated biomedical research support as the de facto prerogative of Congress and delegated the work of nuts-and-bolts policy making to the national institutes.

Nevertheless, in return for their willingness to handsomely fund the National Institutes of Health, congressional principals were becoming more direct in their expectation that the institutes apply these investments to improving the nation's health.[88] As the legal historian Richard Rettig summarizes: "There was essential agreement among all on objectives. Medical research was supported to generate scientific results that would undergird the practice of medicine and lead to the improved health status of American citizens. NIH was a health agency, not a scientific agency, and the investment in scientific research was made because of its health mission. . . . The large issue that divided people the most had to do with the strategy or philosophy of research management. How could scientific research be supported in order to improve the health of the American public most effectively and rapidly?"[89]

While Congress and lobbyists emphasized the health mission of the NIH, federal scientist-bureaucrats' practical commitments emphasized their scientific mission. As the intramural program successfully learned how to address health concerns, efforts to retool the NCI's extramural grants system to support the expansion of medical infrastructure and manpower generated practical work-arounds for operational problems related to the institute's rapid expansion, which led to long-lasting changes in how scientists and administrators interpreted the dual mission of the NCI as a basic research–public health hybrid. Over time, it also encouraged some scientist-bureaucrats to develop organizational means for conceptualizing the general welfare within their routine approaches to both science and policy making.

This chapter detailed how the NCI was modernized through expansive growth driven by a coalition of members of Congress and lobbyists who were persuaded that biomedical research investment could ameliorate health problems in a political environment where national health care reform was no longer deemed politically possible. In its modern form, the NCI was structured as an organization that sponsored, coordinated, and executed the fundamental research that could yield effective cancer interventions. By building infrastructure within the NCI and in extramural research centers, it could seed the projects that would improve cancer outcomes among afflicted citizens. Yet the NCI's growing role in funding academic research and building infrastructure for cutting-edge biomedical science throughout the nation soon enabled it to secure a degree of autonomy and thus greater discretion in shaping its environment toward the agency's own interpretations of its goals. The following chapters detail how the NCI's growing importance to biomedicine allowed scientist-bureaucrats' definitions of the issues and stakes of health-relevant cancer research to feed back into the academic and industrial world of cancer research in ways that enhanced the agency's policy-making expertise and innovative capacity. NCI leadership's early attempts to interpret the organization's mission to serve science and health in light of a melioristic political program would lead it to invest in transformative national infrastructure while also developing a distinct orientation to cancer research policy that would contribute to attempts to target cancer virus and vaccine research in the following decades.

CHAPTER 2

CANCER VIRUSES AND THE PROMISE OF A VACCINE, 1958–1968

I n 1962, the associate director of the National Cancer Institute's intramural laboratory programs, Carl G. Baker, mused:

> The translation of the data of biomedical research into benefits for the sick is often incomplete and always slow. These lags—conceptual, diagnostic, therapeutic—are cumulative and even potentiating. The result is that in some diseases there is little resemblance between what is available to the average patient and to the patient with the same disease at hospitals associated with active research groups. This lag can be excused in a number of ways, but underlying all of them is a failure to accept responsibility for broad application of research information. The scientists and clinical investigators who establish a new finding are best able to recognize its implications, yet are in the poorest position to reduce it to general availability. The discoverers perhaps rightly feel their responsibilities end with publication. But the responsibility deficit is not in communication, for rapid communication of new findings already exists. The responsibility is that for action—to take new findings and to see that they reach the right patients through the complex social, economic, traditional, political and emotional milieu of our free society.[1]

Baker presented the NCI's newly formed Human Cancer Virus Task Force as an effort toward remedying the "lag" between formal scientific knowledge and therapeutic medical intervention by ensuring alignment among the complex social factors that militate against their application. Just as Baker entreated his audience of legislators and scientists to assume their responsibility for ensuring the rapid translation of scientific findings into medical practice, he proposed the NCI as an organization committed to leading the way forward on this front.

Baker's preamble was more than mere patriotic throat-clearing. By 1962, the NCI's intramural research programs were on the leading edge of cancer virology, and emerging findings suggested to NCI researchers the possibility that vaccines might help control the disease in the human population. The origins of the NCI's virus cancer and vaccine programs date back to the institute's rapid expansion during the mid to late 1950s. Initially, cancer vaccine studies were purely coincident with this transformation of the NCI's bureaucratic scope and resources. They developed out of attempts to replicate the findings of a small handful of enterprising biologists such as Ludwik Gross, who in a 1951 publication reported the incidence of tumors in mice whose characteristics suggested an infectious cause.[2] In these early days of virus and vaccine research at the NCI, the costs of necessary apparatus, such as electron microscopes and pure virus material, were expensive for a humble institute, but they paid off. By 1954, the NCI could boast that "for the first time, it became possible to isolate, purify, and characterize the virus that caused a form of leukosis in chickens, a disease that resembles leukemia [and apply] the techniques . . . to human leukemia to discover whether it, too, is caused by a virus."[3] In pursuing such emerging findings, the institute's virus and vaccine efforts would soon become deeply enmeshed in bureaucratic innovations aimed at directly shepherding fundamental biological knowledge through its development into medical and public health technologies.

Scholars of twentieth-century medical science and technology note an enduring tension in postwar (particularly U.S.) discourse around national funding priorities. One tendency, frequently attributed to academic scientists, is toward the elevation of fundamental knowledge derived from investigator-initiated "basic" research as a Jacob's ladder to innovation. Another tendency, often counterposed even as it is implied by its alter, is to perceive "applied" research as the paramount priority for public funding in liberal democracies. This stance is attributed to private interest, policy, and public opinion as reflecting the imperative for research investments to address prevailing societal concerns. There has been great variation within organizations and across time as to which principle should govern research investment priorities. In the NIH, both perspectives coexist. Often, where statutory mandates do not directly implicate NIH scientists' research in improving the health of the general populace, cultural understandings of their obligations as public servants compel them to serve the broader American public in addition to the scientific public.

The NCI's dual mandate to advance both science and health was embodied in this period in the ambitious attempt to design a crash program that would identify a viral cause of human cancers and develop a vaccine to protect the public against this threat. While historians have examined these efforts as expressions of Cold War science planning applied to a civilian health organization,[4] here I focus on how the complex interplay between open-ended cancer virus inquiry and bureaucratic ambitions to develop a vaccine affected the direction of science unfolding in the NCI's intramural program. The virus cancer vaccine programs that developed in this period articulated the broader public health stakes of NCI scientist-bureaucrats' research in bureaucratic planning apparatus, but these stakes had to be iteratively reconciled with their embedded experimental work. In the process of articulating these issues and stakes in experimentation, NCI scientist-bureaucrats justified a profound buildup of the material infrastructure for molecular and immunological work in service of learning how to develop a vaccine against a novel category of RNA viruses.[5] The iterative nature of priority setting in the institute's virus cancer programs opened new vistas for research into the fundamental mechanisms of carcinogenesis at the same time it foreclosed lines of inquiry into alternative viral candidates for human malignancy. The NCI's intramural efforts in this period thus provide a focused case study of how scientific and bureaucratic objectives mutually constitute one another in the process of environed social learning around the objective of developing a human cancer vaccine.

EARLY INTRAMURAL CANCER VIRUS STUDIES

Sarah Stewart (figure 2.1), a Mexican-American immigrant and the first woman to earn a medical degree from Georgetown University, was one of the early pioneers of cancer virology in the NCI. Stewart joined the institute in 1947 as an investigator in the intramural Laboratory of Biology. Whereas her colleagues continued to focus on the kind of fundamental research commonly associated with academic scientists (i.e., exploring morphology and chemical carcinogenesis in animal models and tissue systems), Stewart was an early evangelist of the idea that viruses caused cancer. As colleague Alan Rabson recalled, Stewart set herself

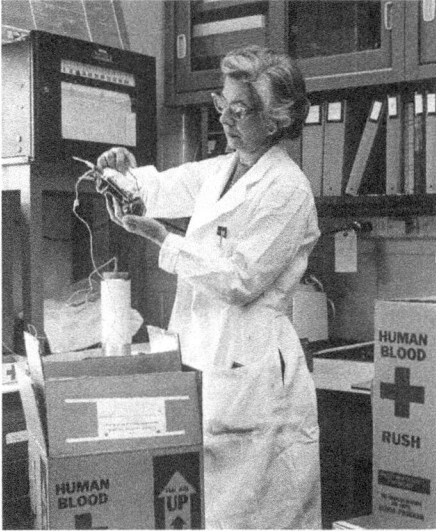

2.1 Sarah Stewart working at the NCI in the 1950s.

Photo credit: G. V. Hecht, Office of NIH History, and Stetten Museum.

at odds with other NCI scientists when "she said she was going to prove that cancer was caused by viruses."[6] Stewart's shift toward defining the issues and stakes of cancer research as one of viruses and their possible vaccines was precipitated by a series of findings generated in her collaborative work with Lloyd Law and others housed in the same intramural unit.

In the first half of the 1950s, Law established a prodigious program exploring the role of viruses in experimental lymphoma in mice. Stewart acted as a co-principal investigator on a series of projects exploring Ludwik Gross's claim that a "cell-free" material, likely a virus, induced leukemia in young mice.[7] From a morass of suggestive experimental trends that failed to yield statistically significant variance in leukemia among control mice and experimental mice injected with "cell-free" material from Gross's leukemic mice, Stewart's attention fixed on one puzzling and unexpected trend: where investigators had anticipated disseminated leukemia, parotid gland tumors occurred in experimental animals at one-and-a-half times the rate of leukemia—and in control mice not at all.

Stewart's colleagues in the Laboratory of Biology proposed a triptych of studies to explore the possible genetic origins of these parotid gland neoplasms in mice and to test the oncogenicity of the Gross cell-free agent in other species. However, in 1954 Stewart's observations colligated around a different line of inquiry. Having experimented in more and different mouse colonies than her colleagues, Stewart observed not only the mysterious parotid gland tumors but also other unexpected neoplasms. Iteratively pursuing these results in a series of experiments, Stewart soon isolated a "filterable agent" (an agnostic category used at the time to suggest the presence of a virus[8]) that consistently yielded early parotid and adrenal gland tumors in inoculated mice. Armed with the hypothesis that gonadal hormones might have an "adjuvant effect" on the development of these cancers, Stewart initiated her own principal project to pursue the possibility that these cancers were caused by a novel virus.[9]

Within two years, Stewart's research had departed dramatically from that still pursued by Law and her former colleagues in the Laboratory of Biology's Leukemia Studies Section. Stewart, now chief of the Laboratory of Biology, began exploring whether the parotid gland tumors she observed in mice were of viral origin in a new series of experiments that drew upon the tools commonly deployed by virologists to isolate viruses.[10] Such a leap from animal studies to propagation of virus in tissue cultures was no mean feat for a physician, let alone one whose efforts were not always vigorously supported by her colleagues. Stewart approached several researchers throughout the NCI who had tissue culture systems that might allow her to continue her research, but all refused her.[11] It was NIH colleague Bernice Eddy, another maverick female scientist working in the Division of Biologics Standards (who made a name for herself by first blowing the whistle on insufficiently treated batches of polio vaccine manufactured by Cutter Laboratories in 1955 and would later help isolate simian virus 40), who eventually provided the tissue culture technologies needed to advance Stewart's experiments.[12]

Another two years of iterative experimentation in monkey and mouse embryo tissue cultures culminated in a 1958 publication where Stewart and Eddy claimed to have isolated a novel virus from murine parotid tumors.[13] The eponymous Stewart-Eddy (SE) virus belonged to a family of viruses they called "polyoma" viruses, so named because these viruses could each produce a number of different neoplasms beyond the parotid gland. The new definition of what was at issue with these parotid tumors—specifically, infection with SE polyomavirus— allowed them to redefine the stakes of their research toward the goal of vaccine development. Encoding these issues and stakes in experimental practice, Stewart and Eddy began immunological studies to test antibody responses to the poly-omavirus in mice, rats, hamsters, rabbits, and humans. Using a protocol initially designed by Eddy, they rapidly developed a live virus vaccine and tested it in hamsters.[14] The results of these studies were promising: 97 percent of vaccinated animals were protected against subsequent viral challenge. As colleague Alan Rabson recalls, Stewart's experiments had been derided by her peers as unrigor-ous, an evaluation abetted by sexism.[15] Yet her discovery of the SE polyomavirus was quickly regarded by "real virologists" as a major breakthrough: "Suddenly the whole place just exploded after Sarah found polyoma."[16]

Stewart's first successful innovation—the identification of a polyomavirus that caused several cancers in animals—quickly led to the development and expansion of new competencies in the NCI's intramural program. Scientifically, Stewart's immunological experiments with SE polyomavirus were now oriented toward demonstrating virus in human leukemia with the end goal of develop-ing immunological assays and prophylactic vaccines.[17] Her scientific goals would ultimately not succeed in producing their target innovation of a human vac-cine. Organizationally, however, Stewart's ambitious vaccine goals expanded the personnel engaged in similar virus projects in the General Biology Section of the Laboratory of Biology where she was housed. Clinicians from the NCI's intramural Surgery Branch, led by Rabson, began efforts to detect virus in brain tissues sampled from humans who died of cancer. Stewart and Eddy recruited John Moloney, a colleague of some note in the world of cancer virus research, to conduct parallel studies of the human cultures they were propagating that were based on Rabson and colleagues' surgical samples. Another colleague, Robert Manaker, assumed the lead on efforts to isolate "hypothetical" oncogenic viruses from these human tissue samples.[18] Many of Manaker's projects proved fruitless and were abandoned, but their failure taught the emerging cadre of cancer virus researchers the importance of developing reliable tissue cultures. There could be no careful planning of such studies in their current resource environment; human tumor samples were hard to come by, and "tissue was utilized as it became available if the necessary tissue cultures were on hand."[19]

By 1958, it was clear to intramural scientists that there was a general dearth of surgical and autopsy samples of human tumors in sufficient quantity to conduct well-designed experiments that could compellingly demonstrate the etiological role of viruses in human cancers. Indeed, it seemed that cancer vaccine stud-ies would not be able to proceed without an expanded network of clinicians and scientists who could supply materials and conduct experiments in search of oncogenic viruses. Another pressing issue was that of space; following the decades-long modernization of the NIH, the institutes' programs had far outrun the capacity to house them at the physical plant in Bethesda.[20] These researchers believed the stakes of their studies, which had the potential to promote human health through cancer vaccines, warranted a major investment in cancer virus studies, for which the NCI's scientist-bureaucrats would need to obtain additional support from their principals in Congress.

CREATING A CANCER VIRUS PROGRAM

As findings mounted, a sense of urgency around cancer virus research piqued NCI leadership. Stewart's groundbreaking polyomavirus studies were quickly joined by Moloney and Frank Rauscher's identification of a number of animal tumor viruses, and both Stewart and her new colleague Mary Fink were earnestly pursuing vaccine systems to combat these newly identified agents. The possibility of establishing a viral etiology to human leukemia and subsequently developing prophylactic vaccines against these viruses seemed nigh. With the aid of the National Advisory Cancer Council (NACC), which included a noted scientist sympathetic to cancer virus research in Nobel laureate Wendell Stanley, then NCI director John Heller successfully petitioned Congress for a special appropriation of $1 million for "vigorous stimulation of research and training efforts in the study of the possible viral origin of human cancer."[21]

Though the NCI and NACC's optimism was largely driven by research emerging from the intramural program, Congress did not focus its funding on an expansion of the NCI's efforts. The one-time influx of federal funds primarily targeted grants-in-aid to train "outstanding virologists, many of whom had made significant contributions to the development of a successful poliomyelitis vaccine and were ready to apply their talents to cancer virology."[22] What remained of the funds after grants were exhausted would be put toward the production of necessary material infrastructure for virus and vaccine research nationwide, including the purchase of the virus antigen and reagent stocks of the National Foundation for Infantile Paralysis, which the foundation was closing out as it planned to shift away from polio vaccine research.[23] While it could not cure the institute of its space and personnel ailments, the special appropriation's use in supporting stockpiles of necessary experimental materials would allow investigators to pursue opportunities in cancer virus and vaccine studies that might otherwise have languished.

In the course of their meetings with the NACC around dispensing these funds, NCI scientist-bureaucrats iteratively reconstructed the possibility of cancer vaccine research around the issue of resource constraints in the NCI. Intramural scientists like Stewart and Fink who had already initiated vaccine explorations found support for this interpretation among scientific principals in the NIH Virology and Rickettsiology Study Section, which counted among its members polio vaccine innovators Jonas Salk and Albert Sabin.[24] These scientists had seen firsthand what targeted interdisciplinary vaccine efforts could accomplish and were persuaded of the need to erect a similar bureaucratic scaffolding to support the NCI's attempts to develop cancer vaccines.

Having colligated around an interpretation of the bureaucratic issues facing cancer virus research as primarily involving resource constraints, NCI scientists and their extramural allies mobilized to encode this interpretation into policies that could address these issues. The study section consulted with NCI leadership and the NACC for more than a year to form a special Panel on Viruses and Cancer that would develop a series of recommendations for expanding the resources and infrastructure necessary to advance cancer virus inquiry toward the identification of possible human vaccine candidates. Though this formulation of the ultimate stakes of resource and infrastructure expansion was compelling to their scientific principals, the NCI's efforts ran up against the limitations of scientific governance in the institute at this time. Although the NACC formally approved projects recommended by study sections, it "lacked the mandate to sponsor specific projects" of its own initiative, including those that might enable the NCI to pay outside laboratories to produce the immunological tools that would allow it to scale up vaccine studies initiated in-house.[25]

The issue of how to target funds to sponsor virus cancer research soon became embroiled in broader administrative and planning issues in the NCI. Together with scientific principals on the NACC, the Virology and Rickettsiology Study Section, and the Panel on Viruses and Cancer, NCI scientist-bureaucrats engaged in a protracted learning process that would end in the expansion of the intramural program's managerial competencies and a shift in the NACC's role in institute governance. The impetus for these bureaucratic transformations was the creation of a new unit in the institute that would fund the creation of large-scale research resources through contracts in addition to grants.

CONTRACT RESEARCH AND THE GROWTH OF BUREAUCRATIC AUTONOMY

Until the mid-1950s, most intramural research at the NCI was investigator initiated and undirected—of a class with canonical "basic research" driven by curiosity and appraised in terms of the fundamental biological knowledge it elucidated. This changed in 1955, when the NCI established the Cancer Chemotherapy National Service Center (CCNSC) as the institute's first large-scale collaborative enterprise. The CCNSC was an attempt to harness scientific and industry expertise around drug screening and clinical trials pioneered during World War II for the purpose of acting as a clearinghouse for testing promising anticancer compounds submitted by scientists from academia, industry, and the NIH.[26] The CCNSC organized extensive networks of intramural scientists, academic clinicians, and industry suppliers around a new approach to moving compounds from screening all the way through human trials. The magnitude and complexity of the enterprise demanded an unprecedented administrative structure and cutting-edge managerial approaches to coordinate drug development and clinical trials. Kenneth Endicott developed these early approaches to collaborative research as head of the CCNSC.

In 1960, Endicott was promoted to become NCI director. As his then deputy Carl G. Baker recalls, "While [Endicott] strongly endorsed the support of basic research, he also believed the NIH research programs should include directed research target programs aimed at solving important disease problems. He brought this philosophy to the directorship of the NCI and would proceed to reorganize the NCI to reflect this philosophy. This change was a shift from a largely *reactive* to an added *proactive* stance on the part of the management style of the Institute."[27] This "proactive" management style was one Baker would later extend in his efforts to adapt Endicott's approach to chemotherapy screening to the problem of cancer virus research and vaccine development in the intramural program.

In his first few years at the helm, Endicott instituted a number of administrative reforms that developed programmed areas of the organization in the image of the CCNSC. When the NACC's Panel on Viruses and Cancer concluded in 1960 that the special congressional appropriations for virus leukemia research should be used to establish a clearinghouse providing research resources for various scientists in the field, the CCNSC offered a clear bureaucratic model for organizing this new unit.[28] The Virus Research Resources Branch (VRRB) was thus established to provide resources (such as virus reagents and tissue cultures) and administrative support to the burgeoning number of researchers within and without the NCI who were investigating cancer viruses.

In addition to building up the material infrastructure necessary for nationwide virus cancer and vaccine research to advance, the formation of the VRRB also led to important scientific collaborations throughout the NIH. The National Institute of Allergy and Infectious Diseases (NIAID), as the resident institute nominally assigned the task of investigating viral diseases, was enrolled in the project of building up the NCI's stores of virus materials from agents identified in the preceding decade. This expensive and laborious task brought scientist-bureaucrats from the NCI and NIAID together to solve problems of logistics and operations for the VRRB as a service organization. These collaborations would enable a formal avenue for NIAID researchers interested in viral oncogenesis, such as Robert Huebner and Janet Hartley, to benefit from the funding largesse that characterized the NCI's virus cancer program throughout the 1960s.

Alongside its collaborative structure, the VRRB also adopted the CCNSC's use of contracts with private entities and academic scientists to acquire the requisite resources and services it would provide to the cancer virology community. While contracting was a common practice in military funding for research and development, it was a relatively novel bureaucratic instrument in civilian biomedical research funding. Agencies such as the NIH or NSF traditionally dispensed grants for independent investigator-initiated research with few if any requirements for these investigators to produce particular outcomes or pursue predesignated aims. The use of contracts in the CCNSC had garnered some resistance from extramural researchers who exalted the intellectual freedom the grant system provided and resisted any measures they perceived as diverting funds toward other programs. They viewed government-controlled research with suspicion and presumed it could not be of similar quality to work that had survived the traditional peer-review grants process.[29]

Endicott had battled with such objections from the scientific community as head of the CCNSC but objected to the notion that all science was best conducted by individual investigators in their isolated laboratories. He argued that efforts to quickly develop cancer virus research into vaccine candidates would require a tightly coordinated program that was best supported through well-delineated tasks specified in contracts.[30] Upon his promotion to NCI director, Endicott restructured the institute's administration to consolidate contracting authority in the hands of NCI administrators. Ostensibly in conformity with President Kennedy's injunction to stamp out conflicts of interest in government support of private businesses, but likely also in response to criticism from congressional principals who alleged the institute lacked accountability in managing grants allocated to university scientists, in 1961 Endicott restructured the relationship between the NACC and the NCI so that the NACC advised on scientific and technical rather than administrative matters.[31] Endicott justified this reform on the basis of an interpretation of contracts as procurement mechanisms distinct from grants, which "vested legal authority and responsibility for contract awards in government officials [which] could not be delegated to outsiders."[32] The council's standing review bodies once tasked with overseeing intramural operations funded by contract were thus abolished and replaced with "three Boards of the National Cancer Institute advisory to the Director, NCI, on programs that utilize research contracts in combination with direct operations for the three major collaborative research programs in virology, chemotherapy, and field studies."[33] Consequently, the authority to review and approve contracts was consolidated at the level of NCI-assembled internal review bodies.[34]

Endicott justified the removal of NACC oversight from the budding virus cancer program by insisting that long-range targeted programs like those proposed necessitated a different relationship between the NACC and the institute's standard governance structure. While Endicott's assessment of the need for contract research was based on his experiences heading the CCNSC, Baker also found Endicott's approach more appropriate to the relationship he thought the NACC should have vis-à-vis intramural research and development. In a memorandum to the newly formed NCI Policy Group, Baker minimized the role the NACC played not only in such contract-funded intramural initiatives but also in extramural grants, as "the Council rarely changes the Study Sections recommendations." He also insinuated that "how closely . . . the collective action on grant applications relate[s] to Institute programmatic interests" was open for debate.[35] Instead of relying upon the judgment of scientific principals on the NACC, the recently established NCI boards would directly advise NCI leadership, which would report on the progress of cancer virus research to a council that was now without standing to challenge its policy decisions around contract research.

Institute leadership's redefinition of the issues and stakes of virus cancer research as necessitating targeted contracts to address resource problems in the NCI thus precipitated a significant change in the relationship between the NCI and its scientific principals on the NACC. The NACC was primarily staffed by "elite members of the academic medical community" who discouraged the NCI from pursuing bold initiatives out of fear of "a backlash from dashed public hopes" when a cancer cure was not forthcoming.[36] Its primary role, as many NCI scientist-bureaucrats saw it, was to offer technically informed advice with an "administrative-mechanics orientation" to NCI leadership, which would consider this advice when allocating funds or developing organizational priorities.[37] Though NCI scientist-bureaucrats ostensibly enacted the 1961 contracting reforms to increase the utility of the "scientific-technical" advising offered by the NACC, some council members bristled at the removal of their authority to review intramural contracts as undermining their role in ensuring agency accountability.[38] The NACC's advising role was thus a subject of intense debate throughout the 1960s over "what and how much information the NCI should provide to the Council."[39]

More to the point, the NACC was stripped of its authority to monitor internal NCI operations and thus could not ensure the NCI satisfied the standards of scientific principals embedded on the council. While other scholars have analyzed the backlash against the NCI's intramural contracting as an expression of its perceived violation of scientific norms around peer review and a valorized model of investigator autonomy, locating the initial objections to these reforms in the NACC's loss of monitoring authority shows that concerns over accountability relative to council members' perceptions of their structural relationship to the NCI were of central importance.[40]

As Strickland points out, the unity among Mary Lasker and her "noble conspirators" in Congress and the medical community also began to break down coincident with these internal reforms: "The NIH directorate was less and less inclined to do the bidding of the Congress or the outside professionals unless that bidding was in accord with NIH aims. The medical science bureaucrats developed strategies of getting around even relatively specific congressional directives.... The Congress, more comfortable and more sophisticated now, used the outside professionals for their own purposes more and more."[41] At the same time as the once cozy relationships between disease lobbyists and Congress began to pull apart, Lasker and her allies increasingly focused their efforts on steering internal NCI policy through scientific allies on the NACC. Yet the changes to the institutional environment that weakened the ties between the NCI and its principals in Congress and its scientific advisors on the NACC would also limit Lasker's efforts to influence the institute from within.

When in 1963 Lasker and her close confidante on the NACC, Sidney Farber, attempted to push contract review as part of council oversight, they mobilized support from the House and Senate Appropriations Subcommittees in the form of directives to the institute to allow the NACC to review both contracts and grants.[42] Instead of complying with these directives from congressional principals, the NCI used NIH director James Shannon's political muscle to push for an independent review of the institute's contracting approach. The Ruina Report that was issued on this matter in 1966 was seen by NCI leadership as vindication of Endicott's decision to remove contract review from NACC oversight. The report seemed to imply that the NACC operated under a "misunderstanding" that "the deep involvement of the scientific community in grant-review and -award process" would necessarily extend to contract review.[43] Instead, the administrative nature of contracts at the NCI, coupled with precedents for contract funding elsewhere in the PHS, justified their use as instruments for fulfilling what procurement needs NCI bureaucrats deemed appropriate through their own scientific and managerial judgment. Going further, the Ruina Report suggested that external peer review was an inferior mechanism given the virus program's goals to target research toward the discovery of human cancer viruses and vaccines and encouraged the NCI to continue cultivating managerial talents among its intramural scientists that would support more coordinated efforts in the future as a means of putting federal monies to good use.[44] Iteratively encoding its autonomy in making contracting decisions through negotiations with the NACC and the results of the Ruina Report, the NCI was empowered with significant autonomy from oversight by both congressional and scientific principals in its management of contract research. Though the institute considered the matter of contracting settled in its favor, the lack of NACC monitoring would precipitate ongoing political action on the part of lobbyists such as Lasker and, later, molecular biologists to permanently enhance the council's position in institute governance.

LEARNING DIRECTED RESEARCH IN THE
VIRUS CANCER PROGRAMS

By 1962, Endicott had centralized contract authorization capacities in the NCI Office of the Director, ensuring that for these programs at least intramural scientist-bureaucrats would have the final say in determining when contracts were scientifically sound.[45] At the same time, Endicott moved "to utilize senior staff more for broad substantive cancer considerations and less for routine issues."[46] Effectively, this meant that day-to-day execution of projects was put in the hands of scientist-bureaucrats who also occupied mid-level administrative positions (whom NCI leadership of this era took to calling "scientist-managers"), such as laboratory chiefs and project principal investigators.[47] Scientist-managers cultivated organizational competencies that marked substantial breaks in routine practice for resource allocation at the NCI. All other projects funded by the NCI through grants required both the imprimatur of administrators high in the chain of command at NIH as well as a stamp of approval in the form of secondary peer review by the NACC. Endicott's move to position contracting authority solely within the NCI established a decentralized administrative apparatus for executing collaborative cancer virus research that was without precedent in federal health agencies. As the budget for virus research continued to grow briskly over the decade, it would also concentrate significant control over research policy and funding in the hands of these intramural scientist-managers whose primary expertise in cancer research would inform their administrative decisions in the institute's specialized targeted programs.

At the same time these bureaucratic transformations were taking place, growing interest in cancer virus research in the intramural program had prompted the establishment of a dedicated Laboratory of Viral Oncology in 1961. The laboratory's chief, W. Ray Bryan, had designs to expand the scope of virus research in the institute substantially.[48] The intramural reorganization that led to the founding of Bryan's new laboratory was meant to reflect emerging approaches to cancer causation, with "emphasis on clinical investigation of treatment, diagnosis, and prevention."[49] Paramount among these emerging approaches in the Laboratory of Viral Oncology were the virus and vaccine studies spearheaded by Stewart, Moloney, Manaker, and Fink, who split off from the Laboratory of Biology to join the new unit.

The Laboratory of Viral Oncology was founded around an explicit goal of uniting research on virally induced cancers in animal models and research on virally induced cancers in human patients, a transformation in the issues and stakes of cancer virus research that they instantiated in studies of human leukemia of possible viral origin. In 1962, Fink reported a successful live attenuated vaccine experiment that protected mice from challenge with Rauscher murine leukemia virus. Unlike many of her peers who believed that efficacious clinical interventions could only proceed on foundational knowledge of the basic mechanisms of oncogenesis, Fink proposed her successful vaccine experiment as an important contribution to immunological theory. She inferred from the detection of circulating antibody that humoral immunity played an important role in viral oncogenesis, over and above "the generally accepted view of a 'cellular' basis for immunity in other experimental murine neoplasms of unknown etiology."[50] For Fink, whose focus would remain stubbornly on the development of human cancer virus vaccines throughout her career at the NCI, the practical accomplishment of cancer prevention preceded and entailed her contributions to abstract knowledge.

As Scheffler and I have noted elsewhere, the explosive growth of cancer virus research anticipated by these early changes in the intramural program were mortgaged against the discovery of a human leukemia virus that had not yet been shown to exist.[51] Accompanying the formation of the Laboratory of Viral Oncology was the first major example of infrastructure building aimed at developing human cancer virus knowledge and preventive technology. As Endicott noted:

> Looking toward the time when highly suspect viruses are obtained from human cancer tissue, the operation of the Laboratory of Viral Oncology was designed, staffed, and equipped to carry out a number of different investigations. For example, a virus preparation and a diagnostic unit were created, as was a pathology and hematology unit, which will handle the routine testing operations that will constitute a considerable share of the work. Two new electron microscopes were procured for use in screening human specimens for evidence of virus. Without the aid of these instruments, the number of specimens that would have to be tested biologically would far outstrip the Laboratory's capacity.[52]

The laboratory's description of human virus testing capacity was not merely promissory; it was encoded in the concrete practices that characterized the projects being performed by intramural scientists and clinicians in anticipation of such results. The stakes of revealing a human cancer virus in experiments were thus tied to the immediate logistical issue of remedying shortages in human tissue samples, laboratory space, and personnel.

From a bureaucratic perspective, Endicott saw the VRRB as an opportunity to unify the Laboratory of Viral Oncology and other disparate efforts in the organization under a more comprehensive program structure.[53] Thus deployed in concert with intramural scientists' experimental practices, the VRRB enabled the generation of scientific capacities unknown before the federal government's investment in cancer virus research. In this respect, the VRRB presented itself as being "roughly equivalent to the quartermaster and intelligence activities of an army general staff."[54] Its responsibility, as NCI leadership understood it, was to determine the unmet needs of a nationwide cancer virus research and development program and provide the resources necessary to accomplish the end goal of a human cancer virus vaccine. Its mission as such was to provide "the services, resources, and materials . . . [previously] unobtainable either because knowledge and techniques were lacking to produce such resources or because of their noncommercial nature."[55] The earliest contracts issued to industry through the VRRB were meant to secure the provision of such resources not only for NCI intramural researchers but also for cancer virus researchers throughout the scientific community.

The VRRB's orientation toward supporting cancer virus efforts writ large justified not only sponsoring novel enterprises but also supporting production that was critically endangered by market forces. NCI scientist-bureaucrats had concluded that the VRRB was urgently needed because "in some cases, the commercial production of resource materials would be so prohibitively expensive that no market would be possible and no profit obtainable."[56] Indeed, some of the institute's earliest virus contracts, issued in the first years of the VRRB's operations, injected lifesaving funds for notable tissue culture and viral filtration technology projects at the American Type Culture Collection Repository and London's Wright-Fleming Institute.[57] In the latter instance, the NCI rescued a small research unit that produced gradocol membranes for virus filtration from imminent insolvency, supporting this UK institute's operations through government contracts to scale up necessary compounds for virus cancer research.

Unlike the CCNSC that inspired it, the VRRB proved to be more than a clearinghouse for outside investigators to send compounds to be tested for their therapeutic effects. By the beginning of 1963, the VRRB was transitioning into a branch that largely served in-house NCI and NIAID collaborative research on cancer viruses. In this capacity, the VRRB was a central administrative unit coordinating and executing research programs endorsed by the intramural Scientific Directorate. After 1965, "future plans for development of viral reagents [were] intimately linked with the special virus-leukemia program of the NCI" and its scientific program.[58] Collaborations courted by NCI scientists were married to the contracts previously developed through the VRRB to create large-scale diagnostic and tissue procurement programs and expand production capacity for viral reagents and culture media. To this end, the federal investment in virus research would focus on experiments using nonhuman primates as well as bovine, feline, and canine models that would allow NCI researchers to test an emerging theory that livestock and pets might be transmitting leukemia viruses to humans.[59]

With cancer virus research in its infancy, the decision to centralize research and development planning in a branch of the NCI would dramatically shape the priorities of intramural projects to come. Moving forward, the NCI and its contractors would focus their efforts on the detection of human cancer viruses and their eventual prevention with vaccines. To aid in setting the scientific program for this effort, the NCI established a Human Cancer Virus Task Force that brought together the institute's interested investigators with select outside researchers to "formulate and detail program activities which will be supported by funds for direct operations, contracts, and grants. Their objective is to obtain answers to important specific research questions within a period of three to five years, at the end of which time a decision will be made on the direction the program in these areas should take."[60] The initial priorities of the task force would be reproduced in each iteration of the NCI's formal virus cancer programs, beginning with a collaboration initiated in 1962 among the task force, the VRRB, Bryan's Laboratory of Viral Oncology, and a group headed by Dr. Robert Huebner at NIAID's Laboratory of Infectious Diseases that sought to fund studies into human leukemia. Under this collaboration, the VRRB was meant to function as a point of coordination between these groups and interested extramural scientists.[61]

In these early years, the most established lines of inquiry in cancer virus research at the NCI had colligated around murine and avian leukemias. Work done by intramural scientists such as Moloney and Rauscher found that viruses associated with these leukemias were RNA viruses, meaning they comprised single strands of nucleic acid (as opposed to double-stranded DNA viruses).[62] RNA viruses were relatively recent objects of analysis, so many of the studies at the NCI were geared toward producing knowledge of the basic morphology and mechanisms of replication of the "C-type" RNA viruses these scientists associated with murine and avian leukemia.[63] The first serious attempt at connecting viruses to human leukemia was conducted by NCI scientists in collaboration with Huebner's NIAID laboratory. The Huebner collaboration, which was carried out through a large contract with private company Microbiological Associates, included "developmental" efforts to type 120 known human and animal viruses alongside searches for unknown viruses that were potentially carcinogenic.[64] Huebner designed and carried out epidemiological studies to collect serological samples for these projects.

Huebner's efforts proved indispensable to the early planning stages of the Human Cancer Virus Task Force.[65] In November 1962, Huebner composed and submitted to Director Endicott a memorandum laying out in great detail projected resources for a full-fledged program of cancer virus research. As Huebner argued, much of the administrative cost of such a program lay in requisite personnel increases and specialized facilities construction that would dedicate 200 personnel and 30,000 square feet to the program.[66] The memo requested nearly $800,000 for fiscal year 1963 and a dedicated facility in Frederick, Maryland, to advance these efforts. However, Congress did not allocate substantial additional funds for virus studies to the intramural program's regular appropriations until 1965, so contracting became the primary bureaucratic vehicle enabling the virus cancer program to work around these space and personnel limitations. The collaboration between the NCI, Huebner, and Microbiological Associates around developmental resources for leukemia virus research was emblematic of such workarounds in the early task force days.

With the objectives of a comprehensive cancer virus program in mind, the Human Cancer Virus Task Force proceeded to formulate broad research objectives between the end of 1962 and the beginning of 1963 that would formalize the issues and stakes of the program. In February 1963, Ray Bryan submitted a formal statement of the task force's priorities to the Scientific Directorate of the NCI. Together, the task force had sorted suspected cancer viruses into different categories and ranked them according to their promise in explaining the etiology of certain cancers:

> Categories of virus-host (or host-cell) interactions associated with neoplasms of animals.
>
> I. Virus-dependent reactions in which specific viruses (or related types of viruses) are the direct continuing causes of certain specific neoplastic diseases. Examples: Rous sarcoma; leukemia of fowls; leukemia of mice.
>
> II. Viruses-initiated reactions in which viruses of different types act as biological carcinogens in the production of a variety of autonomous neoplasms of different tissues and in different species, but the virus is not associated with continuation of the neoplastic reaction (at least in a detectable form). Examples: tumors, or in vitro cell transformations, induced by the polyoma and SV-40 viruses and by adenoviruses 12 and 18.
>
> III. Co-carcinogenic reactions in which not only viruses of dependent neoplasia (e.g., Shope papilloma), but also ordinarily non-tumorigenic viruses (e.g., vaccinia, influenza) act together with chemical or other carcinogenic agents to initiate autonomous neoplasms, but neither type of agent is associated with continuation of the reaction (at least in detectable form).
>
> IV. Other reactions (this category to include future types of interaction not now known or recognized).[67]

Although category I viruses were at the time exclusively found in animals, the task force had resolved to "follow, initially, the avenues of approach that have given success with the animal model systems of category I."[68] Its focus on category I animal leukemia viruses was not meant to preclude further inquiry into other virus types. Members of the task force in the NCI as well as collaborators such as Huebner continued to investigate other viruses, especially category II viruses that were circumstantially associated with some human cancers.[69]

Despite continued investigations into category II viruses, the task force set the primary objective of the NCI's virus program as "determining whether or not viral etiological agents comparable to those that cause leukemia in fowls and mice are associated with human leukemia and lymphomas."[70] The success or failure of the program did not, however, hinge upon the success or failure of detecting a category I virus responsible for human leukemia and lymphoma.

Instead, "[i]f a substantial effort fails after a few years to yield positive results on these problems, the negative outcome will not conclusively prove a lack of association of human leukemia with a viral etiological agent, but will call for a reevaluation of the intensive efforts following these particular presently known animal model systems."[71] The open-endedness of project evaluation supported a diverse research portfolio at the inception of the program. Over the ensuing decade and a half, the diversity of the early task force iteration of the NCI's virus program would give way to intensified focus on C-type RNA viruses in the form of the Special Virus Leukemia Program. This narrowing of lines of inquiry began gradually as soon as the cancer virus program moved into formal planning stages in 1964. Despite scientist-bureaucrats' nominal efforts to develop a unique management approach that could support pursuit of open-ended virus targets, rooting their interpretations of the NCI's planning apparatus in their own experimental iterations of what was at issue in prospective human virus studies would be central to shifting program priorities decisively toward C-type RNA viruses.

DEVELOPING THE SPECIAL VIRUS LEUKEMIA PROGRAM

While the scientific prospects of a human cancer virus and vaccine initiative evoked optimism among intramural researchers, the task of effectively organizing a targeted research program remained to be solved. Shortly before he was appointed assistant director of the intramural program, Carl G. Baker (figure 2.2) had joined a group of administrators in the NIH interested in improving strategies for research management.[72] Through his extensive reading of the management literature, Baker became convinced of "an inherent tension between directed and undirected scientific research that the NIH should accommodate managerially and financially."[73] Baker was particularly impressed with what systems analysis had achieved in the Department of Defense (DOD) and was determined to adapt this model to help resolve these tensions in the NCI.[74]

At the same time, the NCI was facing strident criticism from Congress about its ability to produce medically useful results for the public from its increased investment in basic research. Some members of Congress felt the NIH had not sufficiently addressed earlier criticisms that the NCI lacked sufficient oversight of the millions of dollars it distributed in grants every year. They launched an additional review under the Wooldridge Committee to investigate whether the

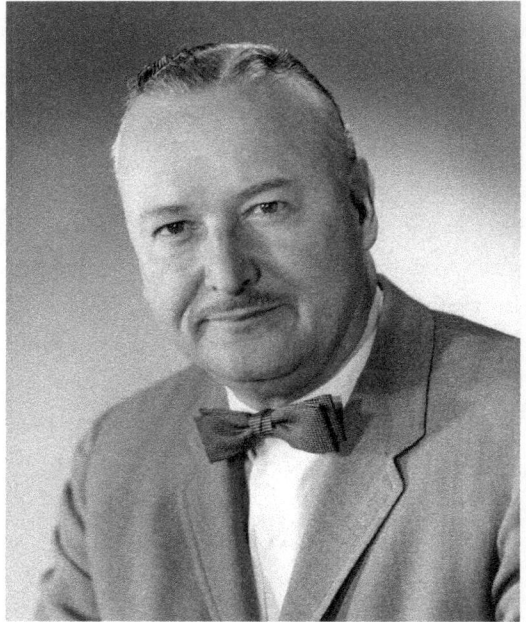

2.2 Carl G. Baker in 1970.
Photo credit: National Cancer
Institute.

NIH—and the NCI specifically—had the management capacity and bureau-cratic will to ensure its investments in science would actually yield improve-ments in health.

At the same time, Mary Lasker and her allies on the NACC continued to insist on greater control over contracting. With Lyndon B. Johnson's ascension to the presidency after the assassination of John F. Kennedy, Lasker gained a close confidante in the White House who could put additional executive pressure on the NCI to realize more medical gains.[75] As pressure from both the Wooldridge Committee in Congress and Laskerites on the NACC mounted in 1964, Baker saw "an ideal opportunity to promote his approach to the administration of bio-medical research" that would make the NCI accountable to both congressional principals and scientific principals on the NACC.[76]

For Baker, the NCI's virus vaccine efforts presented a scientific problem for which systems analysis could provide a managerial solution. While other scholars have emphasized the significance of disease advocates' calls for accountability in public funds as a motivating factor in the development of a vaccine program, this study shows how the vaccine program emerged from a more complex and interactive learning process combining intramural scientists' research ambitions and bureaucrats' managerial approaches to form an endogenous definition of the stakes of cancer virus research in terms of public health.[77] Over the course of almost two years, from 1963 to 1964, Baker and his team colligated extant intramural research programs, the VRRB, and select extramural grants and contracts around a scientific-bureaucratic program unified by a novel approach to targeted research for vaccine development. Though frank about the problems inherent in attempting to plan for a cancer vaccine when no known human cancer virus had yet been detected, Baker and his team had reason to be optimistic. By 1965, intramural scientists had developed successful vaccines against the Friend, Moloney, and Rauscher leukemia viruses in mice.[78] In addition to scientific support, NCI scientists had finally come into vastly increased congressional support for cancer virus vaccine research. For fiscal year 1965, Congress passed an appropriations bill that allocated an additional $10 million for virus research at the NCI.

Baker's earlier studies of scientific management persuaded him of the importance of the "managerial and political" context of research.[79] Attention to both this context and the content of research was focused in the cadre of NCI intramural researchers who would be appointed as scientist-managers in the new targeted program. To Baker's mind, the purpose of an ideal scientist-manager was to mediate between the demands of "authorities" outside the institute and the research endeavors under way in its laboratories and clinics. Struck by the "avalanche of evidence from an unprecedented number of scientific disciplines" suggesting that researchers were on the cusp of identifying a virus responsible for human leukemia, Baker set to work designing a comprehensive plan scientist-managers could use to guide the institute's cancer virus studies toward vaccine development.[80]

By the close of 1964, NCI scientists studying viruses and cancer had invested the majority of their time, energy, and faith in the pursuit of leukemia viruses. Their focus was concretized in the formation of the Special Virus Leukemia Program (SVLP) in late 1964, a bureaucratic unit based in the NCI whose task was to develop an "integrated research and development" program "directed toward the primary objective of prevention through a vaccine or other control methods of virology."[81] This definition of the stakes of the SVLP ensured that "from the moment of its formation, the principal methods of the SVLP's search reflected its mission of developing a vaccine."[82] The vaccine mission profoundly shaped the science SVLP researchers undertook, which mimicked earlier approaches to vaccine development by "drawing on the traditions of immunology and microbiology . . . to associate viruses with cancer rather than to understand the mechanism by which viruses induced cancer."[83] Prior successes in developing vaccines against pathogens whose basic mechanisms of disease action were yet unknown made the pursuit of a prospective human cancer virus vaccine more tractable as both a scientific and organizational feat.[84] Baker's efforts to design the SVLP would marry the scientific stakes of cancer virus research to the organizational stakes of vaccine development by using both bureaucratic techniques of planning and material infrastructures that transformed the landscape for conducting molecular cancer research toward these twinned goals.[85]

The Convergence Technique

Planning for a new management approach began with a series of working-group meetings that drew NCI scientist-managers as well as consultants from the extramural scientific community together to discuss four research foci they considered crucial to a successful leukemia virus program. Having defined the stakes of vaccine development, these research foci specified the remaining issues limiting scientific understanding (such as identifying human cancer viruses and their relationship to animal leukemia viruses) and infrastructural capacity (such as adequate experimental facilities and research materials). Members of the eight working groups (two per area of research) met separately, and their leadership convened with an NCI-appointed management working group headed by Baker.[86] Their combined efforts yielded common operational objectives to be pursued in advancement of each area's goals and a preliminary management approach for the new SVLP.[87]

The management approach developed for the SVLP was dubbed the "convergence technique" by Baker and his administrative aide, Louis Carrese.[88] The convergence technique was inspired by systems planning approaches developed in the DOD's Polaris Missile Program, which approaches were also being applied to aerospace engineering projects at NASA. The version of systems analysis applied to Polaris was known as the Program Evaluation Review Technique (PERT), and it entailed the systematic disintegration of large, time-sensitive programs into discrete milestones.[89] PERT was rigidly hierarchical, characterized by a central planning apparatus and strict project management timelines. Though the convergence technique retained some of the hierarchical structure of systems planning, such as the assumption that projects dispersed throughout collaborative programs should travel through discernible benchmarks on the way to meeting a central goal, the philosophy behind the convergence technique held that these traditional systems planning approaches were ineffective for targeted biomedical research and development. This is because the former counted on well-defined objectives and methods for achieving goals that could be planned at the outset, while the latter depended on foundational scientific insights that had yet to be discovered. In Baker's and Carrese's minds, the convergence technique was an attempt to adapt systems planning to an enterprise where ongoing, discovery-oriented science formed the basis of everyday operational activities distributed across dispersed laboratories and clinics. The challenge was in developing management techniques that could integrate loosely interrelated research projects with open-ended timelines and indeterminate tasks and objectives, all of which unfolded in an environment of great uncertainty. From a management perspective, curing cancer was not rocket science—it was infinitely more complex.

The structure of the convergence technique was developed and approved in a series of meetings between a specially appointed management task force and the NCI Scientific Directorate that took place in 1964. The convergence technique broke up the goals of the SVLP into a series of five phases: "1) identification and study of unknown virus agents, 2) production of large quantities of highly purified virus, 3) verification of the carcinogenic properties of the viruses under study, 4) the planning and conducting of field trials and evaluation of control measures, and 5) control of disease by routine and widespread use of preventive or other control measures."[90] Predetermined criteria for relevance were built into this management structure in the form of "decision points." Decision points were meant to function as moments of discretion where program leaders could evaluate the direction research should take in light of the best available scientific evidence and the program's ultimate goal of controlling cancers through vaccines.

As was customary with the fruits of NCI task force planning, the SVLP began under a five-year deadline to demonstrate scientific results.[91] A special $10 million congressional appropriation earmarked for leukemia virus research in fiscal year 1965 allowed Baker to implement the convergence technique at a scale appropriate to its formulation as a management approach (something otherwise only possible in the institute's handsomely funded carcinogenesis screening program).[92] Many of the initial 150 scientific projects composing the SVLP were funded through both grants to academic scientists and contracts with academic and industry scientists, though the latter predominated. Projects by intramural scientists at the NCI and by Huebner and select NIAID colleagues made up a large proportion of the projects supported and, because of the substantial role intramural researchers played in approving contracts, would have a significant impact on the trajectory SVLP research would take.

Converging on a Viral Candidate

Scientific priorities for the SVLP were cemented in the first six months of 1965 through the activities of the eight topical working groups that met with the management team and Scientific Directorate to help implement the convergence technique.[93] That category I viruses were prioritized during these meetings proved influential in steering work in the SVLP toward C-type RNA viruses. Here the iterative nature of social learning about cancer viruses and vaccines is particularly evident. In the early 1960s, the NCI was home to the most sophisticated research into the role viruses played in animal malignancy, in part because such research had been regarded as illegitimate in mainstream cancer biology for many years.[94] The initial priorities of the SVLP were the product of NCI scientists' focus on C-type RNA viruses, which perforce concentrated much of the nation's extant scientific competencies on this virus family. Whereas scholars and contemporaries have interpreted the NCI's focus on C-type RNA viruses as the product of scientist-managers' career-oriented self-interest, a greater appreciation of the historical context for early cancer virus research in the NCI shows that the processes whereby NCI scientists interpreted the scientific and management stakes of the program in reference to their own experimental work is what iteratively encoded this group of viruses as the most promising candidates for realizing the ultimate stakes of the vaccine program.[95]

The projects funded in the first two full years of the SVLP illustrate the iterative encoding of this focus on C-type RNA viruses over time. For the period 1964–1965, the virus types NCI scientists studied were sorted into categories of "oncogenic" or "non-oncogenic" for the purposes of potential drug and vaccine development, as depicted in table 2.1.

TABLE 2.1 Suspected Oncogenic and Non-oncogenic Viruses, 1964–1965

Oncogenic Viruses	Non-oncogenic Viruses
Rous sarcoma (RNA)	Vaccinia (DNA)
Polyoma (DNA)	Herpes simplex (DNA)
Myxoma (DNA)	Influenza (RNA)
Fibroma (DNA)	Columbia SK (RNA)
Rauscher (RNA)	Poliovirus T_2 (RNA)
Moloney (RNA)	Semliki Forest (RNA)
Friend (RNA)	Lymphocytic choriomeningitis (RNA)
Rich (RNA)	Eastern equine encephalomyelitis (RNA)
Adenovirus T_{12} (DNA)	Encephalomyocarditis (RNA)
Adenovirus T_{18} (DNA)	Guaroa (RNA)
Avian myeloblastosis (RNA)	
Human wart (DNA)	
Simian virus 40 (DNA)	

Source: Reproduced from "Viral Chemotherapy Section," National Cancer Institute Annual Report of Program Activities, 1965 (NARA II, Record Group 443, UD-WW Entry 4, Box 4), 214–15.

Importantly, many of the suspected oncogenic viruses during this early period were DNA viruses rather than C-type RNA viruses. The list in table 2.1 includes not only viruses scientist-managers had assigned to category I but also probable category II and III viruses.

The nature of the work being conducted at this time, which primarily involved pursuing leads into potential oncogenic virus types, was similarly open-ended. As Baker recalls, "once the laboratory methodologies for animal and human cancer virology were worked out (including availability of sufficient quantities of viral and immunological reagents), studies began to correlate the laboratory data with the data from population groups."[96] These population studies, initiated in 1965, included epidemiological investigations of geographic leukemia clusters and epizootiological inquiries into whether suspected leukemia viruses in animals that share close proximity to humans (such as cows, dogs, and cats) could cross species barriers to infect humans.[97] At this time, the leadership of the Etiology Area in which the SVLP was situated also anticipated "a substantial enlargement of the DNA virus-cancer research."[98]

In a material sense, the more open-ended goals of NCI scientist-managers continued to outrun their present capacity to act toward them. While Rouse has made this point about how scientists define the issues and stakes of research generally, the early years of the SVLP demonstrate how a lack of organizational competencies prevented scientist-managers in the SVLP from fully pursuing alternative viral candidates. Restrictions of space, manpower, and funding persisted throughout the 1960s despite budget increases and special appropriations to the SVLP. In some instances, the delays would have serious consequences, as when a shortage of available space suspended Huebner's long-planned DNA tumor virus research programs until 1968. Until this time, serious experimentation on DNA viruses, ranging from suspected oncogenic naked DNA viruses such as simian virus 40 to the membrane-bound "herpes-like" Epstein-Barr and hepatitis B viruses associated with Burkitt's lymphoma and liver cancer, respectively, could not proceed. These bureaucratic limitations led to missed scientific opportunities of great historical consequence.

In a striking example of the above, Mary Fink detected the presence of "Australian antigen" in sera sampled from some leukemic patients in 1964. This antigen was first identified months earlier by Baruch Blumberg, a research physician who had just relocated from the NIH to the Institute of Cancer Research at Philadelphia's Lankenau Hospital. Blumberg collaborated with Fink and shared materials sufficient for a mutual identification of the antigen, but Fink, housed in the Viral Leukemia and Lymphoma Branch with its emphasis on RNA viruses, was unable to pursue her findings beyond the NCI's present capacity to develop established cell lines expressing this antigen and its associated viral particles.[99] These capabilities were self-limiting, as failure to match the Australian antigen with suspected human leukemia viruses brought Fink's project "more or less to a standstill."[100]

Coupled with her stance as a scientist-manager in charge of the Viral Leukemia and Lymphoma Branch's Immunology Section that the laboratory's commitment to program goals around vaccine development "bears great influence on the proposed course of [their] endeavors," Fink's rationale for abandoning the project with Blumberg in pursuit of the leukemia viruses she had been studying for years appeared both scientifically and managerially appropriate.[101] In adherence to the SVLP's long-term goals, Fink was determined to ensure that it could "in the foreseeable future be possible to have the equipment and skills available with the necessary personnel and the necessary space, to develop techniques and/ or adapt all known present techniques to problems within the viral leukemia and lymphoma area. The hope which permeated the entire operation is that we will be able to find workable solutions to the problems encountered in murine leukemia, and will have the potential of immediately transposing these to human leukemia, diverting the entire effort of the laboratory in a very short time to the human problem."[102] A robust research agenda that pursued the relationship between Australian antigen and solid tumors—which Blumberg soon identified as a DNA virus he called hepatitis B virus and implicated in liver cancers—was categorically excluded from planning and materially unlikely given efforts to concentrate the SVLP's experimental apparatus on known murine leukemia and lymphoma viruses.

It thus happened that the SVLP terminated its early involvement in the discovery of the first known human cancer virus in pursuit of experimental programs around RNA viruses for which there was a greater concentration of scientific expertise and material infrastructure in the institute. Blumberg, whose laboratory at the Institute of Cancer Research soon after identifying the hepatitis B virus discovered that the excess surface protein it produced offered protective effects against subsequent infection, would patent a novel hepatitis B vaccine in 1972 and license this patent for development by Merck & Company. In 1981, the hepatitis B vaccine developed by renowned Merck vaccinologist Maurice Hilleman would be the first cancer virus vaccine to come to market in the United States.[103] Though the NCI supported Blumberg's research throughout the 1960s and 1970s through general grant funding and the NIH encouraged him to patent the novel hepatitis B subunit vaccine technology he produced, the SVLP could make no claims on the sole cancer vaccine success that emerged during its operation.[104] The way SVLP scientist-managers defined the issues and stakes of the program would lead them in other, ultimately less successful, directions.

MAKING THE SVLP ACCOUNTABLE

By 1966, the budget for the SVLP had reached $17.5 million. The number of supported projects had expanded to 180, 70 of which were contracted to outside entities.[105] As SVLP researchers could not boast any major breakthroughs in the program's first years, their assessments of the program's status in annual operational reports were based on optimism for future discovery. In formulating these projections, SVLP scientist-managers drew upon both of the alternative systems for evaluating scientific success active in the program—the uncertainty and unpredictability of basic research and the structured and predictable planning of targeted research:

> The very nature of research makes it impossible to predict when certain events will occur. Nevertheless, if the overall progress on this program continues as expected, it is reasonable to believe, at this time, that within four to six years definitive scientific information and technical competence will be attained to establish that viruses, comparable to those known to cause leukemia in animals, are associated with leukemia in man. The program statements developed for fiscal years 1967 through 1970 are based on this belief.
>
> However, it is important to note that if certain key projects now ongoing in several critical research areas continue to develop and provide essential research information, it may be possible to establish a firm association of viruses with human leukemia sooner than stated above.[106]

SVLP scientist-managers suggested an additional $13 million in funding would help achieve their more optimistic timeline. Though Congress did not grant this additional lump sum, the SVLP could look forward to budget growth with each fiscal year. Integrating the SVLP with the convergence technique provided a potent rhetorical resource for NCI leadership to demonstrate accountability in their use of public funds to their principals in Congress.[107]

The convergence technique was meant to embody the spirit of operations research in an organization where networks between tasks were too complex and interdependent to be reliably modeled ahead of time. Instead of providing an actionable strategic orientation toward specific tasks, Baker and Carrese's approach was focused on supporting scientists whose work was assumed to converge over time upon more general program targets, such as developing candidate vaccines that could be tested in animal models and then humans. New discoveries could be integrated into the program's goals as they arose in experimentation. As Baker notes:

> Systems networks provide the basis for key decisions that must be made for a program to progress operationally, i.e., through various Program phases. As a program evolves, outputs of program efforts (data or materials) move to required sites in the planned program, and flows of information and other resources move across the network. The systems approach was a great

improvement over the earlier grid because inter-relationships could be shown, and Program decisions were aided by the systems network. Another advantage is that the network allows reiterative visualization of the total program, and, if changes are made, the effects on other components can be noted more easily.[108]

The use of these systems networks, modified to facilitate the indeterminacy of ongoing cancer virus research, was intended to allow NCI scientist-managers to communicate across projects dispersed among different laboratories, branches, or organizations and to coordinate scientific activities that otherwise took place independently of one another. The explicit role of scientist-managers in this relationship was to "reiteratively" reconstruct relationships between the different component projects in service of the projected goal of vaccine development.

In the absence of strict oversight from congressional or scientific principals, NCI scientist-managers had the autonomy to structure SVLP practices around a relatively endogenous articulation of the issues and stakes of the virus and vaccine program. In so doing, they confronted a tension between routine scientific practices that encouraged the pursuit of emergent findings in experimentation and the more rigid teleology embodied in the SVLP's vaccine goals. While the convergence technique was meant to resolve these tensions by changing the way disparate SVLP researchers worked toward a common objective, its practical application in the SVLP reflected a continuation of scientific practices as usual.[109] Criteria for measuring progress toward convergence were interpreted capaciously by scientist-managers, who had been delegated the authority to issue contracts that could rapidly mobilize what resources they deemed necessary to pursue emerging phenomena of interest. SVLP investigators thus enjoyed tremendous leeway in initiating new projects on the basis of their judgment of scientific opportunities, often with minimal accountability to how they would contribute to the overall goal of vaccine development. Whereas the far-flung prospect of a human cancer vaccine was ever-present in the formal planning apparatus of the SVLP, it was unclear in real time to rank-and-file NCI scientists and their contractors how or whether their experimental results (which routinely entailed ambiguity or failure) compassed toward this horizon point.

Despite the lack of structural supports for ensuring accountability to SVLP goals, some examples from ongoing projects illustrate how the interplay of experimental practice and managerial injunctions from the convergence technique shaped scientist-managers' interpretations of the value of different lines of inquiry to the vaccine objectives of the SVLP. The aforementioned example of Mary Fink's abandonment of hepatitis B research was based on her judgment that this DNA virus was less likely to yield a vaccine than were the RNA viruses implicated in leukemia. Yet in another area of SVLP operations, Robert Huebner was developing a line of research focused on DNA viruses as possible "helper" viruses that interacted with C-type RNA viruses to cause some solid tumors in addition to leukemia.[110] After failing to find evidence that adenoviruses—a family of viruses implicated in many common-cold-like illnesses—were likely helper virus candidates, the major focus of Huebner's DNA helper virus efforts shifted to interactions between C-type RNA viruses and other strains from the herpesvirus family, a variegated group of DNA viruses that exhibit similar structural morphology and include herpes simplex viruses as well as Epstein-Barr virus.[111] Epstein-Barr virus, which was found in Burkitt's lymphoma patients, thus became one of the few DNA viruses the SVLP would invest major funding in, though these activities were primarily contracted to build infrastructure for field trials in Uganda where Burkitt's lymphoma was more prevalent.[112]

As the SVLP matured, some in NCI leadership began to worry over deviations from the bureaucratic ambitions of the convergence technique motivated by scientist-managers' interpretations of the scientific priority of prospective lines of inquiry relative to their own experimental competencies. In the absence of strict oversight, collaborations that formed on the basis of the autonomous assessments of scientist-managers sometimes conflicted with the ultimate goals of the convergence technique in the eyes of Director Endicott.[113] The crux of this conflict was that NCI investigators frequently initiated collaborations and funded them through contracts negotiated between the relevant parties, for which they had to obtain approval only from NCI-staffed working groups.[114] Members of the working groups were assigned formal oversight to ensure these contracts funded work that corresponded to the goals enshrined in the convergence technique, but in practice the contracts allowed principal investigators to determine the direction of program investments without impediment.

As a 1965 memo from the NCI Science/Management Group admitted, these working groups likely did not develop "a detailed knowledge" of the contracts they approved in the early years of the SVLP because of the sheer number of contracts they were asked to review.[115] This meant that working groups often approved work that might have otherwise been flagged as questionable from either a scientific or managerial perspective. Despite the convergence technique's gestures toward central coordination and command of collaborative efforts in the SVLP, most decisions as to which projects to pursue and with whom continued to reflect the priorities of NCI scientist-managers. In the absence of oversight that might ensure integration between the convergence technique's definition of the issues and stakes of overall program research and their own experimental programs, many SVLP scientist-managers ignored program goals entirely. As Baker admits, only one-third of all scientists involved in the SVLP appeared to make a sincere attempt to realize the goals of the convergence technique.[116] In practice, actors at the level of administrative operations (i.e., working-group members) merely passed along NCI scientist-managers' often ad hoc justifications for contracts rather than independently reviewing and approving them according to their priority in the convergence scheme. As *Science* correspondent Nicholas Wade would later quip, the convergence technique was often "regarded as a harmless absurdity by the active scientists in the program."[117]

Ultimately, the convergence technique lacked teeth when it came to holding even NCI scientists accountable to program-level priorities in their routine decision making. Researchers were frequently derelict in reporting basic information necessary to make informed administrative decisions to project officers, effectively cutting this level of management out of substantive decision-making processes.[118] Some scientist-managers simply refused to show up to working-group meetings entirely.[119] As working-group members would later admit to external reviewers, they often felt as if their role was to rubber-stamp decisions that had already been made at the contract level and felt powerless to prevent contracts they found questionable from being approved.[120] This management from below was rarely questioned, as evidenced by a general reluctance to challenge, let alone review in depth, the contracts presented before working groups and program segment chairmen joint sessions.

The sum of these practices was that learning remained operationally at the project level, such that scientist-managers' own research trajectories shaped their definitions of the issues and stakes of a human cancer virus vaccine program toward their own scientific predilections rather than the SVLP's bureaucratic ambitions. The perceptions of the most promising research areas they developed thereby were iteratively reinforced in organizational exercises, such as contract review and annual reporting, that allowed them to justify their research trajectories within the structure of the convergence technique on paper even as many of them failed to integrate overall program goals into their scientific routines. C-type RNA viruses thus remained the favored etiological agents in NCI researchers' analyses by default, and the few forays made into new scientific territory (whether DNA viruses or solid tumor studies) had to be accommodated to how SVLP scientists defined what was at issue in human cancer viruses relative to their own C-type RNA virus studies.[121]

Thus, despite designing decision points into the convergence technique to ensure there would be opportunities for shifting managerial focus in light of new evidence, NCI scientist-managers used their scientific definition of the issues of C-type RNA virus research to downplay mounting evidence of a link between the DNA herpesvirus Epstein-Barr and Burkitt's lymphoma. In compiling the annual operations report, members of the SVLP argued: "The obligation to follow the herpes lead does not mean that efforts with C-type particles will be curtailed. The elusive C-type particle is still considered the prime candidate, and newer leads emerging from model systems will be expeditiously exploited and applied to studies of the human disease."[122] Citing NCI scientists' own research, they noted: "Experiences with animal neoplasms indicate that there are at least 22 different viruses etiologically associated with the induction of leukemia and lymphoma in murine, avian, feline, and probably in canine and bovine species. This and other information suggests that if some human leukemia and lymphomas are virus induced, the most likely etiologic agent will be of the C-type."[123] Thus, despite the SVLP's ultimate goal of producing a vaccine against human cancers, scientist-managers' continued insistence that C-type RNA viruses were the most likely causes of leukemia and lymphoma justified the program's disproportionate investment in these candidates in light of scientists' past success in detecting them in animal systems over emerging evidence of a direct link between a DNA virus and *human* cancer.

A NASA FOR CANCER

In an attempt to manage their growing investment in targeted research programs, the NCI established a Systems and Operations Planning Branch in the Office of the Associate Director in 1967.[124] For Carrese and Baker, the proper management of collaborative research in the NCI prescribed not only a managerial approach that adapted systems planning to open-ended biomedical inquiry. It also involved a particular understanding of the relationship between basic and applied research:

"The applications of the Convergence Technique [in the Cancer Chemotherapy Program and SVLP] were made by treating research as a continuum. This seems desirable if the full range of biomedical research activities is considered, particularly when mission-oriented or problem-solving research involving a wide range of research activities is attempted."[125] The research continuum Carrese and Baker spoke of blurred distinctions between basic and applied science around certain activities, such as inquiry into animal models for viral oncogenesis. Yet it also implied that the relationship between basic and applied science was linear—that applications would proceed from prior discoveries made in the laboratory. The popularity of the linear model during the Cold War period is often attributed to Vannevar Bush, who in 1945 famously argued in favor of a National Science Foundation on the assertion that basic science discoveries would yield the kinds of technological innovations that would serve the national interest.[126] The Manhattan Project exemplified such an approach to the relationship between basic and applied science in Bush's time. But as the Cold War ramped up, NASA's Project Apollo began to supplant it in the public imaginary.

Baker's application of systems analysis to the problem of developing a viral cancer vaccine paralleled the efforts of James Webb to apply the same technique to Project Apollo at NASA. Though champions of the War on Cancer in the 1970s such as Mary Lasker would mobilize space-race imagery in defense of their goal to cure cancer by the American Bicentennial, a similar narrative had emerged earlier in the planning stages of the SVLP on the basis of the program's *bureaucratic* affinities.[127] NCI scientist-managers' interpretations of a NASA-like approach hinged on issues of how to ensure successful collaboration advanced toward medical breakthroughs while accommodating the stark differences in available knowledge base between enterprises such as the SVLP and Project Apollo.

From the perspectives of SVLP scientist-managers, NASA provided an aspirational model for how to use contracts to organize scientists from within the NCI as well as outside the agency into long-term, large-scale collaborative programs oriented toward a central mission of enormous scale and consequence. In addition to motivating the use of contracts, the magnitude of the feat—curing cancers as equivalent to putting a man on the moon—was prominently featured in NASA talk at the NCI. As Robert Huebner remarked:

> The attack we envision on basic etiology and prevention of cancer cannot
> be mounted unless we can think and operate along "Big" science targeted

NASA-like lines. Many of those (including myself) who have been immersed in studies of this problem for many years believe that, like the moon landings, control of cancer can be achieved. It seems equally clear to us that if this is to be accomplished, it can only be done with an effort comparable but not equal to moon shot proportions. We think the effort, viewed in any context, should be worth several hundred million dollars. The talent needed in this effort is available and eager; all that is lacking is the will and support of the Administration.[128]

While Huebner's statement taps into the same public imaginary as Lasker's (and toward the same purpose—securing a larger budget for the NCI at a time when federal programs were throttled by the 1968 Expenditure Control Act), his appreciation of the " 'Big' science" necessary to execute a NASA-like attack on cancer showed a deeper engagement with the organizational requirements such a plan entailed.

Their emphasis on Project Apollo as a bureaucratic achievement is striking given that NCI scientist-managers otherwise balked at the implication that curing cancer was merely a problem of engineering. NCI administrators sought to maintain structures for grant-funded basic science in the same organization, allowing for very different evaluative standards to coexist in the same bureaucratic units. As Baker argued:

> The criteria for evaluating the two areas [grants and contracts] were different, and the responsibilities placed on the program leaders in the former area were heavy. . . . The measure of success in the contract funded areas was whether the contracts were moving the overall program toward the defined objectives, as well as whether progress in extending basic knowledge was achieved. To manage targeted research programs effectively, it was thought that considerable authority ("power") had to be given to those who were charged with responsibilities to execute the programs. . . . Moreover, the various contract efforts must be integrated within the total program, a situation not required with the projects in the grants area.[129]

NCI leadership used NASA as a symbol for directing collaborative research with grandiose goals but were self-conscious and explicit about how a NASA-like approach was limited in supporting the kinds of scientific practices that would ultimately allow them to achieve cancer cures.

Though the imagery of a NASA for cancer was embraced with some hesitation in the SVLP, it nevertheless had a "powerful impact on the practice and politics of cancer virus research," effectively "realigning control among activists, researchers, and managers" around the promise of a targeted approach to research.[130] The savvy Lasker used the enormity of the organizational challenge in curing cancer to lobby congressional principals to revoke the NCI's autonomy in dictating the direction of science and policy in contract-funded collaborative research programs such as the CCNSC and SVLP. Having been frustrated in her attempts to win scientific principals on the NACC oversight for contracts, Lasker seized on negative findings issued by the congressional Wooldridge Report, completed in 1965, to once again challenge the autonomy of these collaborative research programs.[131] While the Wooldridge Committee did include an indictment of the NCI's use of contracts in the CCNSC, which the committee judged were "of lower scientific quality and show[ed] evidence of inadequate central supervision," the threat these criticisms posed for the SVLP's ability to continue utilizing contract research was unclear.[132] Indeed, scientist-managers saw the SVLP as an opportunity to demonstrate to congressional principals that NCI bureaucrats had learned from and improved upon the use of contracts in the CCNSC, and even to offer the convergence technique as a blueprint for overhauling management of the CCNSC in the future.[133] Though Lasker and her allies in the NACC remained committed to gaining oversight over contracts and hoped to use the Wooldridge Committee's findings to open the SVLP up to scrutiny as well, "Endicott converted this planned defense of the NCI's administration [via the convergence technique] into a brief in favor of both the contract mechanism and the discretion of the NCI's leadership to set their own agenda for biomedical research."[134] Congress was satisfied with the NCI's response to the Wooldridge Report and rewarded the NIH with a $30 million increase over the White House's proposed budget for 1966. Lasker's sway in the NACC, once based on her staunch advocacy for science-driven improvements to health, could not in this instance penetrate the NCI's bureaucratic agenda that enshrined scientist-managers' own interpretation of their mission into the organization's programmatic objectives.

THE SVLP BECOMES THE SVCP

In 1967, the Solid Tumor Virus Program (STVP) was launched with Robert Huebner at the helm. The STVP was directly modeled after the SVLP in its administrative structure and drew researchers from throughout different NCI laboratories, especially the recently founded Viral Carcinogenesis Branch (of which Huebner was also head).[135] The STVP was since its inception guided by Huebner's work on the relationship between RNA and DNA viruses, which the scientific community at large agreed should be funded at a grander scale.[136] To the extent Huebner's Viral Carcinogenesis Branch first pursued DNA virus research within the objectives of the convergence technique, these explorations colligated around studies that carefully integrated DNA virus candidates into an overall scientific program prioritizing RNA viruses. As the associate director for viral oncology pointed out, "[d]ivision of tumor virus programs into RNA and DNA components has been a matter of administrative convenience rather than biological necessity and this fact is no better demonstrated than by the frequent and multiple crossing over of administrative lines by the personnel of the Viral Carcinogenesis Branch who serve as project officers on the Special Virus Leukemia Program."[137] Though the SVLP and STVP were formally consolidated under the administrative heading of the Special Virus Cancer Program (SVCP) in 1968, in practice the two already functioned as a coordinated program. This is evidenced not only by crossovers in administrative staff but also in coordination of STVP contract funding in SVLP meetings.[138]

The field of DNA virus cancer research the STVP could support was diverse, as reflected by the great variety of presentations given at an NCI-organized conference on solid tumor viruses held at Arlie House in Warrenton, Virginia, in September 1966.[139] Huebner's work on viruses and cancer in the first half of the decade had reflected a similar diversity of potential etiological agents and approaches.[140] However, once Huebner joined the SVCP, his research quickly came to serve as a theoretical offshoot of investigations into RNA leukemia viruses. Nevertheless, Huebner's more expansive imagination for DNA virus candidates seemed to be the managerial push the SVCP needed to invest in a small number of studies on herpesviruses that had been identified as promising years prior.

As with the SVLP, the majority of funding in the STVP went to animal studies. Nevertheless, DNA viruses had already been implicated in a number of human malignancies. Studies on Epstein-Barr virus (EBV) and Burkitt's lymphoma were thus joined by studies attempting to establish an association between herpes simplex virus type 2 (HSV-2) and cervical cancer. There was widespread agreement that cervical cancer was caused by a sexually transmitted agent, and the NCI could utilize data from existing cervical cancer field studies to gather samples to test the hypothesis.[141] Despite these attempts to encode DNA virus candidates into the priorities of the convergence technique, C-type RNA viruses remained the favored etiological agents in NCI researchers' analyses, and much of the early work in the STVP focused on sarcomas associated with C-type leukemia virus strains that NCI researchers such as Moloney and Bryan had previously discovered.[142]

SVCP scientist-managers defended continued investment in C-type RNA virus research even as new viral candidates emerged that, due to their direct associations with human cancers, could have plausibly been interpreted as more promising in light of the program's goal of developing a vaccine for use in humans. While the SVCP did accommodate research into herpes-like DNA viruses, its leadership was less charitable in their interpretations of the potential of other possible DNA cancer viruses. Ironically, the scientific consensus around the importance of C-type RNA viruses that emerged as a result of SVCP scientist-managers' interpretations of program priorities would neglect some viruses that later proved etiologically significant in human cancers and amenable to vaccine intervention.

Though downplaying the importance of DNA viruses was an early decision that proved fateful in hindsight, the pursuit of C-type RNA virus studies soon precipitated their own problems for the scientific trajectories the SVCP did pursue. Despite years of substantial investment in materials to propagate human C-type viruses, "success [had] not yet been achieved in the continued propagation of such entities in tissue culture" by 1968.[143] Additionally, "Although a few particles resembling C-type viruses are seen in occasional human cases . . . no case has yet been found in which the number of such particles is sufficient to constitute convincing evidence that they actually represent virus."[144] In other words, though some particles suggestive of infection with these C-type RNA viruses were detected, their presence was so limited relative to what would be expected from active viral infection as to present a puzzle for those who wished to explain cancers as resulting directly from viral infection. SVCP scientists interpreted this puzzle as a technical problem reducible to a lack of sufficiently sophisticated experimental techniques for detecting what they increasingly presumed to be "latent or 'silent' infections" by such viruses and committed additional resources to developing even more sensitive immunological techniques for their detection.[145] They determined that further investments to improve the infrastructure for conducting these experiments to produce "more efficient methods . . . for bringing 'hidden' infections to light" was the only way forward from the "needle-in-the-haystack approach" currently in use.[146]

CONCLUSION

The NCI's resource capacity was expanded for intramural scientists and their SVCP contractors just as its generosity toward extramural grantees retracted. By 1968, budget constraints forced the Program Resources and Logistics unit (recently separated from the Viral Carcinogenesis Branch) to refocus its production of experimental resources to primarily address the needs of SVCP scientists and their collaborators. Program Resources and Logistics provided necessary infrastructure for the early expansion of cancer virus and vaccine research, which indirectly enabled new lines of experimentation to emerge. Yet the NCI played a more direct and constitutive role as well. The SVLP's early command over leukemia virus reference material for the American cancer virus research community demonstrates how the NCI leveraged its infrastructural role to develop unique perspectives on experimental trends that drove their policy decisions, such as when to stop production of particular viruses or ramp up production on others. Here, the program monitored "fluctuating research demand in quantity and also kind of virus reagents [that introduce] supply problems detected largely by the Resources and Logistics Section by changing patterns of distribution of the various virus products issued by the Repository. Reagent production reflects issue experience and guidance by the SVLP for anticipated projects." Early in the program's inception, the NCI had granted contracts to commercial laboratories to produce reagents for at least seven different major viruses. However, by 1968, only contracts to produce the two most popular virus types in quantity— Rauscher leukemia virus and Moloney sarcoma virus—remained in effect. Additionally, Program Resources and Logistics contracted for the development of large colonies of germ-free animal models for experiments on tumor viruses. These germ-free lines were cultivated according to the specifications required by SVCP scientists but were also used as models that drove their efforts to "promote their use until constant and economical animal resources of high quality are available."[147] Combined, these principles for producing reference material allowed the NCI to steer cancer virus and vaccine studies toward those viral candidates the program's leadership determined to be most important on the basis of their scientific expertise. Viral reagents were only readily produced for two viruses scientist-managers had deemed the most likely oncogenic candidates, ruling out the production of reference materials for the scientific community at large (outside of specific grant or contract provisions that funded the small-scale production of these reagents for principal investigators' use).

Despite the continued march of research in the program, ongoing scientific and technical barriers to vaccine innovation led scientist-managers to hedge their prospective planning with greater discipline than in previous years. The inevitability of rapid identification of and vaccine development for a human cancer virus gave way to the more equivocal statement that "the assumption that at least one virus is an indispensable element for the induction of human leukemia and lymphoma is accepted as *an* hypothesis."[148] Not only did the notion that some cancers were preventable by virus vaccines seem to be up in the air for the first time in the program's history, but also the conviction that the SVCP was capable of surmounting the organizational challenge of vaccine production faltered. The requirements for meeting the experimental burden of proof for viral causation of leukemia, as well as the conduct of human vaccine trials, was now acknowledged as monumental: far from the "imminent" breakthrough promised in 1964, the program now projected vaccine trials themselves "will require approximately 5–7 years and $30,000,000."[149] Scientist-managers' optimism was curbed not only by the logistical complexity of a cancer vaccine but also by its scientific complexity. If viral cancers turned out to be but one factor in a complex causal chain that led stochastically to cancer, the program conceded, "it may be very difficult, perhaps impossible, to prevent more than a relatively few cancers with specific tumor virus vaccines."[150]

CHAPTER 3

MOVING TARGETS IN THE WAR ON CANCER, 1969–1979

Cancer virus research at the NCI began changing rapidly in 1969, of a piece with major shifts in the broader political and economic environment of the institute. As emerging laboratory findings increasingly suggested that the etiological relationship between viruses and cancer was more complex than originally understood, the Special Virus Cancer Program's originating impulse toward vaccine development came into question. The NCI's bureaucratic approach to organizing targeted cancer virus and vaccine research was also being challenged by principals in Congress, with the longtime skeptic of contract research Mary Lasker continuing to lobby for alternative ways of realizing the NCI's health mission. Scientists outside the NCI, jealously guarding grants-in-aid against fiscal austerity, began to mobilize against the NCI's targeted programs as well.

These tensions were not resolved so much as transmuted by passage of the National Cancer Act in 1971. This legislation, which launched Nixon's so-called War on Cancer, committed Congress to substantial increases in the NCI's annual appropriations at the same time that it modified the institute's governance structures. From these changes emerged a new configuration between the NCI and its principals in the legislature and the extramural scientific community. The impressive cadre of elites who had helped lobby Congress to make the NCI accountable to expenditures for medical research in the form of scientifically driven health improvements were in the end victims of their own success. Over the long term, lobbyists such as Lasker would be cut off from the influence they enjoyed on advisory bodies, which in this period became a means whereby extramural scientists could mobilize to ensure that the interests of cancer researchers at large were better represented in NCI policy. Within five years, scientists would firmly take hold of the reins of governance through the National Cancer Advisory Board, which they cemented as a delegation for scientific principals.

In many ways, the Special Virus Cancer Program (SVCP) would also become a victim of its own success in spurring innovative research. Laboratories initially funded through contracts to conduct work that would lend experimental support to SVCP scientists' "viral oncogene hypothesis" would uncover evidence that what were once suspected to be viral genes were in fact already present in normal cells. Though scientist-bureaucrats in the NCI attempted to interpret these findings in ways that would support their rapidly diminishing hopes of a cancer vaccine, it soon became apparent that the institute's investment had funded discoveries that undermined the ambitions enshrined in the convergence technique. Pincered between dispositive program findings and increasingly powerful scientific principals, the Virus Cancer Program would be dismantled in 1978. Though extramural scientists' establishment of the "cellular oncogene hypothesis" is often credited with showing the folly of the NCI's targeted cancer virus and vaccine programs, this chapter shows how the combined scientific and bureaucratic efforts mustered by scientist-managers such as Robert Huebner to pursue proof of the viral oncogene hypothesis were generative of the cellular oncogene hypothesis that NCI contractors J. Michael Bishop and Harold Varmus ultimately proposed in its place. Interpreting viral and cellular oncogene experiments in relation to the issues and stakes of the program that supported them shows how the scientific and bureaucratic environment produced by NCI scientist-managers' unsuccessful attempts to support the viral oncogene hypothesis ultimately precipitated the conditions in which contractors Bishop and Varmus successfully innovated the paradigm-shifting cellular oncogene hypothesis.

THE VIRAL ONCOGENE HYPOTHESIS

By 1968, Robert Huebner and his colleagues in the SVCP were entertaining the notion that viruses played a diminished role in carcinogenesis of solid tumors, contrary to what the original goals of the Special Virus Leukemia Program (SVLP) had assumed for leukemia. With Huebner's helper virus hypothesis hitting several dead ends, he and his colleague George Todaro began interpreting some of their experimental findings in a new light. A wealth of evidence supporting the apparent ubiquity of suspected oncogenic viruses in mice who did not develop neoplasms, and the evident spontaneity of tumor growth in animals whose neoplasms did not yield evidence of virus particles, led to a growing "skepticism" of the basic tenets of the NCI's cancer virus and vaccine program.[1] Huebner used his expansive network of contractors to conduct studies on several strains of mice and was surprised to find that in one series of experiments where cancer was induced through chemical exposure, mice previously thought to be free of virus began to express antigens associated with tumor viruses. This startling finding necessitated "radical changes in previous concepts concerning the mechanisms by which chemical carcinogenesis is induced in laboratory mice. Instead of the chemical inducing a repression or somatic mutation of a cell gene it now seems likely that it is engaged in converting a silent leukemia virus gene, MuLV (o), into an active one, MuLV (+)."[2] The sudden appearance of virus antigens in these cancers colligated into a new "switch off–switch on" hypothesis that proposed widespread latent infections of C-type RNA virus lurked in cells, actuating malignancies when exposed to other precipitating causes. Huebner and Todaro "intensively explored" this switch off–switch on hypothesis in focused experiments that ran for the next several months.[3]

The switch off–switch on hypothesis necessitated a different approach to studying cancer virus transmission as well. Most investigations into C-type RNA viruses had assumed they spread through "horizontal" transmission; that is, transmission of oncogenic virus from organism to organism via environmental exposure. But as they attempted to make sense of the evidence emanating from several experimental iterations designed to test the switch off–switch on hypothesis, an alternative proposition, originally developed by other researchers to explain the transmissible nature of mouse mammary cancers, began to appeal to Huebner and his team.[4] Under this model, cancer viruses were thought to be transmitted "vertically"—communicated from mother to brood in utero, either through the passage of virus through the placental barrier or via transformed genetic material in the germ cell. Seizing upon the latter interpretation of vertical transmission, Huebner hypothesized that viral material was passed down in the genetic inheritance of cells, where it remained dormant until it was "switched on" by some precipitating factor: "the normal cells contain within themselves the necessary genetic information to produce the cancerous condition which is then, in heritable fashion, passed on to all the daughter tumor cells—a process which in vivo eventually kills the host. Here again we must conclude that the neoplastic information had to be acquired prior to birth and represents part of the genetic inheritance of most or all of the cells."[5]

As a class of viruses we now call retroviruses, C-type RNA viruses were hypothesized to insert DNA into the cells they infected. Until the late 1960s, the idea that genetic information could flow from RNA to DNA was controversial, as it defied the "central dogma" proposed by Francis Crick that held there was a unidirectional flow of information only from DNA to RNA.[6] Huebner was able to propose this radical reformulation of virus transmission because he interpreted the recent much-publicized identification of reverse transcriptase, an enzyme that allows RNA to produce DNA, as offering a plausible mechanism whereby RNA viruses could insert DNA into cells. SVCP scientist-manager Frank Rauscher similarly interpreted reverse transcriptase as "an enormous political, as well as scientific, breakthrough" in that it provided conceptual and technological tools that would allow the program to maintain its focus on the stakes of vaccine development for prospective human cancer retroviruses.[7] Though the precise mechanisms whereby human cells inherited vertically transmitted viral DNA remained unspecified, Huebner and his team were more focused on conducting immunological studies that would firm up support for what they were now calling the "viral oncogene hypothesis." Immunological inquiry was pursued not only because the experimental apparatus of Huebner's vast contracting networks supported by SVCP contracts was configured for this purpose, but also because it would allow Huebner to frame future viral oncogene experiments in relation to the SVCP's goal of vaccine development.[8]

Huebner and Todaro's newly colligated viral oncogene hypothesis was "epochal for SVCP, since [it] led to a testable (heuristic) new hypothesis concerning the basic inherited nature of the RNA viral genome as a general cause of cancer and to a unitary theory capable of explaining spontaneous cancer as well as cancer evoked by exogenous environmental pollutants, endogenous physiological aberrations, genetic defects and mutations, as well as cancer clearly induced by viruses in experimental animals."[9] Extending these insights to the intractable issue of cancer prevention and treatment, Huebner and his colleagues argued:

> The concept of built in virogenes and oncogenes, the expressions of which are recognized by both the whole organism and the individual cells as "self" very likely explain the failure of current approaches to control the majority of cancers. Contemporary therapeutic efforts based on destruction of transplanted

tumors in experimental animals, surgical and radiation treatments and experimental immunological vaccines might now be viewed as largely palliative
and, more frequently than not, temporary in their effects on cancer . . . the
only satisfactory *final* solution will have to start with a recognizable handle on the basic inherited genomic cause of cancer which then leads to the
development of methods (1) to repress the built-in oncogene(s) from 'doing
its thing' in the normal cell; and (2) to devise ways for fortifying and supplementing the body's natural protective immunological mechanisms. We
believe, therefore, that the eventual control of cancer will have to come about
at the cellular level through 'repressor' control of oncogene expression, and
at the organism level through maintenance and/or substitution of specific
immunological 'bullets' aimed at specific tumor cell proteins which inevitably must be produced as a result of abnormal gene expressions which lead to
the neoplastic state.[10]

The viral oncogene hypothesis thus expressed a shift in the issues underlying
SVCP research. The new assumption that virogenes were present at birth in the
form of "endogenous" viral infections vertically transmitted in a deactivated
form until later in life when they were expressed by cellular genetic functions
in response to carcinogenic exposures allowed SVCP leadership to propose that
C-type RNA viruses were "unique enough and widespread enough to account for
the generality of naturally occurring cancer in animals and in humans, including those cancers which are induced by radiation and chemicals."[11] Despite redefining the scientific issues of their ongoing research, the perceived evidence in
favor of C-type RNA viruses as nearly universal cancer viruses allowed SVCP
scientist-managers to preserve the looser stakes of a generic cancer prevention
strategy as a viable scientific prospect.

Though the viral oncogene hypothesis emerged from research conducted to
advance the goals of the SVCP, it profoundly challenged the possibility that
developing a cancer vaccine would be a straightforward project. Scientist-
managers struggled with how the planning apparatus of the SVCP would reckon
with the implications of these findings for their interconnected enterprise. Rauscher, who since 1968 was spearheading an effort to realign the goals of the SVCP
around such recent findings, first reinterpreted the program's stakes at the same
conference where Huebner and Todaro publicly announced the viral oncogene
hypothesis.[12] Emphasizing a more general approach to "cancer *prevention* in man,"

Rauscher argued for methods of identifying populations at risk of certain viral cancers and administering some prophylactic intervention "so that these agents which under some circumstances induce cancer perhaps do not do so in other conditions. This is the basis for hopes that vaccines may prevent cancer induction by some oncogenic virus."[13] As their attention shifted to how to design such a prophylactic approach, NCI scientist-managers debated whether to continue their other research programs into herpesviruses or to axe them in favor of a more sustained emphasis on C-type RNA virus studies.[14]

Beyond adapting SVCP scientific and managerial priorities to the stipulations of the convergence technique, Rauscher and his reorganization team were tasked with developing guidelines for new policy directions around emerging findings such as Huebner and Todaro's. To this end, researchers throughout the program produced white papers intended to advise Endicott on where the NCI's investments would be best focused in the immediate future. Baker bragged that these white papers "demonstrated . . . the value of having inputs from a few knowledgeable experts (without the *compromised* output required of large committees)."[15] In this subtle dig against the National Advisory Cancer Council (NACC), Baker argued for the adequacy of internal expertise in developing and guiding NCI policy. More to the point, restricting policy input to NCI scientists and their immediate collaborators ensured that research policy would be tightly coupled to the issues and stakes intramural scientists-managers interpreted in light of their ongoing experimentation in the program.

A "MOONSHOT" FOR CANCER TAKES FLIGHT

At the same time that NCI leadership was reconsidering the issues and stakes of cancer virus research, Lasker and her fellow travelers were attempting to regain influence over the direction of the nation's cancer research investments. With the war in Vietnam ongoing, appropriations for medical research showed their first signs of a downward trend, while Congress increasingly turned its emphasis toward health care delivery after the recent passage of Medicare. Concerned for the fiscal future of the cancer effort, "Mary Lasker and her associates began casting about for a stratagem to restore medical research, especially cancer research, to its financial *status quo ante*."[16] Inspired by a recent book written by physician Solomon Garb that adopted the analogy of a "moonshot" for cancer, Lasker argued to her friends in Washington that cancer was a problem worth pursuing with the same vigor as efforts to put a man on the moon. With sufficient money and planning, Lasker and her supporters urged President Nixon, the U.S. government could achieve a similar feat in curing cancer.[17]

By 1969, the public discourse around a moonshot for cancer had achieved greater coherence and specificity thanks to the efforts of Lasker's Panel of Consultants on the Conquest of Cancer, a coalition of political and scientific heavyweights that developed talking points and lobbied Congress and the White House for increased investment in efforts to defeat the disease through science. Though NCI leadership had previously drawn parallels between its organization and NASA, not least of all because of the shared commitment to managerial models based on systems analysis approaches deployed in the Department of Defense, NCI leadership's conception sharply varied from Lasker's model of a moonshot. The panel of consultants used the NASA analogy to propose that the NCI be made an autonomous agency that reported directly to the president. Still committed to using investment in biomedical research to improve health outcomes, Lasker had grown disillusioned with the administrative structure that made the NCI's efforts beholden to the NIH bureaucracy and was convinced that direct executive oversight would better enable the institute to focus on applying its knowledge base to develop cancer cures.[18] Left to its own devices, argued cancer crusader and Congressman John Rooney in a concurrent resolution that passed in the House of Representatives in 1970, an independent agency could conquer cancer in time for the nation's 1976 bicentennial celebration.[19]

NCI administrators and scientists balked at Rooney's political prognosis. Jesse Steinfeld, the NCI's scientific director of General Laboratories and Clinics, opined before Congress that Lasker's articulation of a moonshot was unrealistic, promising quick results that could be guaranteed by neither the state of the science nor by the scientific community's best efforts to organize.[20] NCI leadership also struck back against the panel's recommendation to make the NCI autonomous from the NIH, which they argued would sever important ties scientists had formed across other institutes. The restructuring would "tend to be counterproductive by removing cancer research from the mainstream of biomedical research on which it is so dependent. The major limiting factor in solving the cancer problem is a lack of sufficient knowledge in an extremely complicated area. Therefore, there is a strong need for continuing input from a wide variety of scientific disciplines and efforts."[21] As Baker (who succeeded Endicott as NCI director in 1969) pointed out, removing the NCI from the NIH was publicly opposed by most major cancer research organizations, with the exception of the Lasker-helmed American Cancer Society.[22]

Conflicts between NCI leadership and political principals over the moonshot heightened as legislation for a national cancer effort moved through Congress in 1970. Though NCI staff, including Baker, had met with the panel of consultants to discuss the institute's planning approaches, they worried that Lasker and her advocates were overpromising results.[23] NCI scientist-bureaucrats were "concerned that Congress and the public should not be misled to believe that the cancer field is at a stage where the major theoretical problems have been resolved and where a 'Manhattan project' or 'NASA man on the moon' approach would guarantee success."[24] They were particularly concerned that the standards of accountability congressional principals were preparing to hold them to on the basis of the panel of consultants' promises were discordant with their assessments of the state of cancer science. They lamented "an insufficiently clear statement about the intent of [proposed cancer legislation]; is Congress to believe that it can buy a product that requires *only to be manufactured* or is Congress to believe that this is an *investment* in a worthy venture that *may* or *may not* yield the specified goal of conquering cancer?"[25] Lasker's panel of consultants countered in congressional testimony that it intended any parallels with Project Apollo to be administrative and not scientific:

> You will hear the criticism made that the analogy to the splitting of the atom or the space program (where independent agencies were given the job) is not valid because we do not have the basic scientific knowledge in cancer that we had in those fields, and therefore this program is not a program of engineering implementation of existing knowledge as those programs were. . . . The valid analogy is not the scientific analogy but the organizational analogy. The cancer program, in order to succeed, needs the same independence in *management, planning, budget presentation, and the assessment of progress that those programs needed*, and in those respects the independent authority analogy is a valid one.[26]

Despite the panel's insistence to the contrary, NCI scientists and administrators continued to interpret the panel's calls for a moonshot as predicated upon scientific and engineering goals that misapprehended the issues and stakes of cancer science on the whole.[27]

The moonshot debates between NCI personnel and the panel of consultants were ultimately resolved by the passage of a compromise bill that would become the National Cancer Act of 1971. Richard Rettig has expertly recounted the political and legal machinations that led to the act, paying particular attention to the role Mary Lasker and her connections in Congress and the White House played in making such legislation possible. As Rettig stresses, the National Cancer Act was a distinctive legislative achievement because Lasker's panel of consultants was responsible for "writing the report, preparing for its reception, and securing the commitment to action of the key senators" who would sponsor the bill, which was fortuitously aligned with Nixon's desire to support the cancer effort.[28] NCI actors' perspectives on these legislative maneuvers are infrequently analyzed, though the consequences of the act for their organizational routines were sometimes far-reaching. The most immediate consequence was a dramatic increase in funding for research, which was concentrated in the NCI. This funding was meant to expand a National Cancer Program (NCP) that integrated researchers in the academy, industry, and health care organizations around strategies spearheaded by the NCI. To better support this expanded role, the NCI was elevated to bureau status within the Public Health Service (PHS). Though the NCI was still formally an agency of the National Institutes of Health, its bureau status meant the institute submitted its budget directly to the president for approval rather than going through traditional NIH line channels. Additionally, the NCI director was made a presidentially appointed position.

The National Cancer Act also included a key structural change to governance at the NCI. Until 1971, the NACC had played an advisory role subordinate to the NCI directorate, which "exercised great control over" the NACC and "had substantial influence on resource allocation and program management" irrespective of the council's advice.[29] This arrangement had long vexed Lasker, who had expected greater influence over how the NCI allocated funds, especially through contracts. Lasker's lobbying was central to securing a more expansive mandate for the new National Cancer Advisory Board (NCAB), which would replace the NACC after the National Cancer Act passed. This aspect of the National Cancer Act also "decreased NCI operational control by . . . converting the advisory NACC to a board of directors-type NCAB" that reported to its own elected chair rather than to an absentee surgeon general.[30] As an oversight committee of the NCI, the NCAB had "far broader authorities and responsibilities than its predecessor," including "authority to investigate all the activities of the NCI it deems desirable."[31] The board would flex its muscles most decisively in the investigation into the SVCP it initiated in 1973, but it also commenced participating in the review, comment, and approval of all aspects of the NCI's planning and operations out of the gate in 1972.

One of Lasker's central strategies for securing influence on the NCAB involved the portion of legislation that required NCAB members to be appointed by the president. Having lost many of her stalwart congressional allies to death or defeat, Lasker was increasingly focused on the White House as a controlling arm for medical research policy. She was assured enough in her ability to secure a position for herself or one of her supporters on the NCAB if these appointments were controlled by the president. On the other hand, making the White House useful to Lasker necessitated establishing direct reporting channels to the president, as the NCI's nominal principals were in Congress. To facilitate executive branch communication and control of NCI policy, the National Cancer Act established a three-person President's Cancer Panel (PCP) that would report to the White House and serve as "the major locus of policy leadership for the new cancer program."[32] President Nixon appointed Benno Schmidt, a venture capitalist who supported the president and had headed Lasker's panel of consultants, as the PCP's first chairman. Schmidt quickly showed an interest in and aptitude for the science presented to the panel during regular governance meetings with NCI leadership and the NCAB. Despite the statutory authority to operate only as a "monitoring panel and not a managerial body," Schmidt's "commanding presence" allowed him to swiftly insert himself into "deliberations on management issues" that should have been the purview of the NCAB: "Thus, it was sometimes unclear at times which of the three at the head of the table [NCI director, NCAB chair, and PCP chair] was functioning as Chairman of the Board."[33] With a strong détente established between the PCP under Schmidt, the NCAB, and NCI director Rauscher, the PCP established de facto control over the NCAB and the NCI's major policy priorities.[34]

This governance configuration would outlast the individual personalities and informal agreements occupying these positions and have unexpected consequences for the roles scientists and lobbyists would play in policy later in the decade. In 1971, however, Lasker and Nixon had achieved their aims in securing some renewed independence for the NCI from the NIH and ensuring the policies to be enshrined in the NCI's National Cancer Plan would be accountable to a vision that emphasized health outcomes over basic research. The bypass budget structure that saw the NCI submitting its funding requests directly to the White House ensured that the budget would henceforth be "developed without reference to anything but [the NCI's] own plans and aspirations."

A Launchpad for the National Cancer Plan

As the head of the National Cancer Program, the NCI was required to develop a National Cancer Plan, a strategic plan for the nation's cancer research enterprise that integrated all relevant parties, from academic and industry researchers to medical providers, public health agencies, and citizen activist groups. Baker had anticipated a dramatic expansion of the NCI's responsibilities as a federal agency when the National Cancer Act was still being kicked around in Congress, and so he was prepared to spearhead the formulation of a National Cancer Plan in the NCI's first fiscal year after passage of the act. In 1971, as bills for the National Cancer Act were being debated in Congress, "the Institute Director and staff carried forward a series of program reviews and evaluations in preparation for the new, large Federal cancer effort foreshadowed by the developments within the Administration and the Congress. The Institute's senior management staff began a series of seminars on the systems approach to the management of large and complex operations . . . with a view to expanding or realigning them as basic components of an expanded effort."[35]

Baker sought to translate the skills he had learned developing and implementing the convergence technique to his responsibilities in orchestrating the National Cancer Plan as NCI director. He was particularly impressed with emerging evidence in support of the viral oncogene hypothesis and so drew upon the SVCP explicitly in approaching the task.[36] But the National Cancer Plan posed a greater logistical challenge than did the institute's management apparatus, since it required coordination and cooperation among actors from diverse organizations beyond the NCI. Between March and August of 1971, Baker oversaw expanded planning efforts for a National Cancer Plan. His determination to keep scientific input forefront in the planning process resulted in a split structure for the NCP: on the one hand, a Research Strategy that addressed the scientific needs for developing cancer cures, and on the other, an Operational Strategy that mapped the organizational requirements for managing a budget that doubled between 1973 and 1976 (a rise from $508 million to $1 billion) and coordinating efforts across an entire national network of cancer researchers, clinicians, and community actors.[37]

Baker believed that the NCI's role in the National Cancer Program necessitated a managerial approach similar to the convergence technique already in place in the institute's collaborative research programs, including the SVCP. Entertaining an expanded version of the convergence technique that nevertheless maintained a high degree of autonomy for scientist-managers based in the NCI, he argued:

> The managerial apparatus or system required [for the NCP] must be an adaptive organization that can respond quickly to unforeseen opportunities and problems. It must insure continual revision of the program plan and operations as new information is generated, received, analyzed, and acted upon. Organizational adaptability also requires faster decision making; this demands that the use of committees must be restricted to review of broad program activities and that detailed decision making and review must be decentralized, while major decision making and allocation of major blocks of resources remain centralized. For these reasons and to insure the best use of senior cancer R&D managers, much of the work will need to be carried out through a system of lead contractors who will manage segments of the program, including major subcontracting efforts.[38]

Baker's position on management of the NCP evolved alongside the iterative planning efforts that took place in late 1971 and early 1972. In turn, Baker and other NCI scientist-bureaucrats' understandings of targeted research management were altered by their role in the broader NCP planning enterprise.

In October 1971, Baker brought his early plans for the NCP to an expanded assembly of 250 extramural scientists at the Arlie House Conference Center in Warrenton, Virginia. These scientists were tasked with fleshing out the scientific priorities Baker had built into the National Cancer Plan's Research Strategy and hashing out the management, information, and training needs included in the Operational Strategy. Over the next four months, NCI administrators and these 250 extramural scientists developed a draft Strategic Plan for the National Cancer Program oriented around the ultimate goal of "develop[ing], through research and development efforts, the means to significantly reduce the incidence, morbidity and mortality of cancer in man."[39] This goal was broken down further into seven research objectives and eight control objectives, each entailing a number of approaches composing a greater number of approach elements, which were in turn supported by project areas made up of many individual scientific projects. This newly colligated orientation to convergence planning on a national scale is represented in the schematic of figure 3.1.

Despite the apparently hierarchical nature of their planning schematic, NCI administrators insisted its "structure must not constrict the flexibility and adaptability of program operations."[40] Rather, the concentric diagram maintained focus on the ultimate goal of the nation's cancer research efforts—to "develop the means to reduce the incidence, morbidity, and mortality of cancer in humans"—while allowing thousands of researchers in various organizations to pursue independent projects that would eventually contribute to this aim. In this

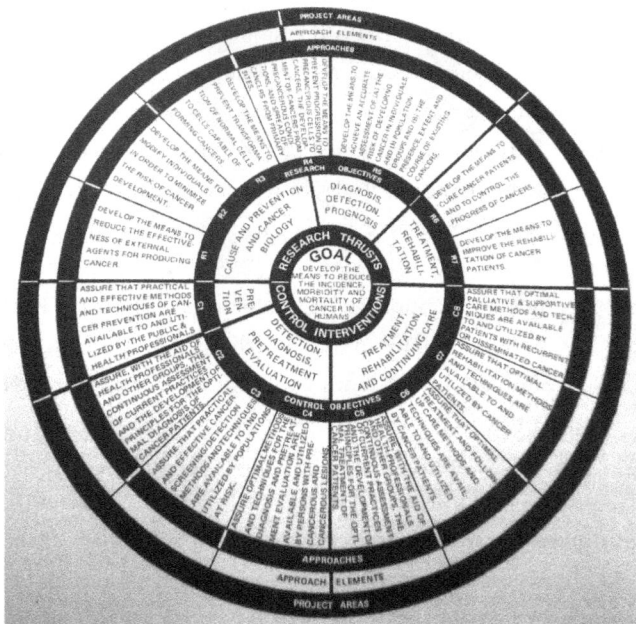

3.1 National Cancer Program Strategy Hierarchy. (Figure I-4 in "National Cancer Plan Operational Plan FY 1976–1980" [August 1974]. National Institutes of Health Office of the Director Central Files [National Archives and Records Administration, College Park, MD, Record Group 443, UD-06D Entry 1, Box 95, Folder 2], I-9.)

sense, the National Cancer Plan preserved much of the open-endedness of the convergence technique as it had been refined in the SVCP.

In the interest of transparency, NCI staff did not participate in meetings among the assembled extramural scientists who determined the approaches the National Cancer Program would use to meet the objectives enshrined in the new management approach.[41] Two problems quickly presented themselves when extramural scientists were asked to participate in detailed planning for cancer research. First, it became evident that many scientists disagreed about which projects were of the highest priority.[42] Second, extramural scientists' disagreements proliferated in number and degree the further down the planning hierarchy they were asked to comment. As Baker remarked, it appeared these scientists lacked a basic orientation to planning and coordinating collaborative research that was familiar to NCI scientist-bureaucrats as a matter of course:

> These outstanding investigators had no difficulty understanding the overall Goal and Objectives nor the Project Areas designation (generally corresponding to grants), but they had some difficulty understanding Approaches and Approach Elements. This difficulty appears to derive from the lack of experience in dealing with blocks of research efforts of the size larger than grant proposals. . . . The concepts of Approaches and Approach Elements developed by NCI staff grew out of experience of preparing NCI budget justifications where larger blocks of cancer research efforts had to be described and justified to the Bureau of the Budget staff, the White House staff, and the Congress. The Approaches would form the basis for the broad research thrusts or major programmatic efforts aimed at achieving the Objectives. Understanding Approaches and Approach Elements was very important since each Panel under leadership of the Chairman was to discuss, and modify if required, the suggested Approaches and Approach Elements before the Project Areas under each Approach were considered.[43]

Put plainly, extramural scientists lacked the bureaucratic competencies that were possessed by NCI scientist-bureaucrats because of their routine participation in agency planning. Baker was thus persuaded that intramural leadership's combined scientific and bureaucratic competencies could supplement extramural scientists' technical expertise such that an appropriate national plan could be devised. The NCI Office of the Associate Director for Program Planning and

Analysis used the Strategic Plan developed during the Arlie House conferences as the basis for an Operational Plan issued in 1974 that would ostensibly guide researchers' and policy makers' decisions around short-term management and long-term planning for the National Cancer Program. Louis Carrese spearheaded this project along with other NCI administrative staff. The focus of the Operational Plan was on developing "balanced coverage of the total research system; new modes of operation; information systems needs; peer review procedures; research data utilization; coordinated efforts; and training goals."[44]

Though a great amount of time and effort was put into developing the Operational Plan between 1973 and 1974, it was never implemented in practice.[45] In May 1972, Baker was informed he would be replaced by the first presidentially appointed NCI director, Frank Rauscher, Jr. Rauscher, who had also enjoyed a long tenure in the NCI's virus cancer programs, continued to support the institute's decentralized administrative efforts in its collaborative programs, though the convergence technique was quietly abandoned during his directorship. By reputation Rauscher "was not a very good administrator," and in his stead he appointed the NCI's chief of medicine, Vincent DeVita, Jr., to testify on behalf of the NCI before Congress.[46] DeVita was acquainted with Lasker and supportive of her lobbying, which he insisted "made sense. If you wanted to be against what she wanted, you'd have to really go against logic."[47] Despite reported tensions between Lasker and Baker, DeVita had seen how Lasker and her allies mobilized Baker's ambition to organize research toward specific health aims as ammunition to ensure the passage of the National Cancer Act and remained persuaded that her political approach would be beneficial to the continued growth of the institute.[48] Lasker and DeVita agreed that Baker was too much an "administrator" and thus lacked the practical scientific expertise to "make the connection between the lab and the clinic," which both felt should be the motive force behind the National Cancer Plan.[49] Where DeVita and Lasker parted ways was in their opinions about contract research. DeVita saw contracts as being one of the few ways scientists could conduct the kind of accelerated interdisciplinary research that would actually yield breakthroughs given how disjointed specialties were in the NCI and in most academic settings.[50] He felt contracts need only be more judiciously administered so that discretion over their distribution was not concentrated in the hands of a small number of intramural scientists.[51] Lasker had long resisted any use of contracts without significant oversight from the NCI's advisors, who increasingly counted among them extramural scientists categorically opposed to the use of contracts.

Criticism of the NCI's contracting practices also emanated from the secretary of the Department of Health, Education and Welfare after the 1969 Sisco Report.[52] In many ways a sequel to the Wooldridge Report, the Sisco Report reflected an effort by Congress to closely examine the integrity of contracting practices throughout the NIH. It formally recommended total centralization of NCI contracting practices in the Office of the Director, NIH, so that all contracting functions would travel through line channels between the institutes, per pre-Endicott protocol. NCI administrators had stood their ground against the report's recommendations, insisting that, though the Department of Health, Education and Welfare and NIH were welcome to set broad policies for contracting, control of actual contracting functions should remain close to the project principal investigators who administered them in the institute.[53] In the interim, NCI scientist-bureaucrats maintained the status quo ante of decentralized contracting practices, a position Baker had interpreted as legally supported by the National Cancer Act of 1971, which had elevated NCI to bureau status in the PHS.[54] The NCI's bureau status created ambiguity over line channels between the NCI and NIH, as it suggested the NCI might be of parallel rather than subordinate status vis-à-vis the NIH. As Endicott's success in implementing and defending decentralized contract administration in the face of criticism from the NACC and Congress attests, this kind of structural ambiguity was not necessary to maintain contracting practices in the NCI's collaborative research programs. Yet it provided additional ammunition for NCI administrators who felt the need to defend a dramatic expansion of funds for cancer virus research in light of the imperative to coordinate interdisciplinary, multi-institutional research efforts as part of the National Cancer Program.[55] It also very decisively shut down Lasker's renewed efforts to put the NCAB in control of individual contract approvals during the new board's inaugural meeting in March 1972.[56]

Where Lasker found her influence on the NCAB increasingly limited, NCI leadership found themselves under the scrutiny of political principals throughout the legislature. After the Sisco Report, the NCI had won over some support in Congress for the institute's decentralized contracting authority on the basis of a study by the comptroller general showing it was a more efficient means for funding targeted projects.[57] A review commissioned by the president in 1973 also found that the NCI's autonomy was appropriate given the institute's role in leading the National Cancer Program and lauded NCI contracting practices as improving participation in the national effort from private industry.[58]

A separate 1973 congressional review of NIH contracting practices also interpreted increases in contract research as reflecting the institutes' responsiveness to public pressure to fund goal-oriented research.[59] Nevertheless, external reviewers continued to struggle with the level of decentralization of contract approval and administration in the NCI's collaborative research programs and often supported the use of contracts contingent upon the NCI's willingness to make concessions toward a more traditional hierarchy of administrative control between the NIH and NCI.[60]

Though significant parties in Congress and the White House were warming up to the NCI's distinctive brand of contracting practices in managing the increasingly complex organization, many extramural scientists remained skeptical of the use of contracts. These scientists continued to insist that only certain types of science (directed or targeted) were appropriately funded by contracts, and that funding basic research through contracts was always inappropriate as it undermined peer review and free inquiry. In the process, they drew distinctions between basic science and directed or targeted research on the basis of the assumption that the latter did little to contribute to basic knowledge.[61] Extramural scientists' assumptions about basic science, targeted research, and contract funding stood in stark contrast with the opinions shared by NCI scientist-managers in the SVCP who argued their contract-funded and targeted research had led to fundamental interventions in basic knowledge, such as Huebner's work on the viral oncogene theory. A general reluctance to impose uniform distinctions between basic, applied, and targeted science in the SVCP allowed for a kind of flexibility in pursuing basic research leads that was discordant with extramural scientists' expectations of such a targeted program.

That contracting in the NCI's collaborative research programs had become a lightning rod for varied controversies reflected some resentment among extramural scientists that such a substantial share of the institute's growing budget was allocated to projects conducted under the discretion of intramural NCI scientist-managers. Between 1961 and 1975, the NCI's annual appropriations increased more than sixfold. These increases occurred even through the lean years of Nixon's early administration. Direct operations at NCI grew at a pace that far outstripped extramural grant awards, with the former increasing eightfold and the latter only fivefold. At the decade's halfway mark, NCI leadership was optimistic that funding would continue to flow toward targeted programs such as the cancer virus effort. In fact, NCI leadership anticipated it would close out the 1970s with a doubling of funding for virus efforts in the institute.[62] This positivity would be short lived, as both scientific discoveries and responses to problems stoked by external criticisms would soon turn the tides against contract-funded targeted research at the NCI.

SVCP CONTRACTORS TRANSFORM
THE ONCOGENE HYPOTHESIS

Already in 1970, scientist-managers such as Huebner were entertaining interpretations of the relationship between viruses and cancers that implied a radically different prevention strategy from vaccines. Addressing the issue of where the SVCP's targeted research would terminate, Frank Rauscher argued that "control of virus-induced cancers in man seems to be heading toward eventual success, [a]lthough some of the pathways are changing from conventional vaccines to newer immunologic and preventive measures still in the developmental stage."[63] Expositing at length before the World Health Organization's International Conference on the Application of Vaccines against Viral, Rickettsial, and Bacterial Diseases of Man, Rauscher argued the following:

> The new measures for possible control might include immunization involving virus-induced transplantation antigens, substances on the surface of cells that have been exposed to a virus and stimulate antibody production against that virus or against their induced cancer cells. Another method might be interference with the action of an important enzyme, the RNA-dependent DNA polymerase found to be associated with RNA virus-caused cancers in animals and in white blood cells from leukemia patients. Still another measure might be the use of natural or synthetic repressors for viral activity, an avenue of inquiry suggested by Dr. Robert J. Huebner of the National Cancer Institute as the next step in cancer research to follow his "oncogene" theory. Or it might be interference with the environmental or hormonal derepressors which Dr. Huebner believes may "trigger" these latent but naturally occurring virus genes in all vertebrates, man included. However, a "standard," or conventional type, vaccine may still be a practical approach to some human cancers . . . [as] cancers in mice and chickens can be greatly reduced by the use of standard virus vaccines.[64]

Attendant upon the shifting focus of experimental work, the formal organization of the SVCP under the convergence technique confronted a need to revise its goals. Together with agents from the Systems and Operations Planning Branch of the NCI Office of the Director, program scientist-managers worked to "formulate a revised program plan reflecting the current key research problems, program decisions, and decision criteria." Despite the radical scientific shift its authors attributed to the oncogene hypothesis, systems and operations agents claimed that "the convergence technique developed by Mr. Carrese and Dr. Baker continues to be the method used for structuring the research logic."[65]

Huebner and his team continued to utilize the contracting functions of the SVCP to steer the nation's now vast infrastructure for conducting RNA virus research toward providing further support for the viral oncogene hypothesis. Of particular significance to this project was a cluster of laboratories Huebner contracted with in California and the state of Washington, colloquially known as the West Coast Tumor Virus Cooperative, which shared resources and techniques enabling the study of Rouse sarcoma virus (RSV).[66] One of the newest and most promising contracts in the cooperative had been given to a laboratory at the University of California, San Francisco (UCSF), headed by J. Michael Bishop and Harold Varmus. Bishop and Varmus focused on detecting the presence of *src*, then assumed to be a gene fragment of RSV, in various animal tumors. As Huebner considered RSV one of the most likely candidates for providing experimental support for the viral oncogene hypothesis, he sponsored their work generously through the SVCP. Bishop and Varmus soon relied on program contracts for 85 percent of their laboratory's funding. Their funding tripled between 1971 and 1974 as leadership in the newly renamed Virus Cancer Program (VCP) identified it as "one of the best" contracts funded by the institute.[67]

As Scheffler and I detail elsewhere, "the experimental systems developed in Bishop and Varmus's laboratory with the purpose of supporting the viral oncogene hypothesis to advance the NCI's vaccine mission produced the conditions for the emergence of very different phenomena."[68] When calibrating a hybridization probe to detect *src* in RSV-infected chicken cells, Dominique Stehelin, a visiting researcher in Bishop and Varmus's laboratory, found that uninfected cells also expressed *src*. As *src* was understood at the time to be part of the RSV genome and thus should not have been present in cells not previously exposed to RSV, this finding posed a profound and urgent puzzle that occupied the laboratory for more than a year. Initially, the NCI confronted Bishop and Varmus's findings as evidence of endogenous virus transmitted vertically in the genetic heritage of human cells. Presenting the VCP's interpretation before the NCAB, NCI leadership argued that emerging findings from Bishop and Varmus's hybridization probes supported the continued search for RNA viruses in humans homologous to those established as oncogenic in other animal models.[69] These findings would suggest continued hope for vaccination as a preventative against oncogenic RNA viruses, though effective vaccines would have to be administered early in life before these endogenous viruses could be switched on.[70] While presenting the Bishop and Varmus lab's findings to the NCAB the next year as examples of how the VCP was funding exceptional basic research through contracts, program scientist-managers maintained that "the major goal of the program remains the prevention of cancer through the development of vaccines."[71]

Yet the scientific leeway the VCP routinely granted its contractors in pursuing their own lines of inquiry allowed Bishop and Varmus to entertain interpretations of what was at issue in their findings that led them to deviate substantially from the stakes defined by the VCP. The Bishop and Varmus lab had spent years fine-tuning hybridization techniques toward the immunological specificity required by a hunt for specific viral genes that might be targeted by a vaccine. Once Bishop and Varmus's research colligated around an alternative explanation—that *src* was not a viral gene, but a *cellular* one—they "revers[ed] the progress . . . they had made toward creating a specific and precise hybridization probe for *src*" to explore this possibility in a series of iterative experiments.[72] In 1975, the laboratory adapted the immunological *src* probe to be *less* specific in order to pursue a hypothesis that c-*src* (their designation for *src*-type genes of cellular origin) had been passed down through cellular DNA from a distant evolutionary ancestor. The team, enhanced by the efforts of postdoctoral scholar Deborah Spector, used the less specific probe to find evidence of c-*src* in phylogenetically related avian species, as well as in urchins and mammals—including humans.[73] They now proposed that what the VCP had considered to be vertically transmitted endogenous *viral* genes were instead part of the normal genetic inheritance of many species' *cellular* DNA. This proposal not only radically reinterpreted what was at issue in the research the NCI had contracted with them to conduct but also turned Huebner's viral oncogene theory on its head. Bishop and Varmus now proposed what they called the "cellular oncogene theory" as an explanation of the common cause of many cancers.[74] Only after the publication of the Bishop and Varmus lab's findings would the NCI's Edward Scolnick, whose research in the SVCP had proceeded under the understanding of viral oncogenes as the predominant issue, nevertheless admit before the NCAB that the stakes of the VCP should be reinterpreted to suggest "vaccines against standard types of viruses are less likely to be useful" than once presumed.[75] (Scolnick would shortly go on to identify the first cellular oncogene implicated in human cancer, *ras*, after shifting the issues and stakes of his lab's research toward the cellular oncogene interpretation as well.[76])

Bishop and Varmus's findings, published in 1976 after years of additional research, would earn them both a Nobel Prize. The cellular oncogene hypothesis would soon come to represent the dominant theoretical perspective on cancer causation in biomedicine.[77] As sociologist Joan Fujimura recounts, the cellular oncogene theory would also unleash a stampede of new molecular oncology studies focused on cataloguing human oncogenes, and the tools refined by those researchers hopping on the "oncogene bandwagon" helped form the basis for the rapid expansion of the biotechnology sector in the 1980s.[78] Yet in pursuing experimental findings meant to support the efforts of SVCP scientist-managers to develop a vaccine against human cancer viruses, the cellular oncogene theory finally presented a problem that could not be reconciled with the NCI's management apparatus.

Fatefully, the NCI's VCP began this experimental trajectory away from its long-held promise of a cancer vaccine at the same time it lost its staunchest proponents for the convergence technique. As Baker was elevated to the NCI directorship (and, shortly thereafter, replaced), he maintained his conviction in the system he had developed for targeting and accelerating research toward cancer preventatives and cures and integrated the convergence technique into planning exercises for the National Cancer Plan. Though advocates of the approach remained in Congress and in Lasker's influential lobbying circles, scientists familiar with the research findings emanating from the NCI's own targeted programs became increasingly skeptical that the institute could deliver on its promises. Concerned for the fiscal fate of investigator-initiated grants, they warily eyed the growth of the National Cancer Plan.

SCIENTIFIC PRINCIPALS TAKE OVER THE NCAB

As criticisms of the SVCP indicate, many scientists outside of the NCI viewed the targeted management system invoked by the convergence technique as anathema to good cancer research, as it clashed with the prevailing institutional norms of small-scale, grant-funded investigator-initiated inquiry.[79] These complaints were registered in an opinion piece authored by *Science* correspondent Nicholas Wade immediately after the National Cancer Act's passage. Wade's investigation echoed the opinions of many extramural scientists but also presaged the condemnation the program would receive from the Zinder Report two years later. As Wade recounts, "[t]he major criticisms made of the SVCP are that it uses a wasteful method of supporting research, allows too much power to individual scientists to channel resources in a single direction, has failed to develop an intellectual base for its overall research strategy, and excludes critics and outside advice."[80] Quoting anonymous respondents from the scientific community, Wade opined on a lack of structural openness around contracting and a culture of deliberate isolation borne of defensiveness.[81] At the heart of these criticisms was a perception that SVCP contracts were approved without adequate peer review. Given the tremendous power and discretion the small group of NCI scientist-managers composing the SVCP held over research priorities with nearly $50 million in funds at stake, one of Wade's respondents warned of "an incredible fiasco should their judgment prove wrong."[82]

The changes the NCI's move toward targeted research had wrought in the broader institutional ecology for scientific research had not gone unnoticed, nor had SVCP scientist-managers' efficacy in defining the political stakes of research alongside the scientific issues at hand. Robin Scheffler recounts how the War on Cancer activated a nascent political movement within the field of molecular biology driven by scientists who appreciated that the continued growth of their academic enterprise was dependent upon generous support through federal grants. Efforts led by prominent researchers such as Paul Berg and James Watson in 1970 to persuade the National Science Foundation (NSF) to establish a dedicated program in molecular biology did little to assuage their anxiety that federal funds would be insufficient to sustain the growth of their materially intensive inquiries.[83] Frustrated by what they perceived as an overemphasis on health in the NCI's mission-oriented programs, these molecular biologists mobilized to advance "a new understanding of cancer and cancer research" that was based on the need to return to the fundamental genetic mechanisms behind biological processes such as cancer.[84]

Political scientists have described the style of congressional oversight for most complex and expert-driven executive branch agencies such as the NCI as "fire-alarm" oversight. Lacking the requisite knowledge and motivation for direct centralized surveillance of agencies by members of Congress, "Congress established a system of rules, procedures, and informal practices that enable individual citizens and organized interest groups to examine administrative decisions (sometimes in prospect), to charge executive agencies with violating congressional goals, and to seek remedies from agencies, courts, and Congress itself."[85] Of course, fire-alarm oversight is only effective insofar as citizens or interest groups can persuade members of Congress that they aren't just blowing smoke. In several instances surrounding NACC oversight of contracts and criticisms of the NCI leveled during the campaign for the National Cancer Act, Lasker and her allies were able to attract congressional attention to bureaucratic practices at the NCI that appeared to threaten political principals' interests. By comparison, molecular biologists were a loosely confederated movement yet to speak in a unified voice and lacking the elite status and personal connections that enabled Lasker and her allies to elicit a response from Congress. Despite mobilizing to protest the National Cancer Act in congressional testimony, molecular biologists won few supporters in the House or Senate.[86] Congress was evidently unmoved by the argument that targeted or mission-oriented programs did harm to the scientific community generally. Scientists' continued grievances about targeted programs at the NCI and the War on Cancer in general failed to attract significant attention despite concerted efforts by professional associations such as the Federation of American Societies for Experimental Biology (FASEB) to coordinate letter-writing campaigns to Congress or to bend the ear of the president.[87]

These hard lessons were not lost on concerned molecular biologists. As their appreciation for the political environment sustaining concentrated investment in mission-oriented research at the NCI grew, they located the institute's governance structure as a crucial site for redefining the stakes of cancer research in their favor. The control the National Cancer Act vested in the NCAB (figure 3.2) over scientific and policy decisions at the NCI opened the possibility that direct appeals to Congress were unnecessary; molecular biologists could represent the scientific community's position from within the institute's own governance structure instead.

As one of the most prominent molecular biologists in the public eye and a staunch critic of the NCI's attempts to use vaccine development to claim public

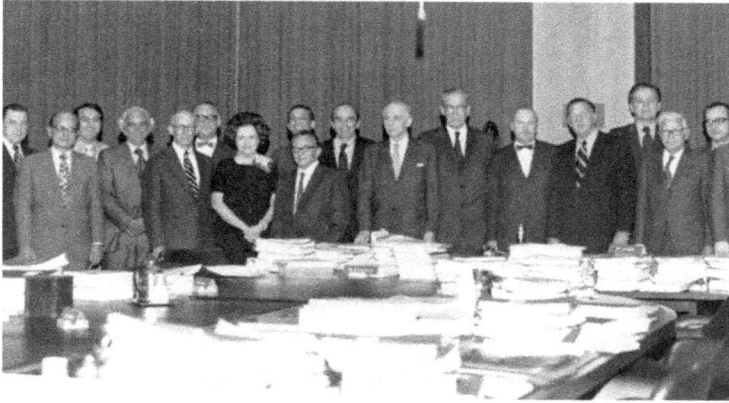

3.2 First meeting of the National Cancer Advisory Board (NCAB) in 1972.
Photo credit: National Library of Medicine.

accountability, James Watson became a figurehead for articulating the common stance among many molecular biologists that "aiming to gain therapeutic payoffs from [basic] research in the short term was foolhardy."[88] He instead advanced the community's view that the interests of the public would be best served by supporting open-ended research that would uncover, through serendipity, long-term solutions to the problems plaguing human health. Watson found a powerful venue for pushing this alternative when he was elected to the NCAB in 1972. In his brief stint on the board, Watson aggressively objected to the "political hacks" who aimed to use the NCI to steer the future direction of biomedical inquiry, warning of the ruin cancer research would find itself in if subordinated to the desires and instruments of administrators.[89] Watson's ire soon became sharply focused on the SVCP's use of contracts to fund and coordinate science.

Though Watson was the SVCP's most vituperative opponent on the board, other molecular biologists on the NCAB were similarly critical of both the scientific value of program efforts and what its contracting practices might portend for a shift away from the academy and toward industry. In 1973 and 1974, declining appropriations throughout the NIH (with the exception of the NCI) were accompanied by Nixon's increasing emphasis on sponsoring private enterprise through contracting, a prospect that particularly threatened academic scientists.[90] To appease dissenting voices on the NCAB and among the research communities they represented, NCI director Rauscher authorized an investigation into the SVCP.

At Watson's insistence, molecular biologist Norton Zinder was appointed to lead the committee. Privately, Zinder disclosed that his motive was to undermine the use of contracts in the NCI and reassert the importance of funding research through peer-reviewed grants.[91] The Zinder Committee's investigation unfolded alongside Watergate, endowing the months-long proceedings with an air of intrigue. The Zinder Committee quickly found its villain in Robert Huebner, whose command of millions of dollars dispensed across an expansive contracting network drew criticism that federal monies were too centralized in the hands of a small group of scientist-managers. The committee did not share the NCI Directorate's enthusiasm for the oncogene hypothesis; despite promising developments from Huebner's contracted research with Bishop and Varmus, the Zinder Committee objected in principle to the concentration of so much fiscal power in one intramural figure. Their criticism questioned the propriety of the SVCP's management structure, leaving aside scientist-managers' own insistence that science and management were unified in the program's priorities.[92]

In 1974 the Zinder Committee transmitted its findings about the VCP[93] to Director Rauscher. Damningly, the Zinder Report found that "because the direct targets have become fuzzy since 1964 . . . the program seems to have become an end in itself, its existence justifying its further existence."[94] Despite agreement that the "scientific rationale for an intensive study of the role of viruses in human cancer is well founded" based on the conviction "of the scientific community at large that a virus etiology for some human cancers is probable," the reviewers objected to the concentration of much of the nation's resources for virus research and the recruitment of so many extramural scientists in the service of whatever projects a small cadre of NCI intramural scientist-managers deemed most relevant.[95] The report argued that at its inception "[t]here did not, nor does there exist, sufficient knowledge to mount such a narrowly targeted program."[96] The Zinder Report singled out the use of contracts as particularly problematic given what was perceived to be an inappropriate system of peer review. Like Wade before them, the committee found that NCI scientists had too much power to distribute funds to friendly contractors, and that the allocation of funds often seemed to "be determined by the interests of and perhaps personal relationship to" one of the program's scientist-managers.[97] Further exacerbating this favoritism, the report noted that the working groups that formed one of the two layers of peer review in the VCP were staffed primarily by researchers who received support through VCP contracts. When the committee interviewed these contractors, they found that many did not feel free to express disagreement with funding decisions in contract approval meetings, nor did they feel comfortable criticizing how NCI scientists reviewed and approved contracts.

The Zinder Report did not attribute these failures in peer review to corruption, abuse of power, or obliviousness on the part of NCI scientist-managers. Instead, it argued that allowing VCP scientist-managers too much discretion in determining how the program would evolve over time resulted in a closed shop:

> The mistake that led to the excesses we describe was primarily one of management. The program was allowed to grow from the inside out. The vision that established the program was sound, but the underlying philosophy that the role of management of fundamental science is the same as the role of management for engineering or development when the fundamental knowledge is available, was sadly in error. Instead of allowing the direction of the scientific program to come from the working scientists by opening it to all, the program appears to have been a closed operation from its start.[98]

To correct the deficiencies they detected, the committee recommended the VCP open its "closed shop."[99] This primarily involved reconstituting groups tasked with reviewing contracts so that at least half were non-NCI scientists, in addition to opening up contract competitions to all. The report also recommended canceling all existing contracts and reassigning funding for basic research to grants, reserving contracts only for those worthy projects that did not otherwise attract sufficient attention from the extramural scientific community.

Many of the criticisms contained in the Zinder Report addressed management practices in the program that NCI administrators had already come to perceive as problematic. Only months prior to receiving the report, the institute had made moves to consolidate the working groups responsible for initial review of contract proposals and discontinue the questionable practice whereby contractors might sit on the same committee that reviews their submission.[100] Earlier in 1973, many of the SVCP's scientists, including Huebner, came under attack by academic scientists who argued before the NCAB that their close control over the direction of research in the program worked "to the detriment of the science."[101]

Rauscher ensured the Zinder Report was not circulated beyond the NCAB and geared the NCI's response solely toward satisfying the board in its governance capacity. John Moloney headed the NCI's response to the Zinder Report's criticisms. He rejoined that there was a "tremendous amount of basic research supported by the Virus Cancer Program" even for those contracts that primarily produced reagents, and that contract "activities resulted in 1,183 publications in FY 1972."[102] More to the point, funding for basic research had been assumed by the convergence technique at the outset of the program, in part because "the Virus Cancer Program has never considered the virus-cancer problem to be one which would be readily resolved, and the breadth of its overall activities across different research specialties shows cognizance of the need for such contributions converging on the major objectives." It was thus incorrect to fault the program for "fuzzy" targets, as it never assumed "that knowledge of the virology and natural history of tumor virus was sufficient to achieve control of virus-induced cancer and that the most basic information was on hand to achieve a definitive result in a relatively short period."[103] In his defense of the scientific integrity of the VCP, Moloney fudged the program's initial ambition to rapidly produce a vaccine and the role this goal played in structuring and securing program development under Baker. In so doing, Moloney lent credence to critics' attempts to redefine the issues and stakes around the legitimacy of contracts rather than the interplay between scientific and managerial priorities that had been generative of so many breakthroughs, including the embattled Huebner's oncogene studies.

After a member of the NCAB leaked the Zinder Report to *Science* reporters who were similarly skeptical of the VCP, a contingency within the broader community of molecular biologists took up the report's critiques in arguing against Congress's 1974 reauthorization of the National Cancer Act.[104] Esteemed biomedical scientists publicly aired their grievances about the handsome funding the NCI enjoyed during lean times, with prominent figures such as Arthur Kornberg and Sol Spiegelman contending that the War on Cancer was diverting funds from grant-funded basic research to the National Cancer Program.[105] Their argument found sympathy with some NCAB members as well, who objected to what they perceived as the redirection of federal monies from investigator-initiated research to cancer control and other applied programs. With several years of threatened budget reductions from the Nixon and now Ford White Houses, many of which jeopardized grant programs, extramural researchers were increasingly leery of programmatic funds, contract or otherwise. The fat days of unsolicited increases for the NCI were gone; in this increasingly zero-sum game, what mattered most to these scientific principals was that the funds available for grants to investigators for self-directed inquiry were maximized.

With pressure mounting from members of the NCAB who positioned themselves as scientific principals holding the institute accountable to its mission to fund the best science, NCI leadership attempted to retool management practices developed around contracts so they hewed more closely to the grant model. In 1974, shortly after the Zinder Report had condemned the NCI's use of contracts, Director Rauscher debuted official plans for the new Cancer Research Emphasis Grants (CREGs) that would replace the funding apparatus covering most of the contracts then issued to scientists at nonprofit institutions. Though the timing suggested CREGs were a response to the Zinder recommendations, the new mechanism had been in development since the prior year. The move toward solicitations for more open-ended research than that funded by contracts addressed what Rauscher recognized was a growing discomfort with contracting among extramural scientists, manifested in part in their reluctance to participate in programs like the VCP.[106] Approved in 1975, the CREG initiative was meant to ensure that "the contract mechanism will no longer be used to support best effort, basic research projects in which NCI does not need to provide frequent direction and control."[107] CREGs were published solicitations for research projects that targeted specific scientific gaps the NCI felt needed to be addressed. CREGs "designate the research desired, but approaches and methodology are left to the creativity of the extramural scientists who apply."[108] The rise of CREGs justified leveling-off trends in contract funding at the NCI, which in the first half of the decade had grown to exceed contracting efforts in all other NIH institutes combined.[109] By 1976, most of the VCP's former contracts that had not been allowed to expire were converted to CREGs. The remaining intramural projects were absorbed into the nontargeted intramural Viral Oncology Program (VOP) in November 1975, leaving little of the original structure of the VCP remaining.

THE DECLINE OF THE VIRUS CANCER PROGRAM

In her role in coordinating the National Cancer Act through machinations in Congress and the White House, Mary Lasker had envisioned the NCAB as an enhanced seat of power from which she might exercise control over the NCI's operations. She had not, however, anticipated that her primary source of power in shaping the congressional agenda would erode soon after the NCA passed. Lasker's most successful efforts to maintain funding for biomedicine had often been bolstered by relationships with senior politicians whose leadership positions on key congressional committees helped them control appropriations for the NIH. The power of these chairs was reduced by a series of Democrat-led reforms in 1973 and 1974 that undermined the role of seniority in House committee chair selection. These reforms were passed in an effort to bolster what was seen as diminished congressional power vis-à-vis the executive and to help break up the "iron triangles" between appropriations committees, lobbyists, and federal agencies.[110] The success of these reforms left Lasker with fewer levers to pull in the House and Senate.

Lasker had heretofore paid comparatively less attention to the White House compared to Congress, in part because most of the presidents' budgets throughout the 1960s had asked for decidedly lower funding levels for the NIH than Lasker could secure by lobbying Congress.[111] Yet by 1973 it had become apparent that Nixon's commitment to control the agenda of the National Cancer Plan was focused on the President's Cancer Panel, which was independent of the NCAB and NCI and reported directly to the White House. The White House had given the PCP enough control over its management of the National Cancer Program that its three panel members selected most of the suggestions for NCAB members who were nominally appointed by the president.[112] Lasker quickly moved to influence the PCP, visiting her old friend and PCP chairman Benno Schmidt in early 1974 to appeal for more rapid health results in treatment and leaving "a briefcase full of material" for Schmidt's perusal.[113] Though Lasker maintained her place on the NCAB for several more years, the friendlier and evidently more influential PCP became the focus of her efforts.

Yet the enhanced oversight powers of the NCAB, which Lasker had helped to enshrine in the National Cancer Act of 1971, remained in place, and though the president could appoint whomever he preferred to the board, he nevertheless followed the advice of lower-level officials to recommend physicians and scientists of good reputation to the NCAB. The lack of attention from the executive and Lasker's diversion of lobbying efforts to the more powerful PCP gave the NCAB a degree of autonomy from these interests that it used to embrace the voice of the scientific public. As the decade wore on and subsequent presidencies showed less enthusiasm for the cancer war effort, the PCP's dominance over the policy agenda at the NCI faded. This left extramural scientists on the NCAB in command of a powerful lever of governance in the NCI—one they were pulling in earnest by 1974.

Despite the NCI's best attempts to defend the VCP against insinuations made in the Zinder Report, the NCAB flexed its substantial scientific muscle to ensure the institute would be held accountable to the criticisms in the report. A subcommittee of the NCAB was formed to oversee VCP operations, including the phase-out of most contracts upon expiration. NCI administrators took the opportunity to extend plans for reorganizing several other units in the organization to the institute's viral oncology operations, including much of the research conducted by principal investigators in the VCP. Yet the coincidence of these restructuring efforts with interpretations by some in the VCP's own leadership that the cellular oncogene theory advanced by Bishop and Varmus ruled out a major role for a vaccine ultimately left the NCI's scientist-managers with few reasons to sustain their optimism about program goals. Huebner, the oncogene's chief champion in the program, was scaling back his duties because of complications from advancing Alzheimer's disease.[114] As several key members of the program would later remark in 1977 on the eve of its demise, "scientists have completely redefined the word 'virus' and no longer think of a tumor virus only as a particle that enters a host cell and causes disease, a particle that can be inactivated and turned into a protective vaccine. Thus cancer causation no longer conforms to old concepts of infection and disease."[115] The scientific agenda that had motivated the VCP now appeared moribund, and there were few on the NCAB who would mourn it.

By 1976, the VCP's fortunes with congressional principals were also fading fast. For the first time in its history, funding for the program dropped between 1975 and 1976. This was not merely the result of the growing atmosphere of austerity that would characterize congressional budgeting throughout the late 1970s. As Moloney contemplated a name change for the NCI's intramural virus cancer unit, the *Cancer Letter* wryly remarked on "the diminishing popularity (in Congress, especially) of viruses and the growing popularity of carcinogenesis."[116] A few members of Congress began repeating some of the talking points first advanced by molecular biologists including the accusation that the NCI neglected basic research and starved other institutes of funding.[117] Unlike the criticisms of molecular biologists, the thrust of congressional criticisms focused on an absence of studies on environmental carcinogens, a popular topic among constituents as the environmentalist movement gained steam.[118]

In November 1976, Rauscher resigned as director of the NCI. For the first time in the history of the modern NCI, a new director was tapped from the academy rather than from within the ranks of the institute. Incoming director Arthur C. Upton, former dean of Basic Health Sciences at SUNY Stony Brook, was not only friendlier to the environmental concerns ascendant in Congress[119] but also shared the skepticism toward contract funding for basic research that characterized molecular biologists' critiques of programs such as the VCP. Upon taking office, Upton was forced to respond to allegations of extreme deficiencies in contract administration made by the Office of the Inspector General (OIG) during a May 1977 review of the NCI's contracting practices, which had been instigated by congressional critic Dave Obey.[120] The OIG accused the NCI of a laundry list of questionable practices, including:

> dominance of program officials over contracting officers; program management not separate from review function; use of contracts as though they were grants; peer review observations not always followed; poor procurement planning, resulting in a heavy year-end workload; poor financial and scientific administration of contracts after they are awarded; need for more competition—many of the Justifications for Non-Competitive Procurement were considered weak; inadequate cost analysis of financial proposals by contractors; not enough Departmental stewardship—inadequate OS and PHS supervision (only one review since 1971); and not enough project officers (one was said to be responsible for 58 contracts).[121]

Though the OIG failed to find evidence of corruption, the review that ferreted out these deficiencies was conducted on the basis of accusations of such by the secretary of the Department of Health, Education and Welfare. The NCI did not challenge the OIG's accusations and instead moved to correct the indicated deficiencies. When Upton took over the directorship in 1977, he enhanced the NCI's response by aggressively pursuing the elimination of contracts for basic research, resolving to phase out one-third of all contracts in favor of grants by the end of the decade.[122]

A shift in research emphasis in the intramural Viral Oncology Program suggested that NCI scientists' interests also moved away from targeted efforts shortly after the VCP was shuttered. Rather than probe the relationship between different viruses and cancers, NCI researchers had turned their attention toward illuminating the basic mechanisms of cellular transformation using cancer viruses as model systems. Interpreting the intramural virus program's mission in 1976, NCI leadership reported that "[t]he emphasis in cancer virology has moved from the search for viruses to the study of virus gene transcription, translation and control mechanisms."[123] No longer beholden to program objectives of finding a vaccine for virally induced cancers, the NCI's research portfolio expanded to include basic research that utilized many of the DNA viruses once excluded from VCP contracts.[124] This included explorations of the human papillomavirus (HPV), which was still considered to have a "tangential relationship to cancer research" by most extramural investigators (with the important exception of once-VCP contract beneficiary Harald zur Hausen, who would soon establish a link between HPV and cervical cancer).[125]

CONCLUSION

Though the VCP closed out the 1970s under a cloud of heavy criticism, the seeds the NCI planted through more than a decade of contracts would soon blossom into the biotechnology sector. Much as the cellular oncogene hypothesis (and the subsequent "oncogene bandwagon") emerged from the extended experimental apparatus erected by the VCP rather than in spite of it, several other key technologies were enabled by the NCI's infrastructure during this period. The immunological objectives motivating the program led to substantial investment in resources and training for protein chemistry and encouraged networks of researchers to circulate materials and findings among the growing community united around these contracts.[126] As the sociologists Studer and Chubin illustrate through their citation analysis of early reverse transcriptase publications, the NCI's virus cancer researchers continued to be central to virus-driven research even after the formal dissolution of the targeted program in the institute. Indeed, the NCI's virus cancer researchers formed a bona fide "research program" motivated by common methodological approaches and a "theoretical unity" that spurred significant scientific growth in the field.[127] Though Studer and Chubin imply that the NCI's VCP "stymied" reverse transcriptase research, a careful analysis of networks of practice—rather than co-citation studies—reveals the close interdependence of reverse transcriptase research upon VCP infrastructure and vice versa.[128] The SVCP famously supplied the avian leukosis virus "to the world research community," which used it and other NCI-contracted virus stocks to establish foundational discoveries in viral enzymology, including David Baltimore's simultaneous discovery of reverse transcriptase alongside Howard Temin.[129]

The rapidly accelerating intramural infrastructure projects mobilized during the War on Cancer also unintentionally created the conditions for former NCI contractors to develop some of the earliest self-standing biotechnology enterprises. Though the landmark legislative decisions in intellectual property law that opened the door for federally funded innovations to be patented and sold commercially happened in the early 1980s, the technologies that drew the attention of financial investors to the first cohort of biotechnology enterprises often had roots in NCI contracts. Fujimura's study of the oncogene bandwagon that yielded laboratory discoveries of a host of human oncogenes and Keating and Cambrosio's analysis of how the NCI's clinical oncology networks developed breakthrough therapeutics attest to the general importance of the NCI's efforts during the War on Cancer in driving innovations often credited to private biotechnology and pharmaceutical companies.[130] Despite the NCI's central role in cancer innovation, sociologists tend to reduce the NCI to a passive funding node in innovation networks.[131] Conceptualizing the direct role the NCI played in establishing the material infrastructures and scientific knowledge that propelled molecular biology in this period shows how the NCI's entrepreneurial approach to cancer research policy in the 1960s and 1970s helped create the conditions for commercial biotechnology to emerge in the 1980s.

But the NCI's impact did not end with infrastructure. Ironically, on the immediate heels of the VCP's demise, intramural NCI researchers would announce the discovery of the first human cancer retrovirus. This discovery was a direct outgrowth of the competencies accumulated in the NCI's intramural programs around the VCP's objectives. It would also prove fateful in allowing the NCI to play an unexpectedly significant role in the HIV/AIDS epidemic that would emerge in the 1980s.

CHAPTER 4

BACK TO BASICS

Human Cancer Retrovirus Research, 1980–1984

The 1980s opened on a dour note for many in NCI leadership. Arthur Upton, an institute outsider, had presided over several years of extensive reorganization that overhauled the NCI's procedures around intramural and extramural support. The National Cancer Advisory Board (NCAB) had been taken over by the NCI's scientific principals, who used it aggressively to ensure a return to the investigator-initiated grant funding they claimed best served the interests of the scientific community at large. As Robert Gallo later quipped, the many candidate oncogenic viruses explored by the now-defunct Virus Cancer Program (VCP) "were not associated with anything, except publication of papers."[1] In response to criticism of the VCP as a monumental failure, the NCI shuttered its targeted vaccine programs in 1978 and reframed its continuing virus research as advancing basic insights into the molecular biology of cancer. Dogged by the failures of the War on Cancer, NCI scientist-bureaucrats retreated to the status quo antebellum of independent, investigator-initiated research.

The NCI's organizational restructuring toward grant support for basic research precipitates the irony that the first human cancer retrovirus, human T-lymphotropic virus (HTLV), was discovered by NCI scientist Robert Gallo in 1979—only a year after targeted support for cancer virus vaccine research came to its ignominious end. Despite a lack of formal support for targeted programs, intramural researchers' commitment to the NCI's dual mission continued to motivate them to informally pursue public health applications for new insights emerging from ongoing experiments on cancer retroviruses. This focus on health-oriented biomedical inquiry became apparent when the NCI mobilized the remnants of its virus program to unmask the culprit behind the burgeoning acquired immunodeficiency syndrome (AIDS) crisis. From 1981 to 1984, Robert Gallo and his colleagues at the NCI pursued cancer retrovirus research and codiscovered the pathogen that would come to be known as HIV.

A controversial figure throughout this period, Gallo's research on the AIDS virus found support in NCI director Vincent DeVita, who had learned through his own decades-long experiences as a scientist-bureaucrat the value of supporting such work in the institute. Gallo's efforts to connect basic retrovirus research and clinical attempts to develop health technologies to stem the AIDS epidemic quickly yielded the first successful screening tool for detecting HIV in the U.S. blood supply. Innovating at a time when formal targeted research was considered anathema to the institute's image, Gallo's laboratory would learn how to conduct basic research of public health relevance through informal collaborations with other mission-oriented scientists in the NCI and NIAID instead. Their success in identifying the viral culprit behind AIDS and developing a working screening tool would buttress DeVita's efforts to rehabilitate the NCI in the eyes of the scientific community. In the process, it would train Gallo and his collaborators in a style of ground-up interdisciplinary collaboration that would lay the foundations for the NCI's approach to translational research in the ensuing decades.

REHABILITATING THE NCI'S MISSION

In 1980, Arthur Upton resigned from the NCI directorship, and Vincent DeVita assumed the position of acting director in his stead. Already a shoo-in, DeVita was officially appointed NCI director in July 1980. Though the National Institutes of Health had felt the squeeze of stagflation since the final years of the 1970s, the Reagan administration (1981–1989) famously brought fresh turmoil to most federally funded agencies. Those institutes whose budgets merely failed to keep up with inflation could count themselves fortunate; for many federal health programs, particularly those tied to public health and medical services, annual appropriations declined sharply by the early 1980s and never recovered. Though the NCI fared well relative to these programs, the institute nevertheless began the new decade under the ominous cloud of a declining budget.[2]

Given this fiscal environment, the NCI was fortunate to open the 1980s with Vincent DeVita at its helm. A product of the NCI's renowned combination chemotherapy clinical team, DeVita was also a staunch defender of the institute's previous investment in cancer virus research. All the same, he was strongly committed to restoring research autonomy to the NCI after the obvious failures of the War on Cancer, which many scientists attributed to the invasive meddling of political lobbyists and congressional principals. In his first years at the helm, DeVita reorganized the institute substantially to refocus intramural and extramural efforts around a return to investigator-initiated biomedical inquiry.

By the time President Carter formally appointed him NCI director in 1980, Vincent DeVita (figure 4.1) had already enjoyed a successful seventeen-year career in the NCI's top chemotherapy programs. DeVita was a singular personality at the institute. First hired as a clinical associate in 1963, he came up in the cradle of mavericks Tom Frei and Jay Freireich in the NCI's Medicine Branch, then under the leadership of Gordon Zubrod. In the heady days of the 1960s, when most medical researchers considered the very idea of a chemotherapeutic "cure" for cancer outrageous, the Medicine Branch realized the first full remissions ever effected through chemotherapy. These included efforts led by Frei and Freireich

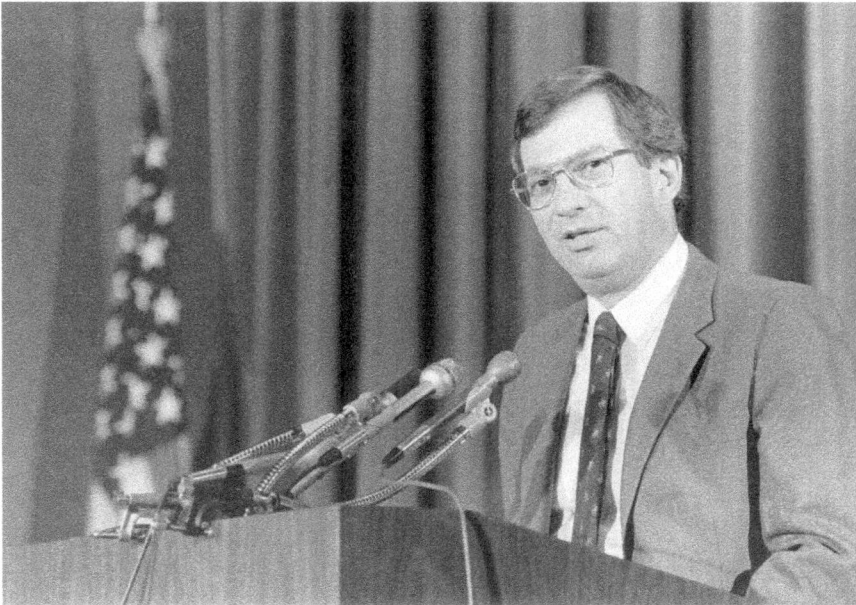

4.1 Vincent DeVita in 1985.

Photo credit: National Cancer Institute.

that used VAMP, the first combination chemotherapy, to cure childhood leukemia; Min Chiu Li's novel methotrexate protocol that cured choriocarcinoma, the first metastatic adult cancer to be fully eradicated through drugs alone; and the MOMP and MOPP combination chemotherapy regimens DeVita developed that sent many patients with Hodgkin's lymphoma into complete remission.

Though celebrated today, in the 1960s the NCI chemotherapists' methods scandalized academic oncologists. Their success simply defied belief. To the average MD, Frei, Freireich, Li, and DeVita were "maniacs"; they were subjected to constant ridicule when presenting their work to professional colleagues, and their commitment to aggressive and novel chemotherapy routinely cost them grants (and, in Li's case, jobs).[3] Oncology was, to DeVita's mind, an extraordinarily conservative academic field. Few organizations would countenance the radical heterodoxy practiced daily on the cancer wards of the NIH Clinical Center. But under the protective wing of the NCI Medicine Branch, DeVita maintained that the "one thing that limited you . . . was between your ears."[4]

DeVita presented the Medicine Branch scientists' successes as a product of their regular cooperative exchanges. Every Friday afternoon a motley crew of clinicians, biostatisticians, and drug researchers led by Frei and Freireich would gather in one of the old chalkboard-lined rooms originally designed by Louis Carrese to accommodate the massive convergence charts used to organize targeted research in the two previous decades. Sarcastically dubbed the "Society of Jabbering Idiots" by one of DeVita's colleagues, this gathering provided a venue where researchers from throughout the NCI who were concerned with developing chemotherapeutics shared and honed their controversial protocols.[5] Reflecting upon how this learning environment yielded such success, DeVita claimed they were "in the right environment, we had the model of acute leukemia, we had [Howard] Skipper's [mathematical modeling] work going on, and then we did the necessary legwork to create the information on the schedule and so forth. We did it, and Frei provided the cover."[6] DeVita credited scientist-bureaucrat Zubrod's stalwart support for their controversial studies in providing the long-term investments in research necessary for the success of treatment protocols that took years or even decades to germinate. Reflecting upon the research that led to his groundbreaking protocol for Hodgkin's lymphoma, DeVita mused: "It takes a long time. I use the development of MOPP as an example that if you want to be a clinical investigator, you have to be patient and live a long time. Because twenty-nine years is longer than most people stay in an institution or a field."[7] This was certainly the case for lightning rods like those in the Medicine Branch. Yet DeVita saw himself as bearing witness to the extraordinary returns the institute could make on such career investments and resolved to continue a legacy where NCI scientist-bureaucrats such as Zubrod "provid[ed] an umbrella for adventurous people" others thought were crazy. As an organization, the NCI protected controversial researchers long enough for them to show their scientific mettle.[8]

Consistent with his image of the distinct advantages of scientific management at the NCI, DeVita was an early and avid champion for the defunct VCP. DeVita saw the NCI's efforts in virus and vaccine research during the 1960s and 1970s as bold and innovative, and he believed the program to be so ahead of its time that its true impact would not be properly appreciated until long after its demise. Immediately after taking the helm, DeVita's chivalry to the program was tested by the prominent Nobel laureate and outspoken NCI critic, James Watson. But by 1982, DeVita and Watson managed to settle into a political truce between the NCI and the faction of molecular biologists the latter helped mobilize against the VCP from within the NCAB.[9] The success of the oncogene hypothesis transmuted from the work of Robert Huebner by VCP contractors J. Michael Bishop and Harold Varmus was an unexpected payoff of the program that extramural scientists were now coming around to recognizing. In a personal communication with DeVita, Watson conceded that "the new strong possibility (fact?) that most if not all of viral oncogenes have their human counterparts" meant "the time is more than ripe for NCI to point out how well the public purse has, in fact, been used."[10] Concurring with Watson, DeVita concluded that, in light of its eventual success, the scientific public's objection to the NCI's targeted virus and vaccine programs could only have "its roots in the governance of science" itself.[11] DeVita's mea culpa came with recognition that the managerial apparatus in place during the early 1970s lacked accountable mechanisms for tracking and redistributing the massive influx of funds proceeding from the National Cancer Act. It should not be cancer virology, DeVita argued, but "the contract mechanism itself" that is "maligned" by its use during the War on Cancer.[12]

Reflecting in a 1984 publication of *Cancer Treatment Reports*, DeVita described the fate of the VCP as coming five years prior. According to this narrative, the Biological Carcinogenesis Program was established in 1979 principally "to take cover from critics of the resources expended on viral oncology."[13]

DeVita argued that the use of contract funds for targeted research provoked scientific ire, dismissing the strong and prevalent criticism inveighed against the quality of program science by cancer researchers and molecular biologists. Intertwining the complicated relationship between the NCI's targeted cancer virus vaccine research program and the cascading developments that led to the cellular oncogene hypothesis, DeVita drew continuity between the NCI's inceptive work on viral oncology (an admitted failure by its own early objectives) and the subsequent success of cancer genetics beyond the institute. Taking the Special Virus Cancer Program (SVCP) as an early precursor to the National Cancer Program initiated by the National Cancer Act of 1971, DeVita argued that the NCI could "take a prodigious share of the credit for kicking off the biologic revolution" in cancer research.[14] The price of these advances in basic research "was the provision of resources and instruments to apply the results of basic research" that would justify the enormous public expenditure on so much blue sky bench-side inquiry.[15]

DeVita saw his role as a scientist-bureaucrat as one of positioning the NCI to ensure the nation's investments could be aggressively put toward promising avenues for biomedical innovation. He did not expect that the scientific community would always agree with the institute's judgments but understood NCI leadership to be best positioned to make them. As DeVita saw it, "the management challenge confronting NIH—not just NCI—is to maintain the flexibility to continue the strategy of rapidly shifting resources to high-priority programs that offer the most promise, regardless of the trauma such shifts cause to the structure of the research apparatus or, for that matter, to the practice of medicine."[16] He opined at length to readers of the leading academic journal *Cancer Research*:

> The decision to allocate resources to different areas of science, even in times of plentiful resources, must always be made by someone. This unavoidable truism is the very crux of the effective governance of science, but it sometimes appears to conflict with the treasured ideal of the spontaneity of investigator-initiated research. . . . These changes have allowed the Institute to support important new programs even in times of tight budget, an essential component of the successful governance of science. The ability to alter course in response to changing conditions and to plan ahead for the next decade will allow NCI-supported scientists to continue to capitalize on the remarkable scientific advances of the 1970s.[17]

Implicit in DeVita's argument is a conception of the time horizon for research findings that prioritizes the organizational realities of research over the political rhetoric of cure. The eventual discovery of a human cancer virus by NCI scientists including Robert Gallo showed that scientific progress could not be bent to political will, lest its merit be "obscured" by misguided criticism.[18] Indeed, as DeVita lamented, the fact that "the success of any complex, multifaceted scientific endeavor . . . depends as much on the governance of science as on its conduct . . . is poorly appreciated by many investigators."[19] Seldom was this clearer in DeVita's mind than when outside investigators criticized prior investments in the NCI's cancer virus initiatives at the same time they depended on the tools developed using resources from these very programs.

While DeVita seemed confident that the eventual success of the NCI's investments in the VCP would win the support of scientific principals going forward, he also needed to appease congressional principals who remained concerned about accountability in the institute's use of taxpayer funds. In 1981, DeVita faced withering criticism from a Government Accountability Office (GAO) report on the NCI's "slipshod" contracting supervision during a hearing of the Senate Labor and Human Resources Committee chaired by Senator Orrin Hatch.[20] Though much of the GAO's report recapitulated criticism the NCI weathered in the late 1970s under Director Upton, new accusations of fraud levied against an extramural laboratory receiving nearly $1 million in grant funding renewed congressional attacks upon the NCI's commitment to administrative accountability. With raptorial focus, Senator Paula Hawkins targeted perceived deficiencies in grant and contract management. The senator excoriated the NCI for its liberty with the public purse and demanded immediate and concrete evidence of improvements from DeVita. DeVita benefited from strong statements of support on behalf of scores of scientists in and outside government who attested to improvements in the institute under his leadership and defended the new director's management ability in the scientific press.[21]

DeVita championed the NCI before congressional principals by demonstrating his commitment to bureaucratic reforms that had been under way since 1980. Learning from criticisms of policy from the prior decade, these reforms primarily involved making decisions over how NCI priorities would affect the allocation of funding for both intramural support and extramural grants more transparent to the public. The first of the NCI's dual layer of peer review for intramural research was revamped around four Boards of Scientific Counselors, comprising panels of nongovernment scientists representing a host of specialties. This broke up the smaller advisory groups that previously informed funding decisions for intramural projects. The decisions of the Boards of Scientific Counselors were now overseen not only by the NCAB but also by a newly founded Executive Committee that actively assessed the institute's entire research portfolio to ensure all sponsored research was meritorious and mission appropriate. Management policy was unified across the institute's various programs and projects and centralized in an office under the directorate. The evaluation and approval of research contracts supporting intramural research was removed to the Division of Extramural Activities where external reviewers would independently evaluate the financial and scientific appropriateness of each proposed contract in a dual-layer peer review system that inverted and mirrored the existing grant review structure.

Most significant for the day-to-day functioning of the organization was a far-reaching overhaul of the assessment and growth of intramural research. DeVita drew upon the governance apparatus cemented after the War on Cancer to overhaul the institute and reallocate resources once assigned to the maligned contract mechanism to investigator grants:

> The new corporate management system, functioning with detailed advice from the four deeply involved multidisciplinary Boards of Scientific Counselors, the NCAB, and the President's Cancer Panel, all in open forum, enabled the NCI Executive Committee to reprogram over $80 million in resources (the majority from contracts), to help absorb a loss of approximately $200 million in purchasing power between 1980 and 1982, and to maintain support for its highest priority basic research in the face of a declining budget. With greater confidence in its review and management, NCI has salvaged the contract as a vehicle of support for research when its use is judged appropriate.[22]

The goal of these management reforms, as DeVita colorfully announced, was to ensure that NCI's management was "squeaky clean."[23] Judiciousness and transparency in the allocation of funding would satisfy congressional principals, while a decisive turn toward grant funding for basic research might persuade scientific principals that the institute operated with their interests in mind.

Despite his recommitment to grant-funded basic research, DeVita's approach to management was not predicated upon a merely ideological faith in individual investigator-initiated science. DeVita had enjoyed an unparalleled practical education in leadership through his informal involvement in the upper echelons of the NCI's executive office. In his beguilingly frank recollections of his career at the institute, DeVita explained how in 1969 his path crossed with that of Mary Lasker. Lasker won over DeVita with her keen political and scientific instincts, and he soon became one of her go-to spokesmen for the NCI at influential dinner parties and state functions.[24] Under Lasker's tutelage, DeVita became accustomed to performing the institute's past accomplishments and future potential before congressional principals. As a scientist whose work at the NCI had already effected one of the few successful chemotherapy protocols at the time, he was the veritable embodiment of the institute's promissory capacity for cure. Soon after Carl Baker was replaced by Frank Rauscher in 1972, Rauscher, too, called on DeVita to represent the institute on Capitol Hill. This practice continued throughout the subsequent leadership of Arthur Upton (1978–1980), who confided to DeVita that "he died a thousand deaths every time he had to testify before Congress."[25] Between Lasker, Rauscher, and Upton, DeVita found himself the public face of the NCI in Congress nearly a decade before his formal appointment to the directorship.[26]

DeVita's approach to administration in the NCI was also shaped by internal reforms he had enacted in his leadership capacities before becoming director. DeVita "had often fantasized about the proper organization of the Division of Cancer Treatment" (DCT) before Rauscher promoted him to the post in 1974.[27] He had formed strong opinions about what was wrong with the DCT and how to fix it, which he aggressively pursued to the great consternation of many of his peers. His double-barreled reform strategy involved consolidating management over intramural and extramural research and creating a more transparent and accountable system of governance for public expenditure on the NCI's treatment programs. He aimed to put an end to the opacity and "cronyism" he felt were rampant in the management of the institute's drug-screening program since its inception.[28] DeVita's solution was to not only open up program review to skeptical extramural scientists but also actively recruit some of the DCT's strongest critics to help oversee the program. His rationale was simultaneously scientific and bureaucratic: "They needed to see how we spent our money. And we needed their ideas, and their critiques, to make sure we were doing our best and were not too attached to approaches that weren't working."[29]

DeVita's reforms incensed many of the personalities he regarded as problematic and led to their exodus from the institute. In part, these changes precipitated one of the first meaningful treatment victories against intractable solid tumors through the National Surgical Adjuvant Breast Project (NSABP), a pioneering effort to improve breast cancer survival rates by strategically combining multiple treatment modalities involving surgery, chemotherapy, and radiation. For years, a coalition of scientists had used relationships with members of the NCAB to obstruct the NSABP's recruitment efforts and starve it of funding. Unfettered from the "vindictive maneuver[ing]" of its foes on the NCAB and under the financial protection of the DCT, the NSABP and its affiliates went on to produce some of the most celebrated clinical trial results of the 1970s.[30] As Peter Keating and Alberto Cambrosio demonstrate, the landmark success of the NSABP-associated trials was the culmination of a decade of previous research originating in DeVita's home clinic at the NCI. These trials "can only be understood as part of the larger research strategy . . . predicated upon the existence of a number of interconnected institutions," emerging professional groups, and "a mounting body of evidence . . . emerging from a *relational system of trials*."[31] This relational system originated in the combination chemotherapy protocols developed for leukemia by Frei and Freireich and for lymphoma by DeVita's trial team and remained continuous with the efforts of extramural researchers funded by the system of cooperative clinical oncology trial grants run out of DeVita's DCT. Management of the DCT was at this time strongly shaped by the changes to the NCI's governance structure effected by the recent passage of the National Cancer Act. Encouraged by Lasker ally Benno Schmidt, head of the President's Cancer Panel (PCP), the DCT was seen as a means to make good on Lasker's wishes that NCI "money was spent on programs for people—not just programs to keep researchers employed."[32] Under the combined leadership of Vincent DeVita and Benno Schmidt, the DCT reconfigured its structure to unite extramural and intramural research on "cancer treatment in ways that would accelerate progress."[33]

The NSABP's success was a learning outcome that was simultaneously one of management and science—an explicit goal of DeVita's reform efforts in the DCT. The NSABP "led the way" in DeVita's clinical trial reforms by "using lab-based scientific logic in reducing the use of surgery and radiotherapy and adding adjuvant chemotherapy for the treatment of breast cancer."[34] DeVita's goal had been to foster a breed of laboratory research that would be readily applicable to the problems confronted in the clinic. At the heart of these bench-to-bedside reforms was an effort to realize on a smaller and more practical scale what he perceived as the motive animating Lasker's approach to the National Cancer Act.[35] DeVita was leveraging developments in basic science to improve clinical outcomes, then using the reach of the NSABP's networks to help integrate this into the policies and protocols of standard medical oncology. DeVita's clinical trial reforms allowed the NCI to lead the field through bureaucratic policy, while the combined scientific and managerial efficacy of NCI's clinical trial innovations served as proof that the institute was fulfilling its dual mission.

"The Twelve Labors of Hercules": Cleaning Up After the War on Cancer

DeVita's success as head of the revamped DCT, both in terms of reforming a troubled intramural program and spurring bench-to-bedside innovation in the neglected NSABP, emboldened the new director to "see what would happen if we used all the resources we had" to fulfill Lasker's intent behind the National Cancer Act.[36] His goal upon assuming the directorship was nothing less than "to reform the NCI and make it fit the vision of the National Cancer Act."[37] In his memoir, DeVita compares the reforms of the early 1980s to the penitence of Hercules in Greek mythology. (He sympathized in particular with the onerous task of cleaning the long-neglected Augean stables of the refuse of a thousand immortal cows.[38]) Driven by a motivation to fulfill the NCI's dual mandate in accordance with his interpretation of Lasker's vision, DeVita went to work "changing the NCI into a tough, well-managed institution—with a silhouette resembling what was described in the cancer act—that could lead the war on cancer."[39]

DaVita's ambition to let the NCI take the reins was inadvertently aided by President Reagan, whose presidential appointees to the NCAB often lacked scientific research experience and seldom "had any appreciable knowledge of the National Cancer Program . . . [or] any experience in the NIH grants system."[40] Diluting the representation of scientific principals on the panel that oversaw NCI scientist-bureaucrats' policy decisions "weakened" the NCAB's role in governance such that familiar observers of institute governance fretted "NCI staff will be making the important decisions since the Board members will not be capable of making reasonable decisions."[41] With the support of the NCAB's remaining faction of basic researchers, such as the vocal Janet Rowley, NCI scientist-bureaucrats took a stronger hand in steering institute policy.[42]

Throughout these first years of the new decade, DeVita's goal was to refocus the NCI's scientific programs to "devote its full energies and resources to the support of basic research and the application of the results of basic research in cancer prevention."[43] Rather than attempt the costly and thankless task of shepherding laboratory findings through the development process, the NCI would instead "emphasize the interrelationship of its basic research programs, such as biological and chemical carcinogenesis and epidemiology aimed at giving a better understanding of the mechanisms of carcinogenesis."[44] Much as the former VCP had been reworked from contract-driven directed research centralized in NCI laboratories, the new NCI would rely on a decentralized but well-funded system of R01 grants that it hoped, with enough money, might lead to useful medical applications.

DeVita was resolute in his faith that the NCI's investments in virus and vaccine research had blazed a trail for the next generation of cancer researchers. His faith rested not only on the promise of finally demonstrating the long sought-after causal relationship between retroviruses and human cancer; DeVita had a finer appreciation for the direct role the institute's VCP contracts played in the discovery of the first human oncogene.[45] The latter development led the "biological revolution" that so excited DeVita and suggested a distinctive path forward for the institute's health goals. Owing to the outsized support the NCI had invested in oncogene research over the previous decade, "the time between discovery and application is shortening, and molecular biology is moving close to the bedside."[46] Testifying before a House oversight committee in 1984, DeVita argued that the quickening pace of oncogene research presented the NCI with a distinctive management challenge. To realize its dual mission, the institute would "allow maximum flexibility for outstanding scientists and make sure that connections are made as early as possible between clinicians and laboratory scientists."[47]

DeVita reassured principals that the NCI's management decisions would "keep the essence of the concept of the National Cancer Program intact as conceived originally, able not only to support basic research but also to apply, when appropriate, the results of this research."[48] To persuade his scientific audience of the importance of both the scientific and health goals encapsulated in the NCI's dual mission, DeVita encouraged them to consider it "an unusual and fragile biological organism with a head at each end."[49] Severing basic research from its application would violate expectations of federal accountability; starving one head would thus inevitably starve the other. One of the hard-won lessons of the NCI's foray into targeted research was that "the delicate balance of sufficient support for basic research and the application of the results of basic research is the very essence of the governance of science and must be carried out in public view by individuals with a broad overview of the program." Extramural scientists should carry over this wisdom to appreciate the NCI's management of the National Cancer Program as a strategic approach to ensuring continued funding through federal grants. "While support of basic research is and always will be our first priority, when the Program shows an unwillingness to apply research results, the public, the Congress, and many scientists as well get cranky."[50]

DeVita's interpretation of the institute's goals helped win back some of the good will lost from academic scientists during the 1970s. No longer would centralized programs focused on producing novel medical and public health applications siphon funds from investigator-initiated research oriented toward scientific knowledge production—a satisfying resolution for many prominent academic researchers. Between 1980 and 1983, the NCI increased the proportion of funding it allocated to basic research from 33 percent to 51 percent.[51] NCI scientist-bureaucrats were left to reconcile the tension this created in their fulfillment of the institute's dual mission. Political support for the National Cancer Program, along with the National Cancer Act legislation that had deputized NCI scientist-bureaucrats into the effort, was clearly waning. In lieu of fulfilling the mandate to improve public health through targeted research and development programs, NCI leadership focused its attention on distributing funding to extramural organizations tasked with distribution and delivery of cancer treatment and control technologies. Yet they had no managerial discretion over how this money would be spent by these diffused cancer centers, and innovations remained slow in coming. Nonetheless accountable for the outcomes these centers were tasked with producing, NCI leadership committed before Congress to reduce cancer mortality 50 percent by the new millennium.[52] This attempt at accountability to the NCI's health mission would ultimately prove unsuccessful.

Though most of the routine focus of NCI governance throughout the decade would be on the arduous task of spurring extramural efforts aimed at cancer prevention and treatment, the intramural program's public health identity crisis would not last long. In 1979, NCI intramural researcher Robert Gallo and his team presented evidence of the first retrovirus discovered to cause cancer in humans. Only a few years later, Gallo's Laboratory of Tumor Cell Biology would thrust itself into the burgeoning public health debate around the etiology of the mysterious new epidemic soon to be known as AIDS. Once again, the prospect of detecting and treating a deadly virus was front and center in the NCI's intramural mission. This time, intramural scientists would lack the concerted managerial efforts characterizing the VCP of the past and would have to develop their own infrastructure for AIDS virology and treatment studies. This ad hoc infrastructure emerged from collaborations forged between intramural bench scientists and clinicians, who would isolate the virus that would become known as HIV and develop an effective assay to detect virus in the national blood supply. These collaborations, which brought Gallo together with Samuel Broder as complementary leaders in laboratory and clinical approaches to the epidemic, would also spur research into the first generation of effective AIDS treatments.

ROBERT GALLO'S RETROVIRUS RESEARCH

Among the programs most affected by DeVita's organizational restructuring was the Viral Oncology Program (VOP) descended from the targeted Virus Cancer Program eliminated in the 1970s. Contrary to popular criticism among extramural scientists, DeVita argued that the institute's two decades of virus research, which cost around $1 billion in taxpayer money, "yielded a trust fund of information, the dividend of which defies the imagination."[53] DeVita firmly demarcated the scientific merit of NCI scientists' viral oncology efforts from the "management problem in the Virus Cancer Program" caused by imprudent use of contracts to fund work that should have been sponsored through grants.[54] He took care to note that the Viral Oncology Program had cut its contract funding and replaced these expenditures with less expensive grants. Nevertheless, DeVita insisted that the scientific community acknowledge how contracts directly led to promising new avenues in oncogene and retrovirus research— successes DeVita argued would not have happened otherwise.[55]

Ironically, the keystone finding of the NCI's VCP—a retrovirus that causes cancer in humans—was finally achieved a year after the program was officially dismantled. The first human cancer retrovirus, human T-cell lymphotropic virus type 1 (HTLV-1), was isolated by Robert Gallo and associates in the NCI's

Human Tumor Cell Biology Branch in 1979. Though an intramural researcher at NCI, Gallo had not been formally involved in the VCP. Like DeVita, he came up through the NCI via Gordon Zubrod's clinic in the Medicine Branch and vividly recalls the excitement of the first generation of combination chemotherapy cures developed by Frei, Freireich, and DeVita. Also like DeVita, Gallo accepted a position at the institute with plans to depart after a brief stint to become a clinician. The allure of laboratory research drew him in despite his formal training as an MD. Gallo found the environment of the NCI particularly well-suited for his research: "if you know you have money for five to ten years, or you are fairly certain of it, then you can ask longer-range questions in your scientific research . . . that security of funding was the best reason for staying at NIH."[56] But the NCI was also "unique in that scientists were able to do research that could be applied to clinical medicine."[57]

Under the accommodating tutelage of Seymour Perry, Gallo was given access to ample resources for pursuing an early interest in molecular biology. He took advantage of both the long-term planning opportunities and the availability of collaborative resources from laboratory and clinic to pursue his early research on the molecular biology of white blood cells. Gallo's trajectory to retroviruses was tortuous, evolving over a decade from his earliest clinical forays on the leukemia ward to bench research on the enzymology of reverse transcriptase. When he took over leadership of his unit in 1972 he renamed it the Laboratory of Tumor Cell Biology (LTCB) to reflect his transition away from the clinic. (At the NCI, "Branches" tend to be focused on clinical research, while "Laboratories" focus on bench science.) Nevertheless, Gallo's lab remained in the DCT's Developmental Therapeutics Program until the mid-1980s. Organizationally, this construed the LTCB's laboratory investigations as "preclinical," a promissory identity not assigned to other laboratory "basic" research units in the institute.[58] Thus, despite the LTCB's emphasis on exploring the biochemistry of cell differentiation and viral carcinogenesis, Gallo described the evaluation of "new approaches to cancer chemotherapy . . . in *in vitro* and *in vivo* systems" as "the ultimate goal of the Laboratory."[59]

Gallo's primary laboratory interests had not originally been with viruses but with transfer RNA. He came into virus research through one of the regular colloquia NCI scientists delivered to their peers. His colleague Bob Ting gave a talk that piqued his interest in animal RNA viruses. This led to a series of collaborations and an introduction to Robert Huebner, whom Gallo came to greatly admire.[60] Though not involved in the central planning apparatus of the VCP, Gallo considered his newly minted Laboratory of Tumor Cell Biology a "sister program"[61] and benefited from funding routed to it by John Moloney, who suspected their early research into human cancer retroviruses would yield a candidate virus.[62] Gallo similarly took advantage of the VCP's promiscuous distribution of reagents, which he used in experiments that would later help establish HTLV-1 as a human retrovirus.[63]

Gallo's recollections include explicit recognition of how the social and material environment he and his team cultivated helped shape their experimental trajectories toward success. Nearly all of his team's innovations originated in episodes where some dimension of the material environment in the laboratory previously coded with an incidental meaning was, over iterative attempts to solve emerging problems, transformed into something salient for driving novel series of experiments. Gallo's first major breakthrough unfolded in this manner, when his lab first found evidence of what would become known as interleukin-2 (IL-2) in the course of conducting a routine experimental set up. At the time, Gallo's team was "using it purely as a practical means for growing human T cells for virological studies and cell biology."[64] Through his organizational connections with clinical researchers, Gallo surmised there were "clinical immunologists in the Cancer Institute who could possibly make use of interleukin-2."[65] Shortly after submitting the lab's first paper describing their findings on IL-2, Gallo contacted NCI clinician Steven Rosenberg to tell him the news and "very rapidly" began seeing IL-2 used in clinical research.[66]

Gallo notes that his laboratory's work on IL-2 depended on a reciprocal relationship with clinical researchers at the NCI. Because of the encouragement of NCI leaders, researchers in the LTCB enjoyed a steady flow of specimens taken from patients being treated at the NIH Clinical Center: "At the time, there was almost a search by the Clinical Center for a scientist to be interested in clinical medicine."[67] Gallo describes the relationship between his laboratory and the Clinical Center as exemplary of "the process of discovery and its applications to clinical medicine."[68] From IL-2 to HIV, Gallo's laboratory maintained consistent interactions and circulation of materials with the clinic; as a result, laboratory staff often sought aid from a pair of clinician's eyes as a matter of course in conducting their research.

In addition to ensuring access to a broad array of materials and collaborators in the clinic, Gallo made it a principle of the LTCB to train the consistent flow of newly minted PhDs coming through the lab in emerging experimental techniques and areas of focus. One of the distinctive organizational qualities of research at the NIH that Gallo cited as significant to the LTCB's innovativeness was created by the lack of teaching obligations commensurate with university research. Academic scientists relied upon the labor of graduate students in training; it kept their budgets low relative to those of the NCI laboratories, which employed postdoctoral labor, but it also meant academic research staff were by and large less skilled than their counterparts in the institutes. Postdoctoral researchers were not only more likely than graduate students to be on the cutting edge of scientific knowledge but also to have mastered the skills necessary to put these into practice. With new theories and methods exploding in molecular biology, Gallo wagered that "anyone who did not make a special effort to keep abreast of a substantial number of these newly developed techniques would, in a few years, fall hopelessly behind even the students at the major universities."[69] As Gallo recalls: "Whenever we read in the scientific literature about some new technique in another lab, we would send [a postdoc] there to learn how it was performed. That person would then come back and teach the rest of us."[70] He described the 1970s as "an active and exciting period in which we, individually and as a group, continually conquered new techniques and incorporated them into the lab's growing technical skills."[71]

Gallo was cognizant of the advantage these learning episodes bestowed upon the laboratory as a functioning scientific unit. He retrospectively claimed that "this early decentralization of expertise is possibly the most important logistical decision I made for the success of our lab over the years."[72] Using this approach, Gallo was able to develop wide-ranging competencies in the LTCB that could be transmitted from postdoctoral researchers to permanent laboratory staff. This enabled postdoctoral and staff researchers to disseminate skills in recombinant DNA technology, gene sequencing, and molecular hybridization early in the adoption curve of these emerging technologies. They were subsequently "able to use these techniques to approach fascinating biological questions at the molecular level."[73]

The intentionality Gallo describes in his approach to managing LTCB personnel contrasts with his descriptions of what motivated innovations. Gallo expounded a personal philosophy where science was driven often by "a certain intuition or a certain belief" as opposed to strict adherence to the scientific method.[74] Why else, Gallo muses, would he have made the "decision to look for a human retrovirus at the worst time, when people were feeling strongly that one could not exist"?[75] By the late 1970s, the NCI's effort to find exogenous human tumor viruses (or, as some had taken to calling them, "human rumor viruses") was considered a disaster.[76] Virologists looked back upon the search for a human RNA cancer virus as "a graveyard of experiments."[77] What little use molecular biologists did have for animal retroviruses was in the form of technical aids for studying oncogenes.[78] The isolation of the first human cancer retrovirus was thus the result of a dogged attempt by the lab to furnish experimental proof of human cancer viruses by poking at the "little holes" they found in their peers' overwhelming criticisms of human cancer virus research.[79]

Uncovering HTLV-1

Gallo finds the origins of his experimental trajectory toward identifying the first human cancer retrovirus in the early years of his laboratory, during which time he "learned to marry white-blood-cell biology to the new developments in retrovirology."[80] Upon the advice of Ting, who had introduced him to cancer virus research at the NCI, Gallo set up his small laboratory with equipment and materials that would help him and his researchers develop an enzyme assay to detect, isolate, characterize, and compare reverse transcriptase across a variety of animal retroviruses. This assay was a means to an end—detecting a human retrovirus in tissue taken from an actual human cancer patient. Achievement of this goal, however, required Gallo and his postdoctoral associates to develop a technique for culturing white blood cells for use in propagating the virus.[81] At the time (1970–1972), this was a particularly challenging technical problem. The laboratory approached this problem by first searching out a growth factor to keep such a culture going. And, because they were seeking the reverse transcriptase of a human retrovirus that had yet to be identified, Gallo's team had recourse only to the "empirical, intensive, old-fashioned" style of problem-solving involving endless iterative cycles of tinkering with the composition and protocol for their assay.[82]

A candidate for human retroviral reverse transcriptase emerged in 1972 from human leukemia lymphocyte studies conducted by two LTCB postdocs, M. "Sarang" Saranghadharan and Marvin Reitz. Together with his colleagues, Gallo interpreted their findings in light of his ultimate aim of finding a human retrovirus. However, in the absence of a complete virus, they failed to persuade the broader scientific community of these stakes.[83] Gallo surmised that achieving their goal would require cultivating large amounts of several fragile blood cell cultures derived from human myeloid leukemia patients. Their first apparent success in isolating a human retrovirus from their new experimental configuration was a disaster—unbeknownst to the team, their cell lines were contaminated with three different monkey viruses, and their findings were ridiculed by their fellow scientists at the annual meeting of the VCP in Hershey, Pennsylvania.[84] This experience motivated a material reorganization of the laboratory space around new cell lines, as well as a distinct "paranoia" that would color Gallo's approach to disseminating findings for the next several years.[85]

The material transformation of the LTCB around these changes enabled two significant elements in the experimental environment to emerge as salient to the laboratory's work in 1975. First, a newly hired hematologist postdoc, Dr. Doris Morgan, persisted in bringing Gallo's attention to some intriguing cell growth in their culture media, despite Gallo's continual dismissal of these cells as probable B cells associated with the Epstein-Barr virus. Second, either by coincidence or as a challenge to Gallo's cavalier interpretation of Morgan's observations, a member of the LTCB sent these cells to a clinician in the nearby NIH Clinical Center.[86] After examining the cells more closely, the clinician noted they were, in fact, T cells. Because T cells and B cells appeared nearly identical when examined using the microscopy equipment available to the team, Gallo only then "realized that we had grown T cells for the first time."[87] These were cutting-edge findings, as immunologists commonly held that T cells did not grow in vitro.

Though salient, the accidental discovery of T-cell growth marked a departure from the planned trajectory of the laboratory's research and thus required a collective redefinition of the issues and stakes of the LTCB's inquiry that colligated around the identification of a T-cell growth factor. Dr. Morgan continued to "nurture" the T cells, and upon the advice of Gallo's trusty technician Zaki Salahuddin, the laboratory soon used human embryotic tissue to isolate a growth factor that enabled the T cells to persist in culture.[88] The newly identified T-cell growth factor soon came to be known as interleukin-2 (IL-2). Gallo eventually interpreted the experimental anomalies around T cells in light of an observation his team made in 1971, when he was surprised to find a growth factor stimulated by T cells in the typically discarded medium of the lymphocytic leukemia cells he had previously studied.[89] Gallo's prior observations of lymphocytic leukemia cultures and the current observations in myeloid leukemia cultures together made

Dr. Morgan's suggestive findings both intelligible and meaningful. In shifting the main focus of one of the laboratory's significant projects toward studying IL-2, the LTCB amplified the stakes of its studies to include the possibility of IL-2's applied clinical utility.

With an abundance of caution after the public embarrassment of their contaminant debacle, researchers throughout the LTCB began using IL-2 to propagate leukemia cells across a series of experimental iterations. After confirmatory research by NCI clinician Thomas Waldmann (who would go on to become one of the first clinicians to diagnose and treat AIDS in the early 1980s), Gallo's team explored these experiments for evidence of a virus.[90] When LTCB researchers observed possible novel reverse transcriptase in a T-cell line they had cultured from a patient with leukemia, Gallo directed the lab to assemble the wealth of reagents they had produced over the years to shore up their claims with a clear antibody test that demonstrated the enzyme was not cross-reactive with any other known virus.

The vast stores of reagents, first enabled by a relationship with the VCP and subsequently facilitated by close networks of NCI researchers at the NIH Clinical Center, helped the LTCB effectively learn from its previous mistakes. The definitive moment in Gallo's recollection was the collaborative relationship formed between postdoc Bernard Poiesz, a recent transfer from the Medicine Branch's clinical wing, and another relatively new clinical unit in the NCI established by John Minna. Poiesz worked with Minna's group to develop a cell line from the tissue of a patient with T-cell leukemia, which subsequently reacted with their suspected retrovirus. For further evidence, Gallo returned once more to Waldmann in the Clinical Center, who furnished a fresh blood specimen from the patient who originated the materials they used in the T-cell line. With rapid turnaround, Poiesz confirmed the presence of their enzyme in this sample.[91] Gallo collaborated with NCI epidemiologist William Blattner in an effort to collect blood samples from healthy and leukemic patients around the world. (The lab would later use these to develop a serum antibody test that would subsequently serve as the prototype for their HIV assay.[92])

Gallo's management strategy was also crucial in enabling the success of these iterative validation experiments. The LTCB, now almost a decade old, boasted a deep bench of researchers trained in a variety of emerging techniques related to different areas of expertise. The material resources and diverse networks the LTCB enjoyed are not uncommon among scientific teams working in academic settings, but these alone could not generate a compelling body of experimental evidence supporting the existence of a novel human retrovirus. Diachronically, several generations of talented scientists cycled through the lab, developing skills in a wide array of experimental techniques and training technicians and newer researchers in their execution. Synchronically, a roster of researchers trained in protein chemistry, enzyme assays, and experimental leukemia therapies contributed to an extended intra-organizational web of expertise that defined problems and tried solutions in simultaneity with one another. The work of discovering the first human cancer virus was thus a strongly collective effort that mobilized scientific and organizational competencies distributed across a large and shifting group of NCI personnel.

Gallo's anxieties about contamination in the lab's experiments contrasted with the enthusiasm of his colleagues around the possibility of detecting a novel virus. The memory of his embarrassing failure five years prior motivated Gallo to handle the publication of the lab's findings gingerly. He thus deployed a tactic he would come to rely on during his early studies on HIV. Cashing in on the diverse skills of its researchers, the LTCB would issue a slate of articles all at once, each detailing a different evidentiary base supporting the claim that they had isolated a novel human cancer virus. After fighting with an editor who refused to publish work on human cancer viruses in principle, they were able to publish all of their core findings by the spring of 1981, two years after they had identified the agent they were calling HTLV.[93]

Shortly after publishing their initial findings, their collaboration with Blattner and other colleagues in Japan and France revealed endemic clusters of HTLV in Japan and the Caribbean. Epidemiological analysis established that HTLV was transmitted through blood transfusion and sexual activity, as well as from mother to child in utero or via breast-feeding; additionally, HTLV-positive populations were more prone to opportunistic infection, suggesting immune suppression.[94] This epidemiological profile attracted the interest of Anthony Fauci of the NIAID and would later influence both Gallo and Fauci's early interpretations of the viral agent responsible for AIDS.

Around the same time that Gallo published the initial HTLV articles, he obtained a sample of David Golde's infamous[95] immortalized T4-cell culture called the MO cell line, originally extracted from a prolific donor with a rare hairy cell leukemia. Researchers in the LTCB subsequently isolated the second human cancer retrovirus, HTLV-2, from this cell line.[96] Marjorie Robert-Guroff, a staff fellow then working under the direction of LTCB microbiologist Carl Saxinger, helped establish the connection between HTLV-2 and leukemia.[97] These twin triumphs provided firm experimental support that some retroviruses could indeed cause human cancers, even if rarely. The timing of their publication would prove fortuitous in the lab's subsequent efforts to meet an emerging public health threat with its own distinct sequelae and retroviral origins.

THE AIDS EPIDEMIC EMERGES

Sociologist Steven Epstein has written on the dynamic interplay between medical, epidemiological, laboratory, and activist expertise contributing to the ultimate closure of the debate around the causal agent behind human AIDS. Epstein notes that the viral origin of AIDS was taken for granted long before the viral culprit was settled among the various competing claimants of HTLV-3, lymphoadenopathy-associated virus (LAV), and AIDS-related virus (ARV).[98] This was primarily a practical achievement; given sufficient warrant to proceed with their research agendas on AIDS, medical scientists and epidemiologists simply forged ahead with their studies in the face of naming disagreements. The "AIDS virus," whatever it may have then been called, was well-enough defined by antibody testing to generate a staggering body of research and prescribe working systems of identifying, ordering, and controlling populations. In other words, practical application of the virus had already achieved social reality before the scientific community settled upon the nomenclature of HIV.[99]

As evidenced by a dearth of applications from extramural scientists seeking grants to study viruses and AIDS, the topic was first pursued aggressively by intramural scientists at the NCI and its sister institutes in the NIH.[100] Gallo traces his own interest in AIDS back to the goading of James Curran at the Centers for Disease Control and Prevention (CDC). He had been among those at the NCI first apprised by Curran in 1981 of a startling new disease affecting T cells that had emerged in small pockets of the gay community. Gallo at first showed little interest in these epidemiological reports as his own research agenda was concerned. In early 1982, Curran returned to the NCI for an update, at which point he chided Gallo on the lack of attention from prominent NCI virologists toward what appeared to be a novel syndrome with viral involvement. It was only after this provocation and another set of chance encounters with two colleagues that reminded him of the tendency of animal retroviruses to suppress the immune systems of their carriers that Gallo saw AIDS as an issue worth exploring using the skills assembled in the LTCB.[101]

Following this moment of colligation, Gallo recalls how early experiments with other leading virus researchers at the NIH shaped how he interpreted evidence from AIDS samples in light of previous work on HTLV and animal retroviruses. Gallo's lab, both together and in parallel with Fauci's lab at NIAID, had been accumulating evidence that the immunological impairments found in those infected with the HTLV family of viruses resulted from the way these viruses targeted T cells.[102] He first turned to the studies conducted by lab personnel Marvin Reitz and Mika Popovic that indicated increased susceptibility to opportunistic infection among HTLV-1 positive members of the communities the lab had been studying in Japan.[103] Gallo wagered that AIDS could be caused by a retrovirus with a mutation in one of its regulatory genes that, as in the case of feline leukemia virus, changed it from a cancer virus to one primarily causing immunosuppression.

A galvanized Gallo gathered interested NIH scientists, including Fauci and NCI clinician Samuel Broder, as well as a small handful of outside researchers and clinicians, and petitioned NCI director DeVita to help him form the NCI AIDS Task Force.[104] DeVita approved the task force to operate under the auspices of the Clinical Oncology Program, where Gallo as "scientific leader" would spearhead "an accelerated effort" to identify the viral cause of AIDS in cooperation with "clinical leader" Broder's efforts to test possible therapies against the disease.[105] As Broder recalled, this interdisciplinary collaboration led to "many interactions, on many levels. This included making sure that the Gallo lab received tissue samples and peripheral blood specimens, which accelerated their discoveries in AIDS. The Gallo group made a number of seminal contributions, and it is my view that their location on the main campus, within easy reach of the Clinical Center, made their lives a lot easier."[106]

Gallo began collaborative efforts by searching human tissue for a retrovirus similar to or perhaps even mutated from one of the HTLV strains the LTCB had lately identified. He recalls having done so with caution, however, as fewer than two years had passed since the lab had publicized its evidence identifying HTLV-1 as the first human cancer virus. Though limiting AIDS virus research to a small subset of the LTCB's activities, Gallo nevertheless drew upon a robust arsenal of materials and competencies that were available in the lab in no small part due to past efforts to innovate leukemia virus techniques. He was optimistic the lab would "make major advances quickly" because "we had the technological expertise—indeed, we had pioneered some of these processes ourselves—and we have the hands-on experience of working with human retroviruses."[107]

Cautious but confident, Gallo began by delegating the first task of using IL-2 to culture three T-cell lines from known, suspected, and control patients to the intrepid technicians Ersell Richardson and Betsy Read-Connole (figure 4.2).[108] The next step was to assay these cells in search of reverse transcriptase cross-reactive with HTLV-1 or HTLV-2. They would then conduct a molecular probe in search of evidence of HTLV infection in cellular DNA. Unbeknownst to the lab chief, a clinical hematologist named Edward Gelman who was working under LTCB microbiologist Flossie Wong-Staal had already begun conducting experiments months earlier, using restriction enzymes to search for evidence of HTLVs

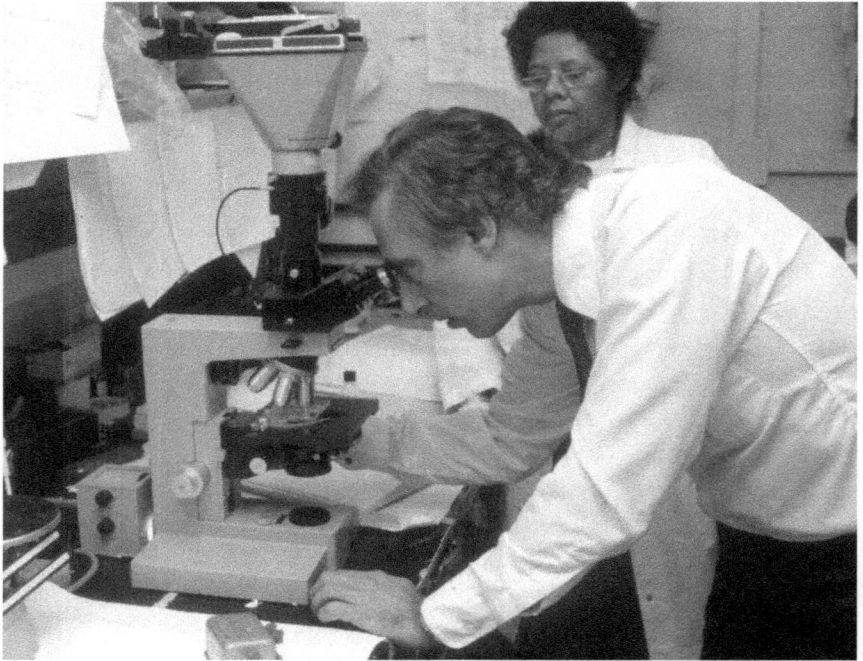

4.2 Robert Gallo (foreground) and Ersell Richardson (background) at work in the LTCB in 1980.

Photo credit: National Cancer Institute.

in the Kaposi's sarcoma of AIDS patients.[109] Gelman soon hitched his wagon to the LTCB's official screening activities, which were now squarely fixed on the hypothesis that AIDS was caused by a retrovirus similar to or belonging to the family of HTLVs the lab had already identified.

The story of Gallo's early experimental forays in the quest to find the viral cause of AIDS is today remembered as one of error and mischance. The LTCB's role in identifying the AIDS virus reflects an instance where colligating around an early hypothesis led to persistent dilemmas in how researchers interpreted the phenomena emerging in iterative experimentation. Gallo also lamented that his mistaken identification of HIV as a member of the HTLV family lost AIDS researchers valuable time: "I really think that, with a little more attention to a couple of details, I could have had the cause of AIDS in hand sooner by a solid year. I was just too much influenced by what I understood from HTLV-1 and 2. I was waiting for things to be happening in exactly the precise way that they would if it was a member of that family."[110]

Successful identification of a virus was forestalled not only by Gallo's commitment to the HTLV hypothesis but by the state of the materials the lab was experimenting upon as well. Both Read-Connole and Gallo complained that materials would often be delayed in getting to the lab for culture; as they only later discovered, the virus quickly killed target cells, meaning tardy samples would frequently yield confounding false negatives.[111] Indeed, their "earliest RT [reverse transcriptase] assay results were ambiguous," detecting viral activity that varied from high to low to nonexistent.[112] These results could be explained away because earlier research suggested human retroviruses left behind few viremia. On the other hand, members of the HTLV family ordinarily propagated well in culture, whereas these cell lines survived for only a brief window, and few showed immunological evidence of HTLV antigen activity even if they tested positive for reverse transcriptase activity.[113] Gallo recalls the lab mucking through these findings in an attempt by the researchers to make sense of what would be novel behavior in light of what they knew of HTLV.

The LTCB's environing conditions began to change when Gallo's French colleague Jacques Leibowitch sent the lab a sample from a Parisian AIDS patient known as "CC." Unlike the materials the LTCB had acquired from American AIDS patients, CC's cell line continued for months despite showing evidence of cytopathic damage. Richardson, who was culturing the cell line, and investigators Popovic and Gallo all noted the aberrant behavior of this cell line relative to the ones they had seen before. Nevertheless, as the CC cultures were more reactive with the HTLV assay than previous sources, the lab chief forged ahead with the HTLV hypothesis. Gallo's hypothesis that AIDS was correlated with a virus similar to the known HTLV strains was echoed by two other major research groups—respectively headed by Max Essex at Harvard and Luc Montagnier at the Pasteur Institute—who collectively agreed to publish their findings together in the journal *Science*. The cluster of publications was meant to serve cautious rather than conclusive evidence that AIDS was caused by a retrovirus, but their reliance upon ambiguous evidence garnered sometimes heavy criticism from other scientists.[114]

Gallo redoubled his efforts to sort through the doubts that now plagued him about the HTLV hypothesis. The lab chief brought more researchers in the LTCB into the fold in an attempt to isolate the virus. It was their integration of clinical information with laboratory experiments that enabled other researchers in the LTCB to colligate their findings around an alternative interpretation that stuck. Marjorie Robert-Guroff would lead this charge with a series of antibody assays targeting all patient sera that showed even some reactivity with HTLV. The probe her team used, which was based on HTLV-1 and HTLV-2, yielded fewer than 10 percent cross-reactive virus isolates and routinely detected evidence of a non-HTLV viral infection.

Robert-Guroff's findings shook the lab, whose chief still entertained the hypothesis that some variant of HTLV would turn out to be the culprit. Genoveffa Franchini, then a visiting associate working under Wong-Staal in the LTCB, recalls the collective process that took place in the fall of 1983 as lab members tried to penetrate the opacity of their separate results. Franchini recalls: "I remember we had the lab meeting, staff meeting, and we had a round table at which everybody was asking at the end, 'Do you believe or don't you believe that an HTLV-1 variant is causing AIDS?' . . . The majority of people really believed that an HTLV-1 slight variant was not the cause of AIDS. The majority thought that it was another virus. Most of it, the negative votes, was because of the Marjorie paper."[115] From across the lab's various sections, a consensus was emerging that went against Gallo's preferred candidate virus. After several experimental iterations seemed to offer up refutation of the HTLV hypothesis, the lab would need to revisit its interpretation of what was at issue in these experiments.

After several replications by different researchers in the laboratory, Gallo's team came to the conclusion that the HTLV-like virus they had been picking up was the result of using cells isolated from a patient who was doubly infected with both HTLV-1 and another virus (CC, the Parisian donor, was HIV-positive, but had also received a blood transfusion in Haiti where HTLV-1 is endemic).[116] Richardson, Popovic, and a team including Markham and Salahuddin were each subsequently able to isolate the unidentified virus from several other samples, which could be distinguished from the HTLV family because it lysed (killed) cells rather than immortalizing them (turning them cancerous).[117] Still convinced that the virus bore a family resemblance to the known HTLV strains, Gallo proceeded in calling the unidentified virus by a name he had been floating for months: HTLV-3.[118]

Further attempts to support or challenge the HTLV-3 conclusion in the lab were slowed by the cytopathic nature of the new virus, which made it difficult to establish in cultures that had not already been immortalized by the presence of an HTLV strain. The new virus was an intractable element in experimentation in the latter half of 1983, when its incapacity to reproduce in their established cell lines led different groups within the LTCB to attempt different solutions to the problem of catching the fugitive virus. Working relatively independently from one another (due in part to a rivalry between two sections in the lab),[119] several teams began constructing experimental apparatuses to successfully isolate and culture the mysterious retrovirus. The first team, comprising Phil Markham and Zaki Salahuddin alongside technician Ersell Richardson, set to work isolating the new virus from clinical samples belonging to known AIDS patients, members of high-risk groups, and healthy controls. The other major effort was led by Mika Popovic with the help of Betsy Read-Connole and involved an attempt to grow isolates of the retrovirus long-term in culture.

Popovic was particularly dogged in his attempts to establish the virus in a cell line, due both to his own failures and the ongoing failure of colleagues in the lab of collaborator Luc Montagnier at the Pasteur Institute to grow a similar isolate they were calling LAV. Vowing to solve the problem of finding a working cell line "no matter what it took," Popovic threw the whole proverbial cryogenic freezer at it. Popovic and Read-Connole began culturing several unanalyzed samples the lab had stored in its freezer.[120] Read-Connole realized some limited success in maintaining cells infected with LAV, which Popovic interpreted as a sign they had the expertise necessary to successfully culture the virus Montagnier and his associates could not make work in Paris.[121] Over the course of several sequential experimental iterations, Popovic was able to sustain virus production by gradually adding additional virus samples into the culture he was nursing. By the time this pooled culture yielded a sufficiently productive infection rate, samples from ten different patients had been added.[122]

Though this creative recombination of in-house resources "contributed to [their] learning to solve the problem of transmissibility to cell lines," it did not by itself guarantee sufficient virus to meet the team's goal of fully characterizing the virus and developing a blood test for it.[123] The lab members thus sought new resources to bring into the experimental environment from their close associates in the NCI. Gallo soon found the LTCB flush with fresher and fresher samples from AIDS patients. Since cell death happened quickly by comparison to the effect of the leukemia viruses they were accustomed to, obtaining new samples as soon as possible was a crucial factor in ensuring enough viral enzymes were left for the team to detect virus. Gallo's ties to epidemiologists and clinical researchers throughout the NIH were instrumental in enabling the quick accumulation of an adequate supply. Gallo recalls receiving several crucial samples that had been "hand-carried from Dr. Broder's office" and from several clinics that had been mobilized by Gallo's pleas for materials before the AIDS Task Force.[124] By the close of 1983, a steady circulation of materials, personnel, and protocols achieved the difficult task of establishing a continuous and productive cell line of the extremely cytopathic new retrovirus. The LTCB initiated its first experiments to develop virus reagents in rabbit models on December 29, 1983.[125]

ISOLATING THE AIDS VIRUS

The antibodies derived from animal inoculations begun in late 1983 provided the key to developing a scalable assay that could be used to screen large amounts of blood for AIDS virus. Based on a similar approach the LTCB had used to screen for HTLV-1,[126] the assay was initially developed for the purpose of preventing infected sera from being incorporated into the national blood supply.[127] The lab combined its approach to an enzyme-linked immunosorbent assay (ELISA) with a Western blot backup that helped minimize false positives, and the combination soon became the "gold standard" serological test for diagnosing HIV infection.[128] The ELISA was not only a practical public health technology but also helped demonstrate that the AIDS virus that researchers were working with around the world was the same entity despite the different names researchers had given it. The stakes of this innovation were no less than ensuring "the epidemic itself could now be monitored for the first time."[129]

Though the breakneck development of the assay system only months after isolating a virus was an immunological success, Gallo "did not believe that serum antibody results, no matter how correlative the positives to the groups within which we expected to find the virus, would be sufficiently persuasive to the main critics in the scientific community with an epidemic disease like AIDS."[130] The issues and stakes of their research shifted to isolating and sequencing the genome of HTLV-3 "to convince the academic community as totally, as widely, and as quickly as possible" that their viral candidate was the cause of AIDS, so that they could avoid any further "loss of life."[131] In the name of expediency toward this simultaneously scientific and public health goal, the initial approach taken by the LTCB was the same as the one they had used to isolate HTLV-1.[132] Using this system for growing T cells in IL-2, Wong-Staal's team sequenced the viral genomes of their isolates and found significant similarity between what they were calling HTLV-3 and what Montagnier's group had dubbed LAV.[133] In the process, the LTCB produced enough virus material not only to begin this project but also to begin entertaining strategies for vaccine development.[134]

These projects were under way, and in March 1984 the lab's findings were in press as a cluster of articles authored by members of the LTCB and of Montagnier's group at the Pasteur Institute. A few weeks later, news that the viral cause of AIDS had been identified was leaked by the international press, and leadership at the Department of Health and Human Services (HHS) decided a public press release was needed to prevent the media rumor mill from going wild. This decision, made by secretary of HHS Margaret Heckler, violated a verbal agreement Gallo had made with Montagnier to forestall announcing that Gallo had found the viral cause of AIDS until Montagnier's collaborative studies could catch up.[135] Heckler's anticipation that a vaccine would be "ready for testing in about two years" unnerved AIDS scientists, many of whom immediately saw the timeline as unrealistic given how they defined their research stakes. Though the "media controversy over who found it first" was immediate, both Gallo and Montagnier initially "played down" any reports of rivalry between the teams by stressing their institutes' long-running collaboration on isolating the suspected AIDS virus.[136] It was only later that tensions between Gallo and Montagnier would erupt into a years-long controversy between the research groups, likely stoked by Gallo's vocal opponent, Donald Francis of the CDC.[137] (The story is well-trod in the print records of the era and in a series of book-length exchanges that revolved around accusations of impropriety and scandal. Readers are amply provisioned with more authoritative accounts of the scandal from varying perspectives.[138])

Another source of tension between the NCI and the Pasteur Institute emerged around patenting the ELISA assay developed by the LTCB. Though Gallo could not financially benefit from the patent at the time, he was asked by the legal teams at NIH and HHS to allow them to file a patent for the technology on behalf of the United States government. Their reasoning was that patenting the assay would allow the government to attract pharmaceutical manufacturers, who were the only source of large-scale production capacity for a test that could be distributed globally, to license the technology and develop the assay for wide distribution in a short period of time.[139] The Pasteur Institute had also filed a patent for an AIDS assay, though this was denied by the U.S. Patent and Trademark Office. In settling the dispute between the NCI and the Pasteur Institute, an agreement was reached to share the former's royalties with the latter. This act of diplomacy allowed for a settlement between Gallo and Montagnier, who coauthored a definitive essay on the discovery of HIV by both groups that established the mutual importance of their scientific contributions to the isolation of the virus.[140]

Though the outcome of the priority dispute over the discovery of what would soon be known as human immunodeficiency virus (HIV) left Gallo and his team out of several major accolades (such as a Nobel Prize), the LTCB continued to forge ahead with an experimental agenda that was based on the research infrastructure they had erected for HIV. Gallo reached out to several colleagues across the NIH and academia to form a collaborative working group on HIV preventatives and treatments in 1984.[141] The group would help formalize ongoing collaborations between Gallo's lab and Broder's clinic, which led to the development of the nucleoside analogs discussed in chapter 5.[142]

CONCLUSION

In reflecting upon his career up to 1984, Gallo credits both the infrastructure of the defunct VCP and his laboratory's own learning process in the development of the findings around HTLV, HIV, and the AIDS assay system:

> No one close to the facts can deny that both basic and applied research, directed toward finding and analyzing viruses that cause human disease, played roles at least equally important. The long-gone Virus Cancer Program of John Moloney and the NCI gave us many of our tools and handles in retrovirology. . . .

My own earlier work on the HTLVs and on the T-cell growth factor (IL-2), for instance, did not come solely out of basic research. It also came out of ideas put to the test, ideas designed to find such viruses in humans and to link them to human disease. In turn, experiences with these earlier human retroviruses gave us the necessary background, knowledge, and credibility to propose a retroviral cause of AIDS and an outline of how to approach the problem.

Throughout the LTCB's investigations into the viral cause of AIDS, the immediate public health goal of identifying the virus and creating an effective screening tool to detect its presence in populations remained a central motivator. Only after the lab had developed these tools did it pursue the task of sequencing the viral genome, and even then in concurrence with efforts to develop a vaccine or antiviral therapies to stop the devastating spread of the virus.

With the management apparatus that once guided the VCP gone, Gallo and his colleagues were left to find their own solutions to the problem of applying their basic findings to health-relevant issues. Gallo's approach to training up postdocs in the latest experimental techniques created a substantial base of scientific competency in the LTCB that not only allowed the lab to keep up with emerging knowledge but also to rapidly accumulate cultures, reagents, and other materials. The lab's collaborations with clinicians and epidemiologists emerged from scientific networks and frequently relied on the proximity of other researchers in the NCI to accelerate progress at a greater speed than other laboratories found possible. The LTCB's collaborations with the NCI's Clinical Oncology Program would help develop a major informal hub for HIV/AIDS research and development within the NCI. Though Gallo's career would not be focused on bureaucratic innovation beyond organizing the AIDS Task Force, by the time the task force was abolished in late 1984 to make way for a more permanent and expanded effort located in the NIH, the ground had already been laid for Broder to extend Gallo's discovery of HIV and development of the assay through treatment breakthroughs around nucleoside analogs.[143] Unlike Gallo but much like many in NCI leadership before him, Broder would continue to inform bureaucratic innovations in the institute as his research into these AIDS treatments advanced.

CHAPTER 5

HIV RESEARCH AND DRUG DEVELOPMENT, 1985–1989

The ad hoc collaborations that developed around the NCI's AIDS Task Force continued after the motive for this group—the identification of the virus causing the epidemic—was satisfied. Much of the urgency NCI scientists and their colleagues in the CDC and throughout the NIH felt toward AIDS research reflected their sense that there was a dearth of interest in attacking the problem among extramural scientists. The NCI's Arthur Levine recalled:

> The intramural programs of the NIH and the CDC responded instantaneously to the epidemic of AIDS and the need for research, both epidemiologic as well as virologic and immunologic, as soon as the intellectual ideas jelled—there had to be some time for people to have a sense of what was going on. As soon as they had performed that feat of intellection, work started. And it started through normal mechanisms; there was no need to pass new legislation. No need to lobby. No need to have peer review. There was a good and vast federal mechanism for immediately responding. I think the response—in retrospect—was, at least for NIH and CDC, astonishingly rapid.[1]

The ability to mobilize quickly using the resources available in the NCI and its neighboring agencies in the Public Health Service created a pocket of focused expertise, infrastructure, and research on AIDS that drove inquiry forward when the broader scientific community remained uncoordinated in its efforts. By 1985, the success of the intramural efforts in the NCI and NIAID finally spurred congressional action to formalize a bureaucratic enterprise in the NIH's centralized apparatus.[2]

As AIDS funding began to pour into the NCI from Congress, both NCI director DeVita and scientific principals on the National Cancer Advisory Board (NCAB) warned against allowing AIDS projects to detract from the institute's cancer mission.[3] DeVita continued to emphasize the NCI's Cancer Centers Program as the best solution to serving the NCI's "dual mandate" by shepherding basic science investments into clinical explorations inclusive of the extramural community.[4] Besides, unlike the prospective cancer retroviruses the institute had invested in during previous decades, NCI researchers had concluded by 1985 that "the AIDS virus probably does not cause cancers . . . but perturbs the immune system, thereby facilitating or permitting the emergence of the tumors" that were characteristically associated with infection, such as Kaposi's sarcoma.[5] Nevertheless, AIDS Task Force member Samuel Broder also offered a principled defense of the institute's intramural AIDS program on the basis of "the scope and urgency of the problem from a public health perspective, NCI's expertise in human retroviral research, the occurrence of cancer as a common feature of AIDS, and the probability that AIDS research will shed light on the relationship between immunodeficiency and cancer."[6]

Though scientists in the NCAB were gradually persuaded of the importance of HIV/AIDS research and drug development to the institute's mission, the NCI's efforts in 1985 continued apparently without recognition from Congress that "most of the important research on AIDS [in the NIH] was being carried out either by NCI intramural investigators or NCI supported extramural scientists."[7] The supplemental appropriations bill that was passed in 1984 to fund AIDS research throughout the Public Health Service (most prominently the CDC and NIAID) omitted the NCI entirely, an "injustice" that incensed NCI leadership given their opinion that the NCI "moved quickly and did all the work" to identify viral candidates, develop and distribute a working assay, and initiate trials into prospective treatments.[8] Though the NCI fought to recover funding for these projects, by 1986 it lost control of the NIH's coordinated AIDS efforts to the NIAID, which Congress deemed a more appropriate bureaucratic home despite the NCI's ongoing scientific efforts. In so centralizing the NIH's AIDS efforts, Congress gave control over vaccine development to NIAID scientist-bureaucrats in 1987.[9] The NCI was left in charge of preclinical basic research and drug development of antivirals. Some observers attributed the decision to distribute efforts among these two NIH institutes, which seemed to consider their missions apart from the strength and substance of their active scientific programs in HIV/AIDS, as an attempt to stave off rivalries between the NCI and NIAID.[10]

Even before these bureaucratic changes took place, the Clinical Oncology Program (COP) in the NCI's Division of Cancer Treatment (DCT; also home to Gallo and the Laboratory of Tumor Cell Biology's efforts in the Developmental Therapeutics Program), had been making quick progress in exploring therapeutic leads into possible AIDS treatments. The COP's collaborative laboratory and clinical experiments, led by NCI researchers Samuel Broder, Hiroaki "Mitch" Mitsuya, and Robert Yarchoan, would yield the first generation of AIDS therapeutics: the nucleoside analogs AZT, ddI, and ddC. An explicit mission of Broder's team involved what he would later commit to calling "translational research": the deliberate and concerted effort to shepherd novel laboratory findings into clinical use as new medical or public health technologies. When Broder's early efforts to realize his vision of translation through AIDS drug development were thwarted by the financial interests of commercial entities they depended on to manufacture those drugs, he and other leaders at the NCI innovated new approaches to managing and licensing intellectual property at the NIH that they felt would counteract the profit motives that had impeded their public health goals. These organizational reforms would persist in the administration of technology transfer throughout the NIH. Under Broder's later directorship, they would give birth to a new interpretation of the NCI's dual mission as a clearinghouse for translational research (the subject of chapter 6). While not directly a story of cancer virus and vaccine innovation, the COP's learning around HIV therapeutics and translational research illustrates how the history of virus cancer research in the institute influenced subsequent scientific and bureaucratic innovations in unexpected ways, which in turn fed back into future efforts to develop unrelated cancer virus and vaccine research toward mission-relevant public health innovations.

LEARNING DRUG DEVELOPMENT THROUGH AIDS THERAPEUTICS

The NCI's clinical program played a significant role in HIV/AIDS research since the very beginning of the epidemic in the United States. In part, this was due to the DCT's major focus on relationships between immune deficiency diseases and cancer. Among the first patients to be diagnosed with AIDS were young men suffering from a rare cancer, Kaposi's sarcoma, along with immune impairment. Metabolism Branch chair Thomas Waldmann was the first physician in the NIH Clinical Center to confront an AIDS patient and make an appropriate diagnosis and was one of the only clinicians willing to work hands-on with cases of advanced disease when paranoia over its mode of transmission reigned.[11] In Waldmann's Metabolism Branch, studies of tumor viruses and their sequelae, such as Epstein-Barr virus and Burkitt's lymphoma, proceeded in collaboration with NIAID staff (some, such as Brian Murphy, who had been involved with the NCI's cancer virus programs in previous decades).[12] These and parallel studies had shifted to focus on T-cell lymphomas, including those associated with Gallo's HTLV, a shift that equipped Metabolism Branch labs with some of the materials and techniques that would become significant to cultivating HIV.[13] The Metabolism Branch had thus amassed scientific skills and resources that enabled Samuel Broder (figure 5.1) to quickly pivot to testing therapeutics against the AIDS virus

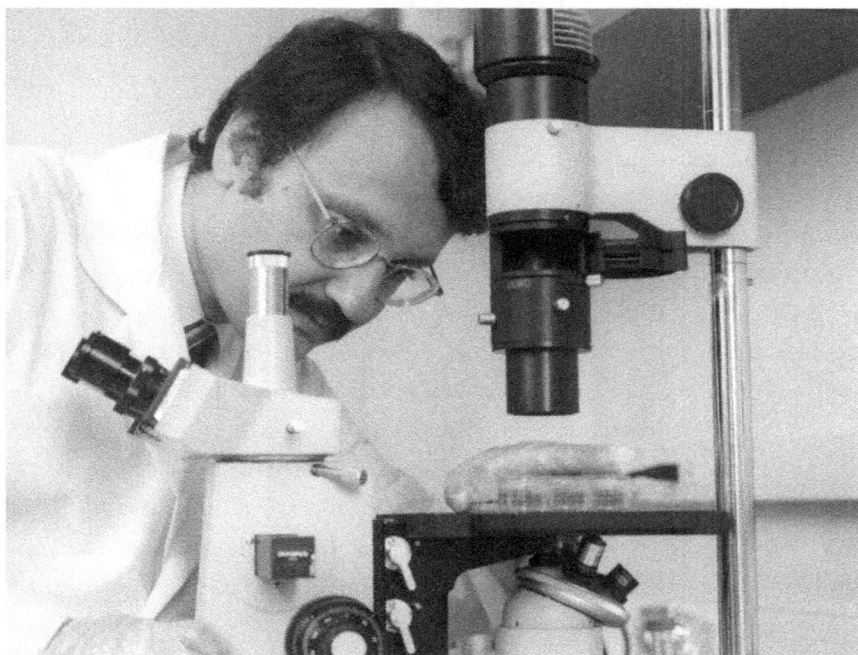

5.1 Samuel Broder in 1986.

Photo credit: John Crawford, National Cancer Institute.

upon his promotion to associate director of the DCT. Promising therapeutic research surged ahead in analyzing potential antiviral compounds, largely driven by Broder and his COP colleagues Yarchoan and Mitsuya.

As the clinical leader of the NCI's AIDS Task Force, Broder's unit in the COP conducted clinical research in parallel or in concert with the work of the Laboratory of Tumor Cell Biology (LTCB) described in the previous chapter. Still collaborating closely with AIDS Task Force scientific leader Robert Gallo and his colleagues in the LTCB, Broder aided in early in vitro experiments to test known compounds for antiviral activity. Materials and analysis commuted briskly between Gallo's lab and Broder's clinic, which helps account for the rapid pace of experimental results on AIDS in the NCI during the 1980s. As coleaders, Gallo and Broder ensured the AIDS Task Force acted as a coordinating mechanism among the NCI's laboratories and clinics that could facilitate further collaborations modeled after their own while enrolling additional support from agents such as Anthony Fauci at the NIAID.

As Broder recalled, these efforts emerged from the initiative of NCI researchers on the ground, who were spurred to action by concern over "what looks like an infectious disease in a public health emergency. In fact, that is a strength of the program. The National Cancer Institute was criticized for doing that. But at the beginning of the AIDS epidemic, NCI resources had to be placed in the service of identifying a cause of AIDS and possible prevention and treatment."[14] The intramural program's sense of public health mission, which seemed to lay dormant after the Virus Cancer Program's demise, was forcefully brought to the fore to address the burgeoning viral epidemic. Broder credited leadership from both DeVita and Bruce Chabner, then chief of the NCI's DCT, for laying the groundwork by supporting rapid drug development as a crucial part of the NCI's organizational mission.[15] The intramural research program of the NCI, and the NIH more generally, was thus an unusual organization where specialized expertise and public health mission met in uniquely productive ways.

Broder also recognized that the distinct extramural leadership vacuum in the early years of the epidemic, which existed because "some scientists and organizations, that might have made a contribution, did not respond to the AIDS emergency," contributed to the NIH intramural program's early scientific and bureaucratic importance in managing the epidemic.[16] When the CDC began reporting on unusual incidence of *Pneumocystis carinii* and Kaposi's sarcoma, scientists working in the NIH Clinical Center took immediate notice. Broder pointed out that "ironically, one of the world's repositories for knowledge about *Pneumocystis carinii* was in the intramural program of the National Cancer Institute, where Vince DeVita was one of the world's authorities. Same goes for Tony Fauci, whose lab was about four floors above the ward. So there was an enormous realm of expertise . . . all within a few floors in one building."[17] Broder considered the presence of so many scientists and clinicians in close proximity to one another, and working in service to a public health mission, critical to the ability to move knowledge and materials between bench and bedside early in the AIDS epidemic. "The NIH, and its unique team of scientists and clinicians, and especially a core of individuals who could wear both hats, made a profound difference. In my opinion, there were no counterparts to Bob Gallo or Tony Fauci outside the NIH."[18] The combined clinical and scientific expertise and bureaucratic mission of the NCI thus converged to enable an unusually rapid and innovative response to this public health emergency.

In the absence of a structured managerial approach such as the convergence technique that might help guide these experts' findings about the virus to clinical studies of potential therapies for AIDS, NCI scientist-bureaucrats would have to muster this expertise through informal coordination. Supporting the AIDS efforts of the COP was what Broder called his "SWAT team": himself, Mitsuya, and Yarchoan.[19] Their close collaboration with associates throughout the NCI gave the team privileged access to emerging data on the epidemic. These data suggested infection with the AIDS virus was endemic in U.S. metropolitan populations of gay men and IV drug users. Yarchoan quickly inferred that years of silent spread of the virus was brewing a "cataclysmic" public health crisis.[20] In proportion to this sense of urgency, Broder "reprogrammed much of [the Clinical Oncology Program directorate's] scholarly activities in response to the AIDS epidemic and the assignment of AIDS as the Department's number one priority."[21] As Yarchoan recalls, "What Sam first did—I think Sam deserves a lot of credit for pulling things together and moving forward—is to hold a small meeting . . . to brainstorm about various and sundry strategies to stop this retrovirus."[22] While some of the initial targets they selected would prove ineffective as AIDS therapeutics, the general problem-solving strategy they pursued—of consulting NCI-supported laboratory research on antiretrovirals and testing whole classes of analogous compounds—would quickly bear fruit.

However, the problem of how to study and treat AIDS without knowing its exact etiology made early clinical investigations challenging. Yarchoan noted the uncertainty prevailing in the COP: "without a causal agent to work with, it was hard to develop rational AIDS therapy."[23] He credited the "unique" environment of the NCI for providing a "critical mass" of leading experts "within walking distance on one campus" whom COP clinicians could consult.[24] Due in particular to his working relationship with Gallo and the LTCB, "there was a lot of interest in Sam's laboratory at the time looking at HTLV-1" as a "good model" for "studying immunodeficiency caused by an infectious agent that you could get your hands on."[25] Thus the same relationship between Gallo's LTCB and Broder's COP that had benefited the former's laboratory in its efforts to uncover the viral culprit of AIDS now provided the materials, methods, and hypotheses to motivate early clinical exploration of antiretrovirals in late 1983. When Gallo provided Broder with the embargoed proofs of the four publications that would support Gallo's claim to discovering the retrovirus causing AIDS, Broder convened his colleagues in the COP and suggested they focus their energies on finding an antiviral agent active against the virus. "Sam sat us down and said, 'Look, there is a small possibility that the idea is wrong, but let us put our marbles on this one.' Sam was quite taken with the idea that you could treat this disease and that this would be our focus."[26] Based on the LTCB's findings, Broder and his team in the COP redefined the issues and stakes of their AIDS research as identifying a treatment that would halt the retrovirus's progress in humans.

With a viral target in sight, the COP could now proceed with a more focused approach to testing prospective compounds. This involved intensive collective discussions about the pathogenesis of AIDS and where and how medicines could intervene in or even reverse its progression. Yarchoan recalls, "The literature on other retroviruses, animal retroviruses, gave us a place to start. We did not know whether it would work or not, but we thought that it was certainly a logical thing to do."[27] Operating under the assumption supported by LTCB findings that the retrovirus infected CD4[+] T cells, the team sought out candidate drugs that could block reverse transcriptase and thereby limit the spread of the virus long enough for the immune system to recover. The problem then confronting them was one of developing a T-cell screening assay that was sensitive to compounds with antiretroviral properties. Struggles in the LTCB to do the same demonstrated the material resistances researchers confronted in early HIV-centered experimental systems. T-cell assays were extraordinarily difficult to propagate on their own; given that HIV infection destroyed these cells, the task of creating a reliable assay that was sensitive enough to detect when antiretrovirals were *themselves* toxic to T cells was even more daunting.

The work of developing an assay that could allow the COP to iteratively test prospective antiretrovirals fell to Mitsuya. Famously dexterous with tissue cultures, Mitsuya was a virtuoso viral pharmacologist whom Broder had recruited from Japan and hired to his staff when populating his new lab in the COP.[28] Mitsuya worked closely with Mika Popovic in Gallo's lab to acquire the tacit skills that enabled the LTCB to pioneer T-cell cultures and assays. Mitsuya had developed a tetanus-specific T-cell clone using his own cells[29] that rapidly died upon contact with the virus to study its cytopathic effect.[30] Yarchoan recalls that "since HIV killed T cells—Sam and Mitch and I all batted these ideas around—it seemed that if you could block the killing of the cell with a drug, that would be a very nice test, because you could show that it was both an antiviral drug and that it was not toxic to the T cells."[31] This solved the problem of evaluating toxicity but left the difficulty of keeping the finicky cell line going. The team seized upon an experimental finding from Gallo's group that distinguished the mechanisms of HTLV-1 and HTLV-2, which immortalized cells in culture, and the identified AIDS virus, which lysed cells. To create a sensitive but durable cell line, "Sam and Mitch got the idea of infecting one of these cells with HTLV-1."[32] Having successfully innovated a screening assay that gave the team new experimental competencies, the COP was now able to conduct further experiments that properly encoded the issues and stakes of antiretroviral development. They dubbed this new screening assay ATH8.

ATH8 was an early example of how close contact between laboratory and clinical researchers could yield innovations quickly. Mitsuya enhanced his existing competencies in developing sensitive cell cultures by learning techniques from the LTCB's own attempts to develop T-cell cultures. The skills necessary to develop such cultures often go beyond the technical know-how and material substrata necessary to set them up and encompass a kind of tacit skill that can only be reproduced through iterative, hands-on training with local experts.[33] Developing this competency and encoding it in the ATH8 cell line was thus an early learning outcome supported by the kind of ground-up laboratory-clinic interactions that Broder would later advocate as a model for translational research.

SEARCHING FOR ANTIRETROVIRALS

The development of the ATH8 line was not merely technical; it addressed an important understanding of the stakes of the COP's research. To expedite the development of a maximally useful and readily deployable public health tool against AIDS, the COP "made a decision in the early 1980s, that we would begin screening for compounds that had several properties: speed, reliability, simplicity."[34] Broder and his team were set on screening established molecules known to have antiviral properties, particularly those shown to inhibit reverse transcriptase, an enzyme that retroviruses such as HIV needed to replicate in hosts. Their early decisions on which compounds to screen also reflected an assessment of how the bureaucratic environment for drug development at the NCI would limit how rapidly their work could progress. Yarchoan explained: "At the beginning, we were most interested in testing drugs that had been used in humans before. The reason was that doing so would cut out what we thought was two years of animal toxicity testing, GMP [good manufacturing practices] production, and all the rest of it, and we could get a trial going soon rather than two years down the line."[35] Researchers in the COP thus mobilized their networks throughout the NIH in search of antiretroviral compounds that had been tested before for other uses, with the intent of moving them into human trials as soon as possible. "Sam thought it was very important to get a clinical trial going. We had no idea how to even test if a drug was working in AIDS. What do you use to follow these patients? . . . So we were struggling to try to figure how to even go about doing a clinical trial to test an antiretroviral drug."[36] Centering the urgency of the public health stakes, AIDS drug development thus presented the COP with additional difficulties that would not have faced a more traditional drug development enterprise based on routine standards of demonstration.

With new information (and misinformation) about the epidemic spreading quickly among the scientific and lay public, the NCI began mobilizing for a more formal approach to organizing its AIDS efforts. For a brief window in 1984 after Gallo announced that the NCI had identified the viral culprit behind the AIDS epidemic, the Department of Health and Human Services designated the NCI the lead institute for finding answers to the epidemic, including vaccines and other treatments. The AIDS Task Force was dissolved and the institute's efforts centralized in the Division of Cancer Etiology.[37] The organizational support provided both formally by NCI leadership and informally by interdisciplinary collaboration allowed clinical trials to proceed at a rapid clip. By the fall of 1984, teams collaborating across Gallo's and Broder's units contributed not only several coauthored publications defending the role of HTLV-3 in causing AIDS but also a slew of promising in vitro studies demonstrating some antiviral activity against the suspected AIDS virus by the drug suramin.[38]

Suramin had previously been tested in humans as a treatment for African river blindness and was recommended to Yarchoan by NIAID colleagues one afternoon when they conversed over lunch about the possibility of experimenting with its chemical analog, rifampin.[39] Brian Murphy, a previous collaborator of Yarchoan's also formerly associated with the Special Virus Leukemia Program (SVLP) at NCI, brought along colleague Jay Hoofnagle, who originally proposed suramin.[40] Suramin had years earlier been shown to be active against many of the murine retroviruses that once formed the backbone of studies in the SVLP. Yarchoan related this news to Broder, who quickly located a supply of suramin and collaborated with Popovic in the LTCB to test its capabilities against the AIDS virus.[41] Upon confirming its activity in the ATH8 assay, Broder and Yarchoan wrote a protocol for phase I suramin trials. Their protocol was approved in a month and a half, a swift turnaround that reflected how the NIH bureaucracy was adapting to the public health urgency of early AIDS therapeutics research.

Broder, Mitsuya, and Yarchoan rushed suramin into phase I human trials even as they were uncertain how exactly to test patient response. Their initial reports suggested suramin performed better in inhibiting viral expression than did other early therapeutic candidates such as ribavirin and HPA-23. However, the possibility of toxicity emerged as a clear issue in these safety trials.[42] Nevertheless, Broder and his team pushed on into phase II trials to determine whether the potential efficacy of the drug would outweigh its toxicity. Yarchoan recalls that the COP team "thought [suramin] was worth looking at further, but we did not feel we were seeing what we wanted to see with this drug, and the thing to do was to try other drugs."[43] By the time the phase II findings were released, the NIH was facing an increasingly restive public, galvanized by AIDS activists who demanded a quicker and more humane approach to drug development and testing.

Making AZT an AIDS Drug

The health goals driving the COP's experimental practices were challenged by the fact that few effective antiretroviral therapeutics existed at all.[44] Broder came to believe "the fate of all future antiretroviral drug development programs would be linked to the success or failure" of early anti-HIV treatments.[45] With this conviction, Broder and his team in the COP "turned [the] laboratory to trying to look for drug discoveries in that arena, knowing that we could have at our disposal all of the things necessary for early drug development, including a ward right down the hall, with the backup of the entire infrastructure NCI had established for new drug discovery and development."[46] Broder continued working with Gallo and his former AIDS Task Force colleagues to target new therapeutic candidates.

The collaborators married two immediate hypotheses to approach the control of AIDS. In the LTCB, the focus was on inhibiting reverse transcriptase to mitigate the immune damage caused by infection with the AIDS virus. In the COP, Broder "initiated a crash program to screen new anti-viral agents using a rapid assay system."[47] To better support the NCI's screening efforts, Broder and his clinical colleagues sent out a call for researchers in academia and industry to share their chemical archives as well. There was a strong historical precedent for soliciting compounds from industry to be screened for their anticancer potential at the NCI, dating back to the Cancer Chemotherapy National Service Center founded in 1955. The COP relied on industry and academic scientists' experience with the NCI's drug-screening programs to heed their call.

If the COP was taking a shotgun approach, its researchers at least felt it was with some analytical warrant. Considering the classes of compounds with established antiviral properties, Broder hypothesized that nucleoside analogs, long ago shown to inhibit reverse transcriptase, provided "an obvious target" for treating AIDS by hobbling the retrovirus.[48] He was aware that Burroughs Wellcome had a nucleoside analog on its shelf and was encouraged by the company's successful development of acyclovir for herpes simplex viruses. Yet this moment of colligation around nucleoside analogs was not merely ideational; in this instance, the NCI's governance apparatus unexpectedly opened distinct possibilities for quickly obtaining samples from the company. NCAB member Dani Bolognesi was a friend and collaborator of Gallo's and a professor at Duke University, a stone's throw from Burroughs Wellcome's complex in North Carolina's Research Triangle Park. In his capacity as an NCAB member and a committed AIDS researcher, Bolognesi wanted to ensure NCI researchers were as well positioned as possible to address the AIDS crisis. He reached out to his friend, Burroughs Wellcome scientific executive David Berry, to orchestrate a meeting with both Gallo and Broder where they might work out an arrangement for accessing the company's stock of nucleoside analogs.[49]

In meeting with Berry, Broder "explained what our capacity was in terms of clinical trials and essentially offered a collaboration with them, with the promise that we would, whatever came up, develop drugs as fast as we could and that they would get a product out of it."[50] In addition to mustering an expansive network for clinical testing, the NCI was one of the few large research centers boasting state-of-the-art biosafety level 3–rated structures at the Frederick Cancer Research Center. Adequate facilities were capital investments pharmaceutical companies would otherwise have to absorb themselves were they to attempt work with HIV.[51] This was no trivial issue for the development and testing of anti-AIDS drugs, as fear of laboratory transmission deterred many scientists from engaging in HIV/AIDS research throughout the early years of the epidemic.

Early on, Broder had taken a principled stance on drug development with industry: collaborations would need to involve a genuine partnership with the NCI, and companies would have to promise to help bring any useful drugs developed through the partnership to market.[52] As Yarchoan recalls, "Sam felt that drug discovery was a complex process; that there were a number of pharmaceutical firms out there that did it; and if he could link up with such a firm, it would help things along."[53] Though Broder would later regard the NCI as something like "a 'pharmaceutical company' working for the public, in difficult areas where the private sector either could not or would not make a commitment," the institute necessarily stopped short of the commercial side of R&D.[54] Yarchoan remembers that "Sam sometimes said that the federal government is not in the business of selling drugs."[55] Carving the institutional environment thus, Broder resolved to "talk to anyone he could get interested in developing drugs. What he found when he spoke to a number of pharmaceutical firms was that they were not interested at that time. In effect, they said, 'Look, it is an epidemic, but there are only 50,000 people with the disease, and we can't justify a big program to our stockholders for 50,000 people.' "[56] Burroughs Wellcome was also initially reluctant to put forth the large investment this new research direction would require without some assurances a profitable drug could be developed. Convinced that the potential for commercializing AIDS drugs was necessary to incentivize industry,

Broder assured potential collaborators that there would be money to make in the epidemic despite the relatively small number of people who had then been diagnosed worldwide.[57]

Broder was eventually able to cajole Burroughs Wellcome into sending the institute a few of their nucleoside analog compounds to screen.[58] Among these compounds, which had been sent to the NCI under codes that concealed their exact chemical makeup, was azidothymidine (AZT).[59] First synthesized under an NCI-grant-funded study by Detroit cancer researcher Jerome Horowitz in 1964, AZT had remained unpatented for decades as Burroughs Wellcome and a few others explored its possible application in cancer treatment and veterinary medicine. Broder sought this nucleoside analog out because of its demonstrated ability to inhibit reverse transcriptase, then the COP's primary criteria for selecting antiretroviral candidates.[60]

Between October 1984 and March 1985, Mitsuya and the few other researchers in the NCI's COP willing to work with HIV/AIDS materials put Burroughs Wellcome's coded compounds through the experimental ringer. According to Yarchoan, Broder "took it very seriously and rededicated a lot of the laboratory effort to testing those drugs during that period of time."[61] Mitsuya famously stayed in the lab deep into the night to ensure the finicky ATH8 could successfully screen for activity against HIV. Because of a combination of organizational logistics related to screening and the material affordances of the novel screening system, it was only in the final two months of these efforts that Mitsuya could demonstrate antiretroviral activity from the compound that turned out to be AZT.[62] Tight laboratory and clinical relationships in the COP-LTCB collaboration led to more results at a more rapid pace. Mitsuya's "techniques were robust, and as events have proven, predictive for success in the clinic."[63] The close relationships between laboratory and clinical research within the COP also made a difference, in that the team "could take [Mitsuya's] discoveries right to the clinic. Even those few people who were screening for new anti-AIDS drugs had essentially no effective clinical arm. . . . [Other researchers] could only work in the lab and then publish some paper somewhere and hope that somebody would pick it up."[64] The NCI's public health mission, bolstered by the work of other motivated intramural collaborators, enabled more focused and prompt attention than NCI scientists expected would ever emerge from uncoordinated research in the academic community.

The COP moved rapidly to transfer their findings around AZT into phase I trials. For this they were dependent upon cooperation from Burroughs Wellcome, who frustrated the team by sitting on Mitsuya's findings for three months before initiating the process to file the Investigational New Drug (IND) application with the FDA that would allow them to move forward with testing.[65] As it turned out, the company used this time to file for a patent for AZT in the United Kingdom, a process it initiated upon first receiving notice of the drug's efficacy from the COP in March 1985. The company's delay in acting upon the NCI team's results has been interpreted as a strategic maneuver to secure exclusive rights over AZT in a country that did not require efficacy to be demonstrated prior to awarding intellectual property rights.[66] Such profit motives, absent among the NCI collaborators who could not have profited at the time even if they had sought the patent themselves, resulted in a delay they found inscrutable in light of their public health goals.[67]

When Burroughs Wellcome finally filed the IND, Yarchoan, whose participation on Broder's team was focused on clinical testing, spun into high gear to initiate phase I trials. Broder worked closely with researchers at Burroughs Wellcome to draft an experimental protocol for the study, which included his insights about "things that we would have done differently based on what we had learned from [the suramin trial] protocol."[68] The COP took the lead under Broder's supervision at the NCI, with another arm planned under Bolognesi at Duke, and a final arm to proceed under the supervision of Burroughs Wellcome in its research facilities in North Carolina. This arrangement was customary in public-private partnerships with the NIH and was an expectation Broder explicitly communicated in negotiations with researchers and executives at Burroughs Wellcome. Nevertheless, Burroughs Wellcome contacted Broder days before the trial was set to begin and announced the company would not conduct any analysis itself.[69] Broder remembered the company being "extremely concerned [about working with HIV]. They refused to accept live virus, and at one point refused to accept patient samples. That was a little unusual. They basically put the entire onus for the phase I pharmacokinetics and related issues on NCI."[70] Broder and his colleagues at Duke forged ahead nevertheless and together treated eighteen patients in the phase I trial.

Perhaps the most marked contrast in incentives among government and industry scientists can be seen in this episode. Fear of working with HIV/AIDS materials was widespread early in the epidemic. Scientists at Burroughs Wellcome refused to work with these materials, which forced their collaborators at NCI and Duke to put in the clinical legwork. In contrast, the recollections of NCI scientists and clinicians at the LTCB and COP are replete with stories of technicians and researchers who took on the additional, uncompensated labor of working with HIV/AIDS materials and patients. Yet the NCI brought more than just motivated actors to bear in spurring rapid drug development. As Broder recalls:

> At one point, [Burroughs Wellcome] could not obtain its own supply of thymidine, a starting block for the synthesis of AZT. We at NCI were able to send them a large shipment. . . . The NCI had a repository of thymidine from another era. We were one of the world's few places where you could get it. But Wellcome scientists were bummed out. I mean, if they were honest, they will recall that they were unable to produce it. There were going to be dramatic delays. And then, voila, a shipment of thymidine arrived in the company loading dock. New drug development is complex, expensive, and not something that just any group at NIH has the infrastructure to do.[71]

The NCI's HIV/AIDS efforts thus enabled it to quickly mobilize the institute's distinctive infrastructural capacity to meet production demands in expedited fashion in response to the urgency of the public health crisis facing the country.

AZT moved rapidly through the regulatory pipeline, as is often the case with lifesaving medications related to public health crises. By the end of 1985, phase I trials had demonstrated to the satisfaction of Broder and his counterparts at Burroughs Wellcome that AZT was of therapeutic benefit. The NCI team met with Burroughs Wellcome to advise on protocol design for the company's phase II trials. In the end, the trial design reflected the firm's priorities rather than those of the government scientists. Yarchoan noted that the studies begun in early 1986 administered "reasonably high" doses of AZT: "My understanding was that the people at Burroughs thought that it was better to be a little toxic but to have the drug work than not to have the drug work. They felt they really only had one shot to show that it was working, and so they designed this trial."[72] Though dissatisfied that the company's regulatory concerns seemed to trump their own scientific judgment, the NCI team nevertheless considered the initiation of phase II trials a great success.

In a pattern that would recur across different projects throughout the NCI, Broder and Yarchoan decided to conduct their own follow-up on the work completed during phase I trials via "a number of extensions . . . and small pilot studies."[73] These follow ups, which proceeded in parallel with Burroughs Wellcome's phase II study and without support from the firm beyond supplying the finished drug, led the NCI team to record declining efficacy of AZT over time. "We were continuing to follow these patients on AZT. What we were seeing was that the CD4 count was going up and then it was coming down."[74] The high replication rate of HIV made it prone to mutation; those mutations that survived in patients administered AZT were then more likely to be resistant to the drug. "For me it was something like *Flowers for Algernon*," Yarchoan mused; "My best guess was that we were buying people twenty weeks with AZT."[75] Once a mutation outcompeted the nucleoside analog that made AZT efficacious, infection could break through from previously infected cells, and disease would continue to advance.

THE OTHER ANALOGS: DEVELOPING DDC AND DDI

However limited, the improvements AIDS patients saw through AZT were encouraging to researchers in the COP. Turning their attention to purine and pyrimidine analogs, Broder and Mitsuya rapidly established the potency and efficacy of ddC, whereupon the NCI AIDS Drug Development Committee advanced it toward clinical trials.[76] By this time in 1986, the COP had a full slate of promising compounds to test for antiretroviral effects. It went to work synthesizing compounds that could "exploit the DDO-nucleoside [dideoxynucleoside] lead to produce even more efficacious analogs."[77] Dideoxynucleosides are compounds that mimic the nucleotides (adenine, cytosine, guanine, and thymine) composing strands of DNA after they are phosphorylated but contain molecular residues that make them incompatible with the structures of other nucleotides necessary for further transcription. As AIDS therapies, they work by outcompeting endogenous nucleosides such as thymidine (in AZT) or cytidine (in ddC), at which point they halt the RNA-to-DNA transcription process that enables HIV to reproduce itself in infected cells. The "chain-terminating" action of phosphorylated dideoxynucleosides, whereby modifications to the residue on the analog prevents DNA synthesis from extending any further, limits the spread of HIV to healthy T cells.

Supported by the extensive testing infrastructure of the NCI's Developmental Therapeutics Program, Broder began by testing another dideoxynucleoside first synthesized by AZT developer Horowitz, dideoxycytidine (ddC), alongside dideoxyadenosine (ddA) and the closely related but only recently synthesized adenosine analog didanosine (ddI). As Yarchoan recalls, Mitsuya began testing these compounds while the laboratory was still conducting the initial tests establishing AZT's activity. Unlike AZT, "these were compounds that, basically, we just ordered from chemical pharmaceutical houses, so they were completely devoid of any drug company support."[78] At Broder's behest, the Developmental Therapeutics Program agreed to test ddC for animal toxicity first ("because it seemed to be more straightforward than ddA or ddI"), followed closely by ddA and ddI.[79]

Though these other nucleoside analogs were being tested in parallel with AZT, Broder's in-house nucleoside analog development was at a disadvantage vis-à-vis AZT because animal trials had not yet been conducted on them, whereas AZT had already been studied before being shelved. "These new ones were really starting from scratch," Yarchoan recalled, with the NCI doing all development and testing until clinical trials were initiated for the first of these compounds, ddC, in early 1987.[80] Yarchoan later argued that "although the drug was eventually licensed to Hoffmann-La Roche, it was really an NCI drug."[81]

Broder and his team continued to benefit from the material support of their colleagues in the LTCB, who provided monocyte and macrophage tissue culture systems for testing the performance of ddC. Using their colleagues' isolates and cultures, they "learned things about AIDS drugs" that were instrumental in testing nucleoside analogs:

> For example, some of the nucleoside analogs we used are inert in their own right and have to be anabolically phosphorylated or activated inside a cell before they begin to work, how they are handled (activated) in monocytes or macrophages is different from how they are handled in T cells. We were learning how to manipulate this system and how to get the maximum activation, if you will, how to pick rational combinations based on biochemical pharmacology. AZT, for example, works especially well in dividing cells. Another drug, ddI, works particularly well in non-dividing cells or resting cells, and, therefore, could block the initial entry into cells.[82]

While other early entrants to nucleoside analog research and development could not demonstrate their efficacy in vitro, the material infrastructure available to NCI researchers was decisive in their success in working with these compounds.

The lessons they learned from working hands-on in their unique material environment was subsequently instrumental in driving the knowledge they developed about these compounds forward. Importantly, NCI researchers were motivated by a newly colligated conception of their mission as one to develop progressively more efficacious anti-AIDS drugs, a goal they could pursue unfettered by profit motive.[83] Their iterative engagement with these materials in extended learning cycles contributed to distinctively innovative collaborations between the LTCB and COP throughout the 1980s.

The experimental apparatus that supported these studies also produced novel findings that led the COP to reconstruct the issues and stakes of nucleoside treatment regimens around combination retroviral therapy using ddI as a complement to AZT. Yarchoan and Broder stumbled upon ddI as a therapeutic after finding that ddA administered by injection was quickly converted to ddI. Using ddI allowed for similar therapeutic benefit without the deleterious renal side effects that resulted from metabolizing the adenine free base found in ddA.[84] Unlike earlier compounds they prioritized for testing, ddI had never before been tested in human subjects.[85] However, Yarchoan and Broder's clinical experience in administering similar nucleoside analogs made them sufficiently optimistic to progress the compound through animal studies and into phase I human trials, which began in 1988.[86] In Broder's mind, the success of AZT had changed "the general scientific perspective on the development of anti-retroviral drugs" such that "the question no longer is *whether* clinically active drugs can be developed for the treatment of AIDS, but *how many* agents will be found and how best to prioritize development of these agents."[87] Early phase I results demonstrated that patients administered ddI showed clinical improvement both in the form of elevated T-cell counts and lower viral load, and that ddI had the most favorable toxicity profile of all nucleoside analogs yet tested.[88] The team thus quickly colligated around efforts to develop ddI as an antiretroviral agent to be administered to patients either in conjunction with AZT or as an alternative to AZT in those who could not tolerate the approved drug.

The COP's optimism around ddI also developed in relation to the findings that were emerging from iterative experiments on their other compound, ddC. As Yarchoan recalls, initial results for ddC showed the compound was "more effective in patients at lower doses than anticipated, but also more toxic and less beneficial overall than AZT."[89] The compound's future lay in combination therapy with AZT, rather than as an alternative. Yarchoan described use of the approach of combination cancer chemotherapy pioneered at NCI as a model for their first study testing AZT and ddC.[90] Another motivating bureaucratic consideration was the need to rapidly move drugs through the FDA approval process so they could reach patients as quickly as possible: "we thought it would take some time to get a trial approved to administer both [AZT and ddC] at the same time but that we could move quickly if we proposed alternating them. We were actually able to do that right within the phase I study of ddC."[91] The development of ddI, with its lower toxicity profile, informed Yarchoan and his colleagues' subsequent trials comparing simultaneous and alternating administration of AZT and ddI. "We found that people did much better combining the two drugs simultaneously at half dose rather than alternating the two at full dose. Over a period of time, people got the same dose of both drugs, but the way that the drugs were given made a big difference."[92] Laboratory work Mitsuya conducted confirmed this was because different cells metabolize the drugs differently. Thus, over several concurrent iterations, the COP homed in on combination antiretroviral therapy as a more effective approach to treating AIDS in the midst of a health crisis that was shifting under their feet.

Combination therapy seemed to suit the changing needs of AIDS patients as the epidemic continued to unfold in the United States. AIDS activists had been particularly vocal about accessing new experimental drugs during this phase of the epidemic. As Steven Epstein has shown, clinical trials for both ddC and ddI were shaped by lay efforts to obtain these drugs outside traditional enrollment criteria. In the case of ddC, some activists went so far as to synthesize the compound in basement laboratories.[93] Yet it was Fauci and the NIAID's AIDS Clinical Trial Group infrastructure that bore the greatest brunt of the activists' frustration. In these episodes, Fauci and the FDA learned from activist insights and demands how to make drugs more accessible, which led to innovations in clinical trial access and approval. In 1989, with the consent of Broder and manufacturer Bristol-Myers, Fauci helped speed ddI through the FDA using the parallel track system of traditional clinical trial enrollment supplemented by access for ineligible AIDS patients, alongside a turn toward using CD4 counts as surrogate end points to measure a drug's efficacy for the sake of regulatory approval.[94] The success of this new bureaucratic approval system with ddI directly inspired a new regulatory paradigm for "accelerated approval" instantiated by the FDA in 1992, the year after ddI was approved.[95]

It was the position of Broder and the NIH Office of Technology Transfer that "a well-established research program" rooted in "capacities developed in the 'War on Cancer' " gave the NCI "a unique capacity to screen compounds for anti-viral activity."[96] If the LTCB's retrovirus studies benefited from the infrastructure developed through directed cancer virus vaccine research, the COP's antiretroviral efforts clearly made good use of the centralized planning infrastructure developed simultaneously around cancer chemotherapy. In this respect, DeVita's arduous rehabilitation of the NCI's controversial investments in health-oriented research paid off to a greater extent than he had initially argued. In addition to an added stock of basic knowledge that proved fortuitous to HIV research, the NCI realized rapid public health benefits in its development of the first generation of AIDS therapeutics. Though the NCI could not have accomplished these outcomes without collaboration across academia and industry, it was the singular infrastructure erected in service to the institute's forgotten goals that made the crucial difference in translating intramural research into useful therapeutics.

Despite the difficulties Broder and the NCI would face after the commercialization of AZT, he credits the drug with spurring a number of other innovations in the NCI and drug development more broadly. He argues that "AZT laid the groundwork for defining surrogate endpoints in other studies, for illustrating that anti-viral agents could work in patients, and for providing a template for moving quickly from a laboratory observation to a proof-of-concept clinical study, and from [there] to a randomized prospective clinical trial."[97] By demonstrating what motivated drug development could accomplish, nucleoside analog research gave birth to a particular conception of translational research in Broder's mind—a conception that would be realized in a number of institutional changes Broder would implement when he became director of the NCI.

LEARNING FROM PRICING AND PATENT CONFLICTS

NCI scientists learned much from their experiences in AIDS nucleoside innovation qua scientists, but some of the most potent and consequential lessons from drug development in this period involved intramural researchers in their capacities as bureaucratic agents of the federal government. The intensity of public scrutiny over HIV/AIDS-related research at the NCI was heightened by the emergence of high-profile activists whose conceptions of agency accountability challenged the settled scripts of congressional and scientific principals. Controversies over access to experimental AIDS therapies were familiar to clinical trial staff and regulators at the NIH and FDA; at the NCI, intramural researchers interpreted activists' concerns over the organization's public mission through practices around patenting and pricing their innovations.

Pressure on these issues first came as public outcry welled around Burroughs Wellcome's announcement that AZT would cost AIDS patients $10,000 USD per year. This was an unheard-of sum for a maintenance medication that had theretofore been provided free of charge on a trial basis, and accusations of profiteering quickly followed. "Perhaps the most galling aspect of Burroughs Wellcome's price tag," the NIH historian Victoria Harden would later note, "was that taxpayers had essentially funded development of the drug but had no control over the pricing."[98] The high price of AZT triggered a congressional hearing chaired by Henry Waxman in 1987, where members of Congress assailed pharmaceutical executives for closely guarding the proprietary pricing formula they used to justify what they were charging for the drug. As analysts pointed out, Burroughs Wellcome spent far less to develop AZT than the average cost of new drug manufacture and licensing. Up to 70 percent of the research, development, and licensing costs of AZT were offset by taxpayer funds in the form of NCI-sponsored research and clinical trials and by tax credits through the Orphan Drug Act.[99] Burroughs Wellcome's decision not to participate in early research and phase I testing also violated the standard expectation for minimal corporate cooperation in public-private collaborations with the NCI. In essence, the company shifted most of the risks of early research, development, and testing onto the federal government while seeking the overwhelming rewards of AZT for itself. So reliant upon federal support was AZT that some regarded it as "essentially a government drug" for which "taxpayers footed the bill . . . at least five times over."[100]

AIDS activists, propelled by the brazen and effective tactics of the AIDS Coalition to Unleash Power (ACT UP), had by this time carved their own policy niche from the unwillingness of federal and corporate agencies to act decisively in the face of the HIV/AIDS public health crisis. In the two years following FDA approval of AZT, a combination of expanding drug indications and the worsening global HIV/AIDS crisis led to a significant increase in the number of the drugs' prospective users that made Burroughs Wellcome's reticence on AZT's high price tag increasingly unconscionable. In 1989, ACT UP staged a series of bold protests that included infiltrating Burroughs Wellcome's executive suites and the New York Stock Exchange. Their concerted and highly publicized actions against Burroughs Wellcome's pricing scheme led the company to lower the cost of AZT to $6,500 USD per year.[101] In addition to protests, AIDS activists explored legal avenues to challenge Burroughs Wellcome's patent rights in court. This put Burroughs Wellcome on the defensive, and the threat of losing its monopoly over AZT rather than the threat of bad publicity may have been the decisive factor in the company's decision to reduce its price.[102]

Public controversy over pricing thus thrust issues of patent rights over AZT to the fore. The publicity generated by AIDS activists in these efforts targeted at Burroughs Wellcome, along with congressional hearings regarding the high prices of HIV/AIDS and cancer medicines such as Taxol developed at the NIH, arguably put the executive branch's feet to the fire on intellectual property issues. Broder, incensed by a letter from Burroughs Wellcome president T. E. Haigler, Jr., that "dismissed the contributions" of the NCI "in deliberate and systematic fashion," cajoled the NIH to hire outside legal counsel to determine whether the federal government had a right to challenge Burroughs Wellcome's patent.[103] The Department of Health and Human Services Office of the General Counsel soon launched a prolonged investigation into the circumstances underlying the NCI–Burroughs Wellcome collaboration. After several years of depositions, it became clear that "no one within the pro-business administration of George H. W. Bush wished to challenge a corporation in court, and the NIH was not willing to do so without support from the White House."[104] Broder later lamented:

> The government was not prepared to defend its position. It did not want to. The Commercial Litigation Branch of the Justice Department seemed very unhappy with the whole litigation and did not put forward, in my view, a spirited defense, or sufficient energy and resources. . . . The adversarial process in a legal setting is predicated on the assumption that you'll allow parties who are equals to contest one another. The government, for whatever reason, did not choose to act as an equal in the litigation. The interesting thing is that Burroughs-Wellcome did not win. That is a misnomer. The Court of Appeals for the Federal Circuit actually upheld one of the counts, or at least, rather, sent it back for further trial. It was just that people did not want to pursue it. If you read the decision, Burroughs-Wellcome had declared my laboratory a "pair of hands," but the Court of Appeals took the unprecedented step of saying, "They definitely were not a pair of hands," in their decision. . . .

The Supreme Court actually was asked to take this case, and they wanted to know what the government's views were. The government asked for the case to be dropped, and I am told that this was against the advice of the NIH. Why they took this position is still not clear.[105]

Broder's palpable frustration with the White House's inaction would impress upon him the importance of a proactive approach to securing the NCI's intellectual property rights.

Burroughs Wellcome (and, later, GlaxoSmithKline, which acquired Burroughs Wellcome's intellectual property rights via merger) was subject to ongoing challenges until its AZT patent expired in 2005. The latest of these cases, filed in 2004 by the AIDS Healthcare Foundation, was open until the patent's expiry. The specific challenges brought in each suit were based on the notion that the initial patent filed by Burroughs Wellcome should be overturned for violating patent law by refusing to acknowledge the role of NCI-sponsored research in discovering the compound and establishing its efficacy in treating HIV-related disease. Resolutions to U.S. patent law disputes can appear notoriously arbitrary to commonsense reasoning. In this instance, despite clear evidence of the NCI's instrumental role in developing and testing AZT as an anti-AIDS drug and strong support for the assertion that its known role went unacknowledged, several legitimate challenges to the patent persisted without resolution.[106]

In defense of the NCI's decision not to seek legal protection outright for the work it conducted on AZT, Broder notes that the collaboration with Burroughs Wellcome was initiated before the 1986 Technology Transfer Act provided the NCI with a robust institutional defense of federal scientists' intellectual property rights. Working in a spirit of "partnership" with the company and without a formal framework for patenting, he and his colleagues did not consider patent protection as a natural or necessary framework for scientific collaboration. Burroughs Wellcome's surprise rebuke of the federal government's role in AZT research and development indelibly stamped the institutional environment for subsequent extramural collaboration throughout the NIH. The NCI would take this lesson to the bank when Broder was appointed director in 1989. In a "controversial" move that was later reversed by NIH director Harold Varmus, Broder inserted a "reasonable price clause" into the institute's Collaborative Research and Development Agreements (CRADAs)—the collaborative mechanism under which Broder and his team conducted their work on AZT with

Burroughs Wellcome.[107] Though time in the private sector after his NCI tenure would soften Broder to industry incentives for innovation, he remained committed to the need to leverage "the NIH's prestige to make sure that the public does not feel that it is paying more than what is fair for drugs that emerge from the NIH programs."[108] To his mind, there were countless "unsung heroes" among the researchers, technicians, and nurses working throughout the NIH. On this point he was less sanguine: "I think that dollar for dollar, the taxpayers got their money's worth out of that intramural commitment. And I think that that would not have happened in any other setting."[109]

Broder and his colleagues were, for their part, ready to bring the lessons of AZT to bear on patenting and licensing for the other nucleoside analogs they were still developing. As commentators recounted, "Broder showed he had learned a lesson from Burroughs Wellcome's approach to AZT, and did not intend to get burned again."[110] Broder, Mitsuya, and Yarchoan all filed for a patent for ddI under their names "to make it clear from the outset that government researchers had been involved in ddI's development—and that, ethically and legally, they retained a degree of control over its marketing."[111]

As with AZT, Broder and his colleagues at the NIH acted aggressively to develop ddC and ddI with industry partners. Though the NCI held the patent for both ddC and ddI as effective HIV antiretroviral treatments, it was nevertheless dependent on industry collaboration to scale up medicines for wide distribution. However, NCI and NIH leadership's experience with AZT had changed their understanding of the stakes of such collaborations for the new nucleoside analogs. As the NIH Office of Technology Transfer put it, "the technology transfer challenge [with ddI] was to negotiate a license that would provide a strong incentive for a drug company to make the significant investment necessary for the rapid development of a new drug while ensuring the long-term public health benefits."[112] The solution was to negotiate a license with pharmaceutical giant Bristol-Myers for a limited term of patent exclusivity, after which time the NIH could exercise the right to make the license nonexclusive and invite other firms to manufacture competing products. Additionally, Broder made sure the licensing contract with Bristol-Myers included a "reasonable price" clause to ensure ddI was affordable, arguing that "the government has a legitimate interest in the final price of a product, not only because government research is involved but because the government is a major customer for drugs."[113] When ddI hit the market in 1991 as the second FDA-approved anti-AIDS therapy, the branded drug was under one-fifth the price of AZT at $1,745 USD per year.[114] In 2001, the NIH exercised its rights to make the patent nonexclusive, at which time ddI became the first generic anti-HIV drug and the most affordable on the market. It was rapidly picked up in developing nations that had been priced out of most other patented therapeutics.

The bureaucratic innovations Broder helped effect around licensing for the ddI patent reflected his team's efforts to develop the drug as a tool that could be of greater use than AZT in controlling the public health threat of HIV/AIDS. Yarchoan echoed the sentiments of his COP colleagues in expressing pride in ddI as one of "their" drugs. For the NCI team,

> ddI was yet another drug that was developed here, and that was also very satisfying because it induced greater immunologic changes than ddC and it was a drug that we really saw through from the very beginning, from the laboratory concept, through its preclinical development, through the phase I testing. The NIH holds the patent on this drug. . . . It was very, very satisfying that ddI is probably, of the single nucleosides, the most active and, for reasons that still are not clear, works for the longest period of time. It is also, I believe, the cheapest on a patient-year basis, and thus it is more affordable for patients in third world countries.[115]

In these respects, ddI fulfilled some of the central organizational commitments that made NCI intramural innovation distinctive from industry and academic research and development. It was a purposefully designed public health intervention that was affordable, efficacious, and propped up by interdisciplinary cooperation.

CONCLUSION

As the NIH historian Victoria Harden has noted, the initial cohort of AIDS researchers, which included members of the LTCB and COP, represented an informal collaborative effort that "arose from individual initiative rather than in response to any top-down administrative directive."[116] Clinicians in the COP learned from developments emerging from these cooperative laboratory efforts how to detect and develop the first generation of effective HIV antiretrovirals.

As they shepherded the first nucleoside analog shown to significantly target HIV, AZT, through industry-supported trials, COP scientist-bureaucrats such as Broder also learned hard lessons about how their health motives differed from the motives of their pharmaceutical partners. Redefining the issues and stakes of nucleoside analog innovation around a need to optimally price these compounds so they could be useful to AIDS sufferers throughout the world, Broder also helped innovate a new approach to ensuring technologies licensed from NCI inventors would be priced competitively by the pharmaceutical companies they relied on to bring these drugs to market. These serial learning episodes show how intertwined scientific and bureaucratic concerns can become as NCI researchers navigate a broader institutional terrain ill-suited to helping them achieve their dual mission of scientific and health-relevant innovation.

Despite their success in stemming disease early in the epidemic, Broder and his colleagues at the NCI had been quick to point out that AZT and its sister compounds ddI and ddC were not "cures." Broder insisted that "there is nothing magical or anointed about AZT. The key issue in that era, really my obsession, was to find something practical that would be shown at a clinical level to work."[117] The nucleoside analogs were the first class of working drugs to extend survival, with known imperfections and exclusions.[118] Most seriously, problems with toxicity continued to plague nucleoside analogs as AIDS treatments. Other patients appeared to develop immunity to the drugs, and their effectiveness in blocking HIV's harmful effects on T cells gradually declined. Nucleoside analogs were also unable to reverse the damage that infection had already done to a patient's immune system, which limited their efficacy in those with advanced disease.[119]

As Steven Epstein notes, researchers such as Broder, Mitsuya, and Yarchoan were well on their way to exploring other classes of compounds by the time the nucleoside analogs were going through clinical testing.[120] The problem was rather that "scientific knowledge about the virus far outstripped an understanding of the immunopathogenesis of AIDS in the human body."[121] Savvy AIDS activists, like those involved in ACT UP's Treatment and Data Committee, soon realized that the future of effective AIDS therapies depended on a drug pipeline that was substantially leaky upstream of clinical trials. Despite a long list of prospective drugs that had shown early promise in vitro or in animal studies, at the dawn of the 1990s the NIAID's AIDS Clinical Trials Group reported a scant few phase I trials under way. Broder and colleagues at the NCI could boast an enormously productive research agenda focused on understanding the fundamentals of the virus, but this wealth of knowledge was of little service in the clinic. Over the next five years, the NCI continued to screen tens of thousands of compounds for treating HIV infection and AIDS complications in an effort to find drugs that were better suited to combating AIDS on a global scale.[122] Physicians still waded through the mire of individual immune responses in an attempt to piece together a clinical picture of how HIV infection progressed to AIDS (or in some cases did not).

Compounding all of these technical issues was the astronomical market price Burroughs Wellcome charged for their branded AZT. Similar market concerns that motivated high pricing for AZT would affect the next most significant innovations in improving survival and quality of life for AIDS patients. As combination antiretroviral therapy continued its development in the private sector, a strong slate of anti-HIV protease inhibitors emerged from Hoffmann-La Roche, Abbott, and Merck beginning in 1996. In combination with nucleoside analogs such as ddI, this new class of drugs contributed to the combination highly active anti-retroviral therapy (HAART) cocktail that provided the most effective regimen in treating HIV infection and advanced AIDS yet seen. But as the epidemic progressed globally and HAART was priced out of reach of all but the wealthiest patients, it became increasingly obvious that death from the disease would be "primarily a problem of underdeveloped countries and people of low socioeconomic status."[123] These populations would be better served by a prophylactic innovation than they would by antiretrovirals that remained largely out of reach.

Though the LTCB had been targeting vaccines as a long-term objective as soon as it narrowed in on a virus, NCI scientists had to accept a diminished bureaucratic role in federal HIV/AIDS vaccine organization and planning after losing primacy in the NIH effort to the NIAID in 1986. The ethical considerations for development and testing of compounds that would best serve populations of low socioeconomic status, such as HIV vaccines, were also starker compared with those presented by the first generation of nucleoside analogs championed by LGBTQ activists of generally high socioeconomic status.[124] Whereas U.S. disease activists stressed individual rights to access experimental drugs, the populations now suffering the most from epidemic outbreaks depended on a more communitarian ethics that prioritized low-cost population-level interventions.[125] Though the NCI had a long history of involvement in virus and vaccine studies in places like Uganda,[126] the concerns of global populations had always been markedly secondary to those of the American populace in the institute. In part due to the problems surfaced by the global AIDS epidemic, the NCI began a slow shift toward conceptualizing public health on a greater scale. With an AIDS vaccine still not forthcoming, the agency's emerging emphasis on global health would develop alongside studies testing its newest viral vaccine candidate against the oncogenic human papillomavirus. The NCI's success in HPV vaccine development would build directly upon the model of translational research Broder hoped to spread throughout the institute as its new director.

CHAPTER 6

LOST IN TRANSLATION, 1990–2001

Talk of "translational research" became ubiquitous in American biomedicine at the turn of the twenty-first century as a way to reference the goal of moving scientific innovations from "bench to bedside" through collaborations among laboratory, clinical, and population scientists.[1] The increasingly complex relationships between academy, industry, and government that now sustain translational research initiatives have led many science and technology studies (STS) scholars to consider translational research in light of a shift toward neoliberal regimes of science policy, whereby market influences colonize domains of research and development previously populated by publicly supported science.[2] Given the coincidence of federal translational initiatives with a particularly market-friendly policy regime in the United States, these scholars consider the problem of closing the "translational gap" to be one of reconciling the goals of market actors and universities. While it is well established that universities have become decidedly more market friendly in the twenty-first century, Elizabeth Popp Berman notes that narratives unifying recent policy trends toward economizing science under the banner of neoliberalism elide the complexity of national policy initiatives, many of which contain strong critiques of market failure.[3] At the same time that the institutional environment of universities has made these organizations increasingly isomorphic with private firms, some policy makers have begun to view government science as fulfilling a role that market forces fail to adequately address.[4]

Though STS scholars frequently locate the origins of translational research in the 2003 National Institutes of Health Roadmap for Medical Research, the tendency to conflate translational research and neoliberal political economic imperatives largely glosses the role the NIH played in establishing translational research as a biomedical policy paradigm in the first place.[5] Not only do scientists and policy makers at government organizations such as the NIH or its constituent National Cancer Institute perceive industry as reluctant to adequately invest in basic research and cancer drug development, they also argue that private R&D efforts can undermine the public good. To the extent the NCI's translational research initiatives critique and even challenge the market's role in R&D, they do not square neatly with narratives of translational research as neoliberal science policy. The primary assumption of a neoliberal framework—that public science is being marketized for private profit—must be qualified in the face of countervailing trends that allow federal agencies to impose patenting, licensing, usage, and pricing restrictions upon products developed from government innovations. Far from a laissez-faire attitude to market expansion, the sociologists Vallas, Kleinman, and Biscotti argue that the U.S. government has, through bureaucratic agencies such as the NIH, deployed a "de facto industrial policy" that facilitates state-backed innovation while escaping the critical eye of market fundamentalists.[6]

Much in the way the historian Philip Mirowski described a growing gulf between how economists utilized the "linear model" of innovation in social science debates and the manner in which scientists themselves understood the relationships between science and technology as more complex, there may be reason to believe that the manner in which translational research is envisioned by social scientists varies from how it is practiced by cancer researchers.[7] At variance would also be the relevant understanding of the relationship between science and the state. Whereas neoliberals have critiqued state approaches to innovation as inefficient compared to market approaches, this analysis of the NCI has shown that a particular version of accountability to political and scientific publics, via stewardship of taxpayer funds toward observable health gains, has long built an alternative means of evaluating the effectiveness of innovations into the governance structure of the NCI.

Efforts to develop policies that meet this standard of accountability at the NCI were central to the spread of translational research policy throughout mainstream biomedicine.[8] Policies that emerged from the efforts of NCI scientist-bureaucrats to connect interpretations of translation to collaborative research practices contributed both to a distinct organizational culture of translational research in the institute and to efforts to build infrastructure for nationwide translational research projects through novel extramural grant mechanisms.

A better understanding of the development of these translational research efforts in the decade preceding the NIH roadmap locates the much sought-after origin of the global translational research paradigm in specific rules, policies, and programs that connected discourse on translation to routines for governing research at the interface of the NCI, Congress, industry, and academic science. Unpacking the origin of translational research at this interface allows greater clarity in discussions of the fugitive "ethos" of translational research that STS scholars have struggled to anchor in scientific practice.[9]

The entrepreneurial role the NCI played in establishing dedicated infrastructure for translational research is crucial to understanding the emergence of this policy paradigm. Funding practices led to the development of functional understandings of translational research among NCI scientist-bureaucrats and their scientific principals on the National Cancer Advisory Board (NCAB) that spoke to demands for accountability originating in Congress. NCI administrators created new funding lines, such as the SPORE grant and RAID program, to target translational research in a manner consonant with scientist-bureaucrats' own ideas about innovation. The growth of translational funding mechanisms was also spurred by perceptions among these bodies involved in institute governance that translational research, much like clinical work, was disadvantaged by the culture of basic research permeating the peer review process. Early on, translational funding mechanisms served in part as compromises that allowed the NCI to maintain an emphasis on basic research, something both NCI directors who reigned during the 1990s believed to be the institute's paramount mission, while ensuring that the knowledge they produced would be put toward satisfying long-standing public demands for measurable disease reductions.

As these new funding mechanisms were being established in the early 1990s, the NCI found itself at the center of a number of critical external organizational evaluations. The relentless oversight focused on inefficiencies in the intramural research programs of the entire NIH prompted dramatic organizational reforms in the NCI. As a consequence of these organizational reforms and the attention paid to new funding mechanisms, the contours of a heretofore wooly construct of "translational research" began to take shape. While scientist-bureaucrats used the concept to defend the high-risk work being done in the intramural program from the agency's multiple principals, the NCI's local vision of translation was transmitted to extramural scientists through its embeddedness in funding mechanisms such as the SPORE program. NCI scientist-bureaucrats were also particularly effective at using intramural projects with translational elements to perform agency accountability before principals in Congress, the NCAB, and the President's Cancer Panel (PCP).

As promising translational projects emerged from NCI-sponsored research, understandings of translational research became more robust among the agency's own bureaucratic-scientific personnel. The development of a vaccine against the human papillomavirus in the NCI's intramural program presents concrete evidence of how local understandings of translational research were refined in relation to experimental and administrative conduct. At the NCI at least, the rhetorical force of the translational metaphor was won in part by tying it to ongoing scientific and bureaucratic practices. These practices included a distinct interpretation of how the NCI could fill important gaps in vaccine research and development left by commercial industry players who had lately withdrawn from what they perceived to be high-risk, low-reward innovations.

BRODER'S TRANSLATIONAL RESEARCH VISION

The first half of the 1990s unfolded in the NCI under the directorship of Dr. Samuel Broder, whom President Reagan appointed to succeed Vincent DeVita in 1989. A clinical oncologist, Broder had spent most of his professional career at the NCI. As discussed in chapter 5, Broder's work was instrumental to the NCI's development of drugs to combat HIV/AIDS, including AZT, ddI, and ddC. By the time Broder took office, these nucleoside analogs were considered some of the institute's greatest drug-development successes.

Despite such apparent successes, the NCI closed out the 1980s in worse financial shape than it had been for decades. After adjusting its budget on the basis of the biomedical pricing index, the institute showed a consistent loss of purchasing power throughout the 1980s, as it failed to keep up with inflation throughout the decade. Whereas various pieces of AIDS legislation, the Human Genome Project, and other initiatives allowed its parent, NIH, to recover and show linear growth up to its then 15 percent over 1980s funding trends, the NCI's growth rate had fallen 6 percent by 1991 before a slight increase put it back to its 1980 purchasing power in 1992.[10] In the ensuing half-decade, the NCI would come under pressure to do more with its stagnant budget. Early efforts to fund translational research emerged from NCI scientist-bureaucrats' attempts to reconceptualize institute accountability in this tight fiscal environment.

The legal and political environment of the NCI had also changed indelibly during the first decade of the HIV/AIDS epidemic in the United States. The history of nucleoside analog research and development illustrates how NCI scientists leveraged the institute's post–War on Cancer infrastructure to advance undirected collaborative enterprises with colleagues in government, academia, and industry. The influence of patent disputes with Burroughs Wellcome over AZT on the subsequent development of ddI and ddC demonstrates how quickly research and bureaucratic practice could creatively respond to hard lessons issuing from the changing national research ecology. Samuel Broder and his team were central to the direction this learning took around HIV/AIDS treatment research. Broder's experiences helped him to develop a distinctive philosophy of innovation that would influence his articulation of translational research paradigms in the upper echelons of the NCI.

Broder's interpretation of translational research extended the philosophy he espoused in collaborating with Gallo's Laboratory of Tumor Cell Biology (LTCB), whose objectives were ultimately focused on leveraging laboratory findings "to develop new concepts of chemotherapy and apply them to animal model systems as rapidly as possible as new information is derived from basic experimental studies."[11] The position Broder's Clinical Oncology Program enjoyed vis-à-vis Gallo's LTCB was reflected in his later discussions of how the institute could foster translational research. Even at its inception, Broder understood the "crash program" he initiated in the Clinical Oncology Program during the early years of the AIDS epidemic to be "illustrative of the kinds of drug-development efforts that are possible in the intramural program."[12] It was, after all, this program that located AZT as among the first promising compounds to test and which secured access through Burroughs Wellcome. On the basis of his experiences (both positive and negative) in developing AIDS therapeutics, Broder had begun to conceptualize the NCI as a " 'pharmaceutical company' working for the public."[13]

Informed by these substantive scientific and bureaucratic experiences, Broder's formulation of translational research colligated around his understanding of the transformations taking place among researchers in the cancer field. Broder recalled: "As the 1970s and 1980s unfolded, we saw a compartmentalization of clinicians versus laboratory scientists. Part of this was based on the reality that laboratory science became extremely specialized, requiring skills in molecular biology not available to the ordinary physician."[14] Though molecular biologists had been successful in carving out a political identity and positioning themselves strategically in NCI governance through the NCAB, there were signs that medical practice was becoming more distant from the research world that produced these new findings. Prominent figures in the NCI worried that the brand of clinician-scientist the NIH had been so skilled in training during the 1960s and 1970s was dying out, particularly as the revenue-driven institutional environment of medical practice discouraged clinical trials as too costly for them to support.[15] Broder envisioned the NCI as one of the few places where clinician-scientists could continue to thrive, remarking that "many of the individuals at the NIH . . . made a very effective transition into the new world of molecular biology. I had the good fortune to work with many such people . . . who were very effective at bridging the gap."[16] Nevertheless, Broder was concerned that "the intramural program does not function at that same level in terms of the interplay between the lab and bedside" as it potentially could because "NIH leadership clearly has not assigned full value to this function historically."[17] It would take determined action within the institute to realize an environment where this type of collaborative research could thrive.

Despite his motivation to transform the NCI into an organization that encouraged such innovative collaboration, Broder's leadership style was, by his own admission, conservative. Throughout his tenure as director, Broder's stated commitment was to science and to the NCI as a scientific research organization. Interpreting bureaucratic challenges in light of his past experiences as a clinician working closely with laboratory scientists to develop HIV/AIDS drugs, Broder firmly believed that the flow of knowledge between the lab and clinic should be bidirectional.[18] He aimed to create an environment in the NCI conducive to this vision of the relationship between fundamental and applied research, which he had taken to consistently calling "translational research." Constrained by his reluctance to alter the formal structure of the intramural program, Broder focused on developing a number of funding changes that would be instrumental to securing a commitment to translational research from the NCI's scientist-bureaucrats and dual principals during the 1990s.

Broder was by all accounts an early adopter of the concept of translational research. Though the term had been in sporadic colloquial use in the NIH and NCI for decades, most researchers outside the institute did not take its definition for granted. For instance, the prominent professional publication *Cancer*

Letter began referencing " 'so-called' translational research"[19] independently of respondents' use of the term only in 1993 and used the term in scare quotes until the mid-1990s. In 1995, J. Michael Bishop, who shared a Nobel Prize for the oncogene research he conducted with former colleague and then-NIH director Harold Varmus, expressed in a letter to Varmus that "the definition [of translational research] still eludes me."[20] Broder's systematic use of the term in the NCI's annual professional budgets and in NCAB meetings appears particularly influential, as the audience for these documents (the NCAB, Congress, the PCP, and professional organizations such as the American Society for Clinical Oncology) subsequently adopted the construct in their own reports.

Broder gave his interpretation of translational research concreteness by iteratively integrating translational research criteria into the review procedures of two extramural funding mechanisms: the extant P01 Research Program Project Grant and the novel Specialized Programs of Research Excellence (SPORE). Translational P01 and SPORE grants challenged the status quo favoring basic research, which had been strongly in place since the early 1980s. By creating circumstances for negotiating distinct approaches to supporting translational research, these extramural funding practices enabled NCI scientist-bureaucrats and their principals to iteratively encode the construct of translational research in peer review and grant management until it was cemented in two bureaucratic innovations. Understandings of translational research that developed in the NCI's governance structure around these funding mechanisms would subsequently inform efforts to implement translational reform in other parts of the NCI. Together, the extramural and intramural efforts to give translational research concreteness in bureaucratic practice led to the enduring changes that helped the NCI become an innovator in translational research policy.

P01s Make Translational Research Competitive in Peer Review

For decades, the grant mechanisms most favored by extramural scientists and their representatives on the NCAB were R01 Research Project Grants. Comprising the major emphasis of the NCI's Research Project Grants (RPGs) portfolio, R01s are competitive grants awarded to individual extramural investigators that allow them maximal freedom to pursue projects deemed meritorious by peer reviewers in Study Sections and on the NCAB. The freedom to pursue inquiry led to a durable association between R01s and basic research, which scientists construed as inquiry focused on the growth of knowledge for its own sake rather than for its possible utility in future application. Yet NCI leadership recognized that the long-running emphasis on R01 grants in the absence of concerted policies around applying research findings threatened to overshadow the institute's dual mission of ensuring emerging research was put to use in improving health. Under Broder, the issues involved in translational research were defined around the problem of changing peer review and grant processes to reward collaborative research that would shepherd basic insights into health-relevant application.

Within the NCI, concern about the possible overemphasis on R01s had been brewing for years. Then-director Vincent DeVita commissioned an external review completed in 1987 that tracked the role different funding mechanisms had played in some of the most recent major biomedical advances supported by the NCI. The study, *An Assessment of the Factors Affecting Critical Cancer Research Findings*, showed that R01s played about the same role in these breakthroughs as intramural projects (supporting 20.1 percent of advancements as opposed to 19.8 percent), and just slightly more than contract research (16.9 percent).[21] More tellingly, another RPG mechanism, the P01, funded 30 percent of all clinical advancements, as opposed to R01s, which accounted for only 10 percent.

P01 Research Program Project grants were developed as a standard funding mechanism for collaborative efforts to supplement individual R01 awards in the NCI's overall strategy toward managing its RPG portfolio. To be eligible for a P01 grant, a project had to include multiple investigators, often but not always at the same institution, who would share common resources and whose individual projects were geared toward a bigger, collaborative goal. Often such projects were purely based on laboratory or clinical science conducted by teams of extramural researchers. A modest adjustment, first proposed to the NCAB by DeVita in 1984, would involve tailoring P01s to clinical research only, thus neatly dividing the institute's RPG strategy into these two separate grant mechanisms. Over time, however, Broder came to see the P01 as a grant the NCI could use to foster interdisciplinary work on a short-term basis (in contrast to longer-term and larger interdisciplinary collaborations in Comprehensive Cancer Centers, which were funded by a separate mechanism).

Because of their use in large projects (and particularly clinical trials), P01 grants consistently consumed a generous share of the RPG budget relative to the more voluminous slate of R01s. Though each P01 grant funded multiple investigators working on multiple projects related to a broader collaborative effort,

NCI administrators counted each P01 as a single grant. This accounting practice meant that, on paper, each P01 grant was magnitudes more expensive than any of the other R01 grants in the RPG pool. In 1990, a single P01 grant cost an average of six times as much as a single R01.[22] Every year, by congressional mandate, the NIH set targets on the number of grants the NCI should award based in part on its share of the overall RPG pool. In fiscal year 1992, this target demanded a $210,000 per grant average, about 5.5 times lower than the average P01 grant actually awarded that year.[23] Broder voiced his suspicion in 1991 that bureaucrats in the NIH were using this discrepancy to crack down on the growth of P01 grants.[24]

Threats to the share of P01 funding were particularly troubling to those on the NCAB who had been persuaded by NCI leadership that the P01 grant was the most promising mechanism for funding translational research. In 1991, NCAB member Dr. Sidney Salmon urged leadership at the NCI to extend its support beyond the traditional R01. Salmon argued P01 grants should be rescued from the "tyranny of the accountants" who wish to count their contribution singly, as P01s "are perhaps the best example where you see the translation from the laboratory bench to the bedside."[25] Salmon became a staunch advocate of P01 grants early in his stint on the NCAB, defending them as the only extant funding mechanism that actually supported translational research.[26]

NCI leadership had been similarly successful in persuading congressional principals on the Senate Appropriations Committee of P01 grants' significance, and the committee expressed like consternation at the thought of the NCI scaling back on P01 grants. The committee's report for the Senate fiscal year 1992 funding bill (released in July 1991) stated: "The committee is distressed that NCI is considering eliminating program project grants in an effort to demonstrate an overall greater number of awards. The P01 mechanism has played an essential role in the transfer of basic research findings to bedside practice."[27] In attempting to adjudicate between the need to allot larger budgets to P01 grants and the need to hit funding targets, the Senate committee felt "that numerical goals for grants should not force the elimination of useful mechanisms of research."[28]

In pondering the source of these bureaucratic tensions, some members of Congress began to suspect the problem with peer review had less to do with the structure of study sections and more to do with the culture embedded in the peer review system itself. As the congressionally appointed Subcommittee to Evaluate the National Cancer Program concluded in its 1994 review, the NCI needed to make changes in its peer review system so that translational research (as well as clinical research) applications could compete on "equal footing" with basic research projects.[29] In leveraging the institute's health mission against its scientific mission, congressional principals put the NCI's scientific principals on notice that peer review in the NCI would need to be made more accountable to both sides of the institute's dual mission.

Much as Broder advocated for translational research as both scientifically and bureaucratically relevant to the NCI's mission, select scientific principals on the NCAB echoed the sentiment that peer review would need to accommodate approaches to scientific innovation beyond the basic research that had been embraced by scientific principals since the end of the War on Cancer. In a May 1992 meeting of the NCAB, Salmon pushed (unsuccessfully) to reserve P01s solely for translational projects. Salmon justified his motion by stating that current funding policies "make it difficult for investigators that have translational research elements to compete successfully against basic research P01s without translational research elements."[30] Per standard practice for RPGs at NCI, each P01 application was assigned a priority score that reflected the merit of the application according to study section reviewers at the first level of peer review. When these applications reached the second level of peer review, where they were voted on *en bloc* by the NCAB, that board determined a particular cutoff score that would fund the top-rated applications up to a particular percentile (called the "payline"). If, as Salmon and others argued, the peer review system favored basic research over translational research, then it would be more difficult for a P01 grant application with a translational research component to win the award.

Though Salmon failed to persuade other NCAB members that the P01 grant should be converted to a translational-only funding mechanism, Broder took the NCAB's recalcitrance as license to exercise his prerogative as director to reexamine P01 grants that failed to make the payline (i.e., applications that were deemed excellent by reviewers but did not receive priority scores that put them in the percentile of applications that would be funded).[31] As director of NCI, Broder and his Executive Committee had the power to grant exceptions to the payline in order to fund meritorious projects that advanced the goals of the institute. Broder determined that any excellent but unfunded applications with translational research components could be funded by exception, a process for which the NCI set aside a small pot of funding in each budget. While the NCI had not hesitated to grant exceptions in the past, Broder for the first time instituted a policy whereby exceptions would be used specifically to increase funding for translational research.[32] In the first three years of the NCI under Broder, 72 percent of all funded P01s included a translational research component.[33]

As Broder points out, the thrust of the NCI and NCAB's efforts by early 1993 was to ensure that the priorities of the institute were balanced across different disciplines. As a result of the learning that occurred around these funding mechanisms, P01 grants became an innovative means through which supporters of translational research could ensure that their interpretations of the institute's programmatic goals would be supported. Yet problems with allocating resources within the RPG pool, as well as retooling the peer review system to meet the needs of P01 grant applicants, limited the potential impact of P01 grants as mechanisms for encouraging translational research throughout the country. Before the NCI's interpretation of translational research could gain sufficient traction among the broader community of extramural scientists, the institute needed to build a more concrete infrastructure for translational research beyond the agency. NCI scientist-bureaucrats accomplished this by creating a new funding mechanism that robustly integrated the goals of translational research into the scientific and administrative operations of collaborative groups housed outside the institute.

SPORE Builds Extramural Translational Infrastructure

Implicit in the debates about using the RPG pool to fund translational research was a tension between the multiple principals the NCI served. The general population of extramural scientists were, presumably, always hungry for more R01s. As the single largest expense at the NCI and the mechanism used to pursue one of its core missions of funding the best science, much of the NCI's governance structure was designed around satisfying the needs of prospective grantees in the scientific community. Yet some NCAB members and especially members of Congress pushed the institute toward its second mandate of ameliorating the national burden of cancer. In advocating for the application of knowledge to improve cancer outcomes, they bore the standard of accountability to the broader constituency of the American public. Though NCI scientist-bureaucrats such as Broder had a strong hand in steering debates over how to fund translational research, these debates should be understood as answerable to the enduring problem of how to manage tensions between the interests of political and scientific principals at the heart of cancer research governance in the NCI.

By all accounts, the SPORE grant could resolve many of the major problems facing translational efforts in the RPG pool: it constituted a dedicated funding mechanism for translational research and included provisions that explicitly required interdisciplinary collaboration. When the NCI approved the SPORE program in June of 1991, it removed it from the RPG funding pool by utilizing the long-defunct P50 funding line. The P50 grant was grouped with the "core grant" line that supported big-budget programs such as P30 Cancer Centers grants but would command an independent pool of funding allocated directly from Congress. Thus, though the SPORE concept originated in the institute, the new funding line was dependent on Congress to authorize funding for particular SPORE projects on the basis of judgments of merit and mission-appropriateness at the discretion of congressional, as opposed to scientific, principals. When the first round of SPORE grants was announced, Congress had approved funding only for three specific disease sites: lung cancer, prostate cancer, and breast cancer.[34]

The three SPORE grants reserved for breast cancer received the most attention in both Congress and the press, likely due to the fact that women's health advocates and breast cancer activists were making the government's efforts toward this cancer site a hot-button issue.[35] As Broder noted, Congress and the White House put pressure on the NCI through language included in their budget reports advising the agency to fund research that would decrease morbidity and mortality associated with breast, cervical, ovarian, and prostate cancer. Nevertheless, these soft earmarks were not accompanied by additional funding that would enable the NCI to conduct this kind of research.[36] The SPORE program thus provided an opportunity to apply the NCI's concept of translational research to an area where congressional principals expressed particular interest in accountability to the institute's health mission, as spurred by patient and disease lobbyists.

Beyond the specific disease sites authorized by Congress, the NCI maintained its familiar policy-making autonomy that allowed it to design the SPORE funding mechanism itself and determine the criteria whereby applications would be judged meritorious. While NCI leadership intended all SPORE grants "to promote interdisciplinary research and to speed the bidirectional exchange of basic and clinical science," the breast cancer SPORE grants in particular pushed a comprehensive agenda of translational research for all funded projects.[37] Per the original announcement, "each SPORE must be dedicated to research on prevention, diagnosis and treatment of human breast cancer and the translation of basic research finding [sic] into more applied, innovative research settings involving patients and populations," and must develop training and tissue resource programs for translational researchers.[38] In addition to these scientific requirements, the SPORE grant required applicants to meet a number of administrative demands for eligibility. Among these was the existence of a "critical mass of both basic and clinical scientists dedicated to the translation of basic findings into more applied, innovative research settings involving patients and populations with the ultimate objective of reducing incidence and mortality to the disease."[39] Further, the goals of the SPORE program must be fully integrated into the institutional commitments of the funded organization.[40] The NCI was asking peer reviewers of SPORE applications to evaluate both the scientific merit of the applications as well as their institutes' commitment to translational research.[41] Acknowledging the SPORE program's unusual accountability to the health demands of congressional appropriators, Broder described the SPORE program to scientific principals on the NCAB as an "administrative experiment."[42]

As NCAB member Frederick Becker pointed out, the SPORE program's focus on cancer sites made many scientists wary that the institute was turning away from funding investigator-initiated research to instead fund organ-site research at the behest of the institute's political principals. Broder stressed that not only were SPORE grants not taking money away from the RPG pool that funds individual, investigator-initiated projects, but also the SPORE program was itself not an organ-site-based effort. Despite the language of the congressional authorization, Broder insisted that the NCI designed SPORE grants with the intent to fund collaborative, interdisciplinary research on the most common cancers in America by using a mechanism that required awardees' research to make "some national impact."[43] PCP member Geza Jako found this framing persuasive and lauded SPORE grants as striking "a fair balance between the National Cancer Program's investigators and new ideas and the public's need for research in high-incidence and high-mortality cancers."[44]

In addition to addressing the anxieties of scientific principals, Broder found himself defending the program in the face of criticism from within his own agency shortly after the first round of applications closed. Balking at the proposed budgets, many of which topped $1.5 million, Deputy Director Daniel Ihde announced that the institute would be funding only seven SPORE grants rather than the nine originally proposed. Ihde's announcement scandalized members of the Board of Scientific Counselors (BSC) for the Division of Cancer Treatment, not to mention Broder, for whom Ihde was standing in at the BSC meeting. Broder blasted Ihde's reduction as "premature," insisting the NCI would treat SPORE grants as "an extremely high priority activity."[45] But work remained to ensure other scientist-bureaucrats in the NCI could be brought aboard the director's vision for translational research.

Perhaps most challenging for the fate of the program was NIH director Harold Varmus's skepticism about SPORE grants. In a 1994 meeting of the NCAB subcommittee to evaluate the National Cancer Program, Varmus backtracked on previous statements supporting the program and proclaimed, "I remain to be convinced of the efficacy of SPORE grants. . . . They're very expensive, they're big. I, myself, do not propose that we have more of them until we see whether the ones we have are actually doing their job."[46] Varmus's statement was in response to the proposed budget for SPORE grants in the fiscal year 1995 Bypass Budget, which requested a fourfold increase to the SPORE budget over its first-year budget in 1992 as well as an expansion of the cancer sites the program covered. Varmus objected to funding directed collaborative efforts at a time when the NCI was "turning down 85–90 percent of our [R01] grant applicants who have their own ideas."[47] He claimed that big-budget awards under the cancer centers lines (with which SPORE grants are grouped) "[tend] to make my colleagues behave like sharks who smell blood in the water. They say, 'There's money out there, let's go after it!' It's not that we have an idea, the money is sitting there."[48]

Varmus severely criticized Broder's defense of SPORE grants as translational research mechanisms. Whereas Broder saw SPORE grants as a "catalyst" for translational research and hoped the program would provide a model for future translational efforts,[49] Varmus saw them as trumped-up cancer center construction projects. "We don't have the drugs that are going to be used in these bedside experiments. We're just going to build these large, clinical/basic research entities that don't really have much to do yet, except provide support to build buildings and take the money that should be used to do the next phase of research, that will actually develop the things that will get to the bedside."[50] As such, the translational mission of SPORE grants was disingenuous: "If we say we're going to set up these big SPORE programs to be sure [that] what we understand about the cell cycle is now beside the bedside, frankly, that's horse manure."[51]

Proponents in the scientific community disagreed with Varmus's insistence that using SPORE funding to buttress cancer centers was putting the translational cart before the horse. Dr. Margaret Kripke, president of the American Association for Cancer Research (AACR), argued before the NCAB that the biggest barriers facing translation had to do with lack of infrastructure and funding for bench-to-bedside efforts in the extramural environment.[52] "To get science to think about how to apply existing knowledge requires interaction with clinicians who understand the problem. . . . It takes translational researchers. It will not happen overnight. It will certainly not happen without nurturing, time and money," Kripke asserted.[53] Other NCI scientist-bureaucrats were quick to defend this interpretation of SPORE grants as translational infrastructure before the institute's scientific principals. As Brian Kimes, director for NCI's Centers, Training and Resources Program, argued in the same meeting where Varmus criticized the SPORE program, "Most of our academic systems reward and provide recognition only for two types of people: the basic scientist[s] that get R01s, and those clinicians that bring in our income. . . . The people who sit in the middle, who are involved in translation . . . don't get the same standard of recognition."[54] Until the culture of peer review changed, there were few other mechanisms for ensuring investigator-initiated translational research would be properly supported.

In the meantime, Broder argued, the SPORE program's ability to bring researchers together in an effort to collaborate and translate their findings was an accomplishment in and of itself. Broder maintained that soliciting interdisciplinary projects, even those that went unfunded, could "galvanize" researchers toward further collaborative work: "I've learned that sometimes the act of asking for certain types of projects induces the formation of collaborations, even if a particular funding instrument is not given to an institution. They've gone through a process of becoming cohesive, and sharing ideas to put in the application and they say—hey, okay, you're cool, we'll get together."[55] The stakes of translational research funding initiatives, which were no less than shifting the way cancer researchers collaborated so their research more effectively yielded health-relevant results, could be realized even through apparent scientific failures if the NCI provided the right bureaucratic opportunities to bring interdisciplinary minds together.

The prevailing narrative throughout many of these debates was that if translational research was going to succeed, those who support and conduct biomedical research needed a push in the right direction. In his final address to the NCAB in January 1995, Broder reflected upon his efforts to maintain balance between basic research, clinical research, and cancer centers funding, particularly by ensuring that each group was aware of and supportive of the efforts of the others.[56] Former NCAB chairman Paul Calabresi and AACR president Kripke lauded Broder for his balanced approach, making particular note of his efforts to foster translational research in the institute. As chairman of the PCP, Harold Freeman pointed out that the recent expansion of translational research was almost entirely funded by the set-asides initiated under Broder.[57] With NCI-issued Requests for Applications (RFAs) still the principal vehicle for funding SPORE grants and the exceptions process crucial to ensuring P01 grants primarily funded translational research, a strong commitment to translation from the administration to succeed Broder's would be necessary. However, as Kimes argued, "You can't sustain any kind of research through RFAs and more directed programs in an institute."[58] Translational research would have to mature in the coming years into a self-sustaining enterprise among cancer researchers, but it remained unclear to the NCI's scientific principals whether the institute would be up to the task of governing this transition.

HPV VACCINE INNOVATION IN THE INTRAMURAL PROGRAM

At the same time Broder was attempting to seed extramural infrastructure for translational research, Douglas Lowy, MD, and John Schiller, PhD, of the NCI's intramural Laboratory of Cellular Oncology (figure 6.1) were innovating the technology that enabled the development of the first generation of human papillomavirus (HPV) vaccines. Lowy had first come to the NCI through the Virus Cancer Program, where he worked on joint efforts between NCI researcher Janet Hartley and her former NIAID colleague Wallace Rowe to study leukemia viruses in the program's twilight years. In the ensuing decades, Lowy established his own laboratory that increasingly focused on the role the papillomavirus (PV) family played in carcinogenesis. Schiller joined Lowy's laboratory as a postdoctoral researcher and, under the principal investigator's advisement, began investigating PVs in 1983. Lowy and Schiller aimed to contribute to the growing body of evidence that indicated infection with certain HPV strains was a necessary cause of many cervical cancers.[59] Schiller notes that when he and Lowy initiated their inquiry into PVs, the idea of a vaccine was far from their minds. A few researchers had previously attempted to develop PV vaccines in animal models, but such

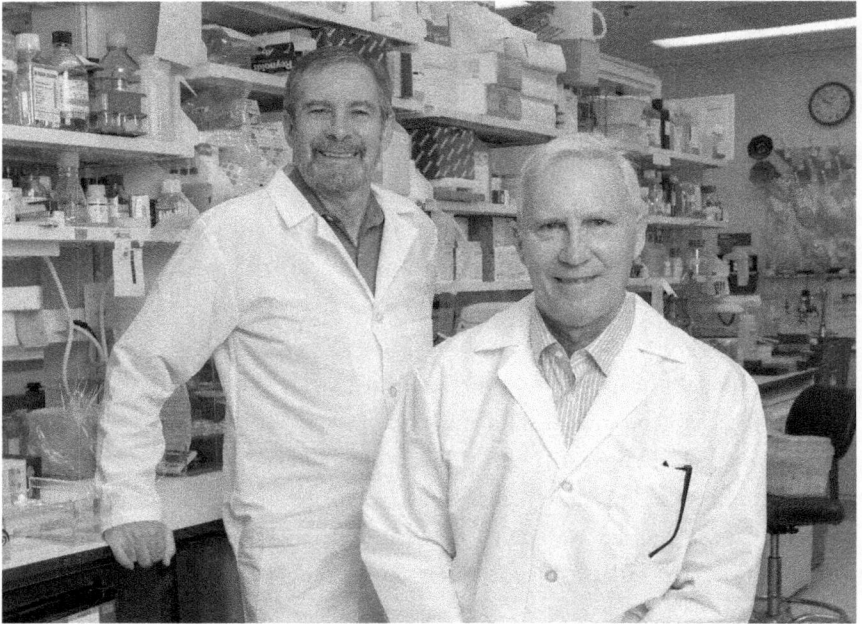

6.1 Douglas Lowy (left) and John Schiller (right) in 2017.
Photo credit: Darr Beiser, National Cancer Institute.

attempts had proven "miserable failures."[60] These earlier studies used denatured PV proteins to elicit immune responses in hosts, but epitopes against PVs are conformation dependent. This means that in order for the immune system to respond to a PV infection, PV proteins need to be properly folded. Any effective PV vaccine would thus have to introduce structurally complete PV proteins, but any safe vaccine would have to do this in a way that did not risk active infection with the oncogenic virus.

In 1991, Schiller and Lowy's laboratory made an important breakthrough that would enable development of a safe and efficacious PV vaccine that could be translated into a public health strategy to prevent cervical cancer. It began when the NCI scientists decided to follow up on a recent publication by Australian scientists Ian Frazer and Jian Zhou. Frazer and Zhou's laboratory had designed a vaccinia model that successfully expressed L1 proteins, but these proteins were defective in structure.[61] This result puzzled Schiller and Lowy, as their prior research on both bovine papillomavirus and HPV oncogenic proteins E6 and

E7 showed these proteins should have self-folded with ease.[62] They soon found a publication suggesting the strain of HPV most commonly used by laboratories around the world contained a point mutation in one of the viral genes and hypothesized that Frazer and Zhou's experiments were unsuccessful because their L1 strain also contained a mutation. Obtaining a fresh sample of HPV from a patient with cervical dysplasia who was being treated by clinician colleagues at the NCI, Schiller and Lowy designed in vitro HPV experiments that demonstrated cellular transformation of tissue cultures with "wild-type" (i.e., naturally occurring) p53 but not mutated strains of p53.[63] The virus-like particles (VLPs) they produced were structurally identical to L1 proteins found on complete PVs and elicited a substantial immune response in host cells.[64]

Schiller and Lowy colligated their experimental trajectory around a new interpretation of the issues and stakes of their PV research program: L1 VLPs were highly immunogenic and, because they could be manufactured apart from the nonstructural viral proteins (E6 and E7) that induced oncogenic cellular transformation, could be used to develop safe and effective subunit vaccines against HPV-16 associated cervical cancer.[65] Subunit vaccines delivered only small portions of a microbe into the body in order to elicit an immune response, unlike the older and more common vaccine technologies that utilized live, attenuated, or inactivated microbes. The recombinant hepatitis B vaccine, which was developed to prevent liver cancers associated with the hepatitis B virus, was the first subunit vaccine developed using VLPs and one developed against a human cancer virus.[66] On the basis of the alignment between this cancer virus vaccine and the stakes of their research, Schiller and Lowy used the recombinant hepatitis B vaccine as a model for their VLP-based HPV vaccine technologies.[67]

A strong exemplar for vaccine development was particularly important to Schiller and Lowy, as neither researcher had any prior experience in immunology or vaccinology. As Schiller recalls, they initially approached the problem of PV VLPs from a perspective oriented toward learning about the "basic biology" of virally induced neoplasia.[68] Schiller saw their work as developing enabling technologies for both basic and translational research efforts and perceived such projects that "straddled the fence" between basic and translational research as ideal.[69]

Despite Schiller's desire to hedge his commitment to translational research in his own experimental practices, the stakes of translational applications for findings such as Schiller and Lowy's were quickly brought to the fore by other NCI scientist-bureaucrats and their scientific and congressional principals. In September 1992, Congress singled out the development of an HPV vaccine as a particularly high priority for the institute.[70] NCI scientist-bureaucrats also presented evidence that strongly suggested the potential to develop effective HPV vaccines to scientific principals on the NCAB.[71] By 1993, NCI leadership was touting the institute's HPV research as a "significant initiative" in its long-term planning strategies.[72]

Early findings from Schiller and Lowy's lab stoked their optimism about vaccine development. As Schiller recalls, their first attempts to inoculate rabbit models against PV, begun in 1992, returned astonishing results. In these experiments, the lab produced sera that contained self-assembled L1 VLPs expressed through insect cells. Over the course of nine months, Schiller and postdoctoral fellow Reinhard Kirnbauer injected the sera at different doses and tested the blood of infected rabbits for neutralizing antibodies. The first injection, which was diluted 1,000-fold, showed extremely high titers of neutralizing antibodies. Kirnbauer ran two more tests, one at a 10,000-fold dilution and the next at a 100,000-fold dilution. To their surprise, even the latter dose proved highly immunogenic.[73]

Schiller and Lowy were quick to act on their optimism around these results. In 1993, after patenting their L1 VLP technology, they began soliciting every large pharmaceutical company and manufacturing firm they could to license their patent for development. Yet the pharmaceutical industry's enthusiasm for HPV vaccines failed to match theirs; Schiller recalls being confronted by a general skepticism that a vaccine for any sexually transmitted infection could succeed. Even in the face of consistent and unequivocal evidence of immunogenicity, most pharmaceutical companies were convinced that vaccines for sexually transmitted infections would ultimately fail in the face of repeated exposures to pathogens. In this context of industry skepticism toward vaccines against sexually transmitted viruses, the basic aim of securing an organization with the resources to develop enough vaccine to test and distribute was Lowy and Schiller's primary goal. They defined the stakes of such a vaccine, if it proved safe and efficacious in clinical trials, as the eventual prevention of cervical cancers.

As Schiller recalls, the laboratory was able to continue into testing when Merck decided to take a "leap of faith" on the vaccine.[74] Schiller credits a meeting with Merck's famed vaccinologist Maurice Hilleman to the company's decision to license the patent. Schiller and Lowy presented their results to Hilleman, who was still operating as an emeritus researcher at Merck. Hilleman interpreted Lowy and Schiller's results through the company's successful hepatitis B efforts and decided, "this is gonna work and Merck's gonna do it."[75] The next day, Hilleman persuaded Merck to contact the NIH legal team to license Schiller and Lowy's patent.

Learning to License HPV Vaccine Technology

The NIH licensed the NCI-developed patent for HPV vaccine technology in an environment that had been definitively changed by experiences with industry in the previous decade. Broder, now NCI director, had learned a hard lesson about working with industry after Burroughs Wellcome's maneuvers with AZT. He and the NIH legal team were determined to improve the institute's approach to intellectual property to better ensure the public, and not merely private firms, would benefit from federal innovation.

After the Burroughs Wellcome debacle, the NCI's policy for patent licensure included a stipulation that patents be licensed to multiple entities in order to ensure nonexclusive use of intellectual property produced using taxpayer funding. This policy had been put to use by Border himself in licensing ddI, but it was particularly important to deploy in the HPV vaccine case as congressional principals were now closely scrutinizing the alignment between patenting and licensing practices and the NIH's dual mission. In 1993, the high prices of drugs such as AZT and Taxol that were developed from enabling technologies invented at the NCI led Congress to criticize the NIH's inability to reign in drug prices as reflecting a failure to protect public investments in biomedical R&D. NIH director Bernadine Healy defended the institutes' approach to technology transfer, arguing that the competitive co-licensing agreements now in use were one of the most effective strategies the NIH could leverage to keep drug prices low while ensuring discoveries were translated into medical interventions.[76] In light of concerns that the NCI had "given away" the publicly funded discovery of Taxol by licensing it solely to Bristol-Myers, it was particularly urgent that new drug development in the intramural program adhere to such competitive cross-licensing practices.[77]

Schiller and Lowy's earliest efforts to develop the HPV vaccine took place during these debates over the relationship between government innovation and private drug development. In order to maintain nonexclusivity in licensing patents and to ensure market competition, both of which served a new definition of developing drugs accessibly priced for public use as the major bureaucratic issue at hand, the NCI cross-licensed the L1 VLP patent to a local biotechnology firm, MedImmune. MedImmune conducted animal trials around this and other HPV vaccine technologies and by 1997 initiated human trials testing one of its HPV vaccine variants.[78] (Co-licensee Merck also began its clinical trials in 1997.[79])

In addition to the privately funded Merck and MedImmune trials, Schiller and Lowy initiated government-funded trials to test the vaccine technology they developed.[80] Because Lowy held the Investigational New Drug license for the L1 VLP technology, the NCI was able to conduct trials on the vaccine in parallel with industry.[81] According to Schiller, he and Lowy were concerned that either Merck or MedImmune could make business-related decisions to discontinue clinical trials for any number of reasons the inventors had no control over. Furthermore, Schiller believed an NCI-funded trial had the potential to "collect a richer base of specimens and understand things" better than could drug company trials, which he believed were unlikely to explore interesting data tangential to the goals of quickly developing a marketable vaccine.[82] Schiller thought that information gleaned from the clinical application of his laboratory's findings could inform further research that might improve cancer outcomes in the future.

Yet Schiller and Lowy's absence of formal training in either vaccinology or clinical trial design, and the NCI's limited experience in producing vaccines and biologicals, presented barriers to straightforward translation that necessitated collaboration outside of their laboratory. Schiller and Lowy consulted NCI epidemiologist Allan Hildesheim, an early advocate of translational viral research in the intramural program, as well as Brian Murphy, an experienced vaccinologist at the NIAID. The NCI-NIAID team contracted with local biotechnology firm Novavax to develop the L1 VLP vaccine in sufficient quantities for a small-scale phase I human trial. They then teamed up with the Center for Immunization Research at Johns Hopkins University, which specialized in conducting human vaccine trials. The Johns Hopkins team designed the protocols and recruited subjects for phase I trials while Schiller and Lowy integrated epidemiological and clinical trial findings into their understandings of how HPV could be studied in their laboratory. This multidimensional approach to collaboration at NCI was at the same time innovative in its ability to unite academia, industry, and government science in short-term voluntarist collaborations and in consonance with the approach to translational research the new NCI director, Richard Klausner, hoped to foster in the institute.

SHAKING UP THE INTRAMURAL RESEARCH PROGRAM BUREAUCRACY

In the decade and a half that marked the renaissance of basic research under NCI directors Upton and DeVita, centrally planned and directed research programs had fallen out of popularity in the NCI. The NCI AIDS Task Force was an exception that proved this rule, and even these efforts had their origins in ad hoc collaborations formed prior to congressional commands to develop formal HIV/AIDS programs elsewhere in the NIH. More commonly, intramural researchers felt the NCI's focus on independent and investigator-initiated inquiry discouraged rank-and-file scientists from consistently collaborating across laboratories and clinics in the institute. Lack of communication and coordination among intramural researchers led many of them to feel isolated.[83] Some considered the formal structure of the NCI as one that supported a feudalistic model, with laboratories and branches serving as fiefdoms and the Scientific Directorate as powerful lords.[84] By the mid-1990s, internal strife over the structure of the NCI's Intramural Research Program converged with external criticism of the institute to usher in dramatic bureaucratic reforms.

In 1992, then NIH director Bernadine Healy assembled a task force to inquire into the quality and efficiency of the NCI's Intramural Research Program. The task force, chaired by the National Institute of Child Health and Human Development scientist Richard Klausner (figure 6.2), summarized the task force's findings in what became known as the Klausner Report. The recommendations contained in the report at first seem uncontroversial; the Klausner Report primarily suggests improving recruitment efforts, making tenure policies more explicit, and reorganizing scientific staff "into a series of trans-institute discipline-based faculties" that would conduct research and make policy recommendations.[85] This latter suggestion, however, was perceived by some as Healy's

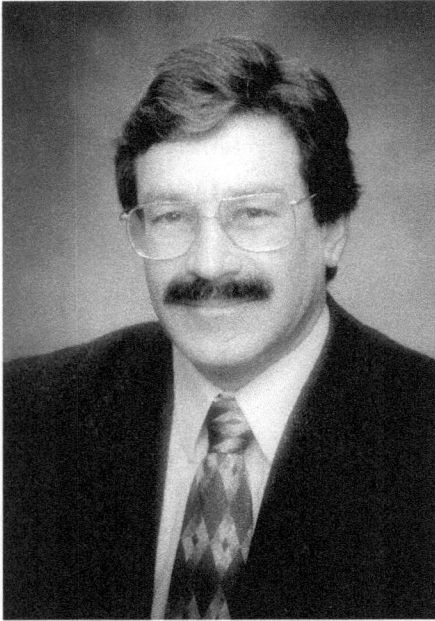

6.2 Richard Klausner, circa 1990s.
Photo credit: National Cancer Institute.

coup to seize power from the long-standing Scientific Directorate system within each institute of the NIH.[86] Healy stated that many of the "morale problems" plaguing the institutes had come from the gradual entrenchment of a top-down management system where a scientific director appointed by the BSC reviewed and made decisions on all intramural research—a system Healy characterized as "positively dictatorial."[87] Healy and her committee imagined trans-NIH faculties as a way to get senior scientists who were shut out of decision making under the Scientific Directorate system involved in bureaucratic work that would give them a role in guiding the future of the NIH as well as their home institutes. Though the Scientific Directorates promised to implement the recommendations set forth in the Klausner Report, they insisted the proposed faculties not compete with their authority.[88] Many rank-and-file scientists in the NIH, however, feared the Klausner Report would accomplish little besides adding another layer of bureaucracy to the institutes.[89]

Immediately on the heels of debates over the Klausner Report, the Senate recommended in its report for fiscal year 1994 that the NIH commission a more far-reaching review of its intramural program.[90] NIH director Harold Varmus, who succeeded Healy in 1993, established an Extramural Advisory Committee (EAC) chaired by extramural scientists Paul Marks and Gail Cassell to examine the intramural activities of the entire NIH. The EAC's final report, issued on April 11, 1994, criticized the "balkanization" of research in the NIH. The report attributed this balkanization to a lack of close relationships between institutes, which resulted in "unevenness in quality, quality control, and productivity" across in-house research efforts.[91] The report was also highly critical of the NIH's failure to adequately implement recommendations made by previous reviews of its intramural structure, such as the Klausner Report.[92] Pointing out that federal funding was faltering and the cost of doing research was rising, the report asked how the NIH could streamline itself in order to translate an increasing number of breakthroughs in biology into clinical application. One major recommendation was to improve the peer review process in the intramural program so that underperforming labs could be shut down and their resources reallocated to projects of greater scientific merit.[93]

Importantly, the staff tasked with implementing the EAC report's recommendations interpreted its discussion of a need for consistent planning procedures for the allocation of resources between intramural and extramural programs as a call for periodic review of each institute's intramural program.[94] These periodic reviews began with the NCI, where Varmus assembled an ad hoc working group chaired by NCAB members Paul Calabresi and J. Michael Bishop to review the institute's intramural program. Though initially tasked with reviewing both the scientific program as well as its organizational structure, the working group soon switched gears to focus solely on how the peer review system, scientific leadership, and decision making around the allocation of resources among intramural and extramural projects could best support high-quality science.[95]

When the ad hoc working group presented its findings in what came to be known as the Bishop-Calabresi Report in mid-May 1995, it proved a bombshell. The report found the intramural program to be full of administrative redundancies, fragmented across divisions in ways that stifled collaboration, lacking in vision for prospective planning, lacking in rigorous peer review, and burdened with a hierarchical structure that led to an "inbreeding" of narrow scientific and managerial attitudes.[96] The most radical suggestion contained in the report involved splitting up the intramural and extramural administrative functions, which were then comingled within the same divisions, and consolidating the intramural program into only two smaller divisions.[97] One of the two new divisions would focus on basic biology and cancer etiology, the other on prevention and treatment.[98] Translational research would be one of the basic tenets of the new intramural structure.[99]

The NCI was in a unique position to implement such a radical plan for reorganization. Just as the Bishop-Calabresi committee was conducting its study, three high-ranking scientist-bureaucrats left the NCI. The first to depart was Richard Adamson, director of the Division of Cancer Etiology, in August of 1994. Next was Bruce Chabner, director of the Division of Cancer Treatment, who resigned in October. Finally, NCI director Samuel Broder announced his resignation in December of 1994. Even before Broder announced his departure, NIH director Varmus cited the "leadership vacuum" left by Adamson and Chabner's resignations as an important opportunity to reorganize the NCI pending the findings of the Bishop-Calabresi committee.[100]

When J. Michael Bishop dropped out of the running for the NCI directorship in April of 1995, it became clear that Richard Klausner was likely to be nominated.[101] Klausner's position on "reinventing" the intramural program in his eponymous report suggested he would be amenable to major bureaucratic restructuring. Klausner did not disappoint; on August 2, 1995, one day after taking office, Klausner announced his plans to consolidate the intramural program in a town hall meeting on the NIH campus.[102] Klausner's plan involved restructuring the NCI's formal organization by moving from a structure where the vast majority of both intramural and extramural research programs were shared across four divisions (Cancer Etiology; Cancer Biology, Diagnosis and Centers; Cancer Treatment; and Cancer Prevention and Control) to a structure where the intramural program was split between two divisions (Basic Sciences and Clinical Sciences), the extramural program distributed across three thematic divisions similar to those that had existed before (Cancer Prevention and Control; Cancer Treatment, Diagnosis and Centers; Cancer Biology), and where one hybrid intramural/extramural Division of Cancer Epidemiology and Genetics would be established. Klausner described these changes, which would be effective October 1, 1995, as following the spirit of the NCAB's Bishop-Calabresi Report.[103] Furthermore, he argued that separating the wet labs of the intramural program from work in the clinical center and enabling bureaucratic decision making further down the hierarchy within these divisions would foster collaboration and build the "intellectual infrastructure" necessary for realizing translational research innovations.[104]

To accomplish these reforms, Klausner recommended breaking apart the "increasingly hierarchical" structure under the institute's Scientific Directorate and replacing it with "a flat structure in which many administrative functions will be performed in the laboratories and branches."[105] Under the new organizational structure, the Office of Administrative Management was separated into two distinct offices, one for the Intramural Research Program and the other for extramural affairs. Intramural projects would be overseen by one advisory BSC, comprising one basic science subcommittee and one clinical science and epidemiology subcommittee. The extramural program would retain a more variegated Board of Scientific Advisors (BSA) to review grant applications from external scientists and oversee new policies proposed by the institute before they reached the NCAB. The restructured BSC and BSA would improve representation for clinical and translational researchers in the peer review system at NCI, a move that further cemented translational research into the routine practices of scientist-bureaucrats as well as the membership of governance committees staffed by scientific principals.

A "Culture of Planning" Under Klausner

Though Klausner's vision of the NCI's mission similarly embraced translational research, it differed substantively from Broder's. Whereas Broder had emphasized the communication of findings between laboratory and clinical researchers, Klausner aimed to create environments where teams of scientists from different disciplinary backgrounds regularly collaborated on projects together. Nevertheless, the changes Klausner instituted throughout his tenure as NCI director responded to the work Broder had completed in fundamental ways. In particular, Klausner challenged Broder's practices of funding extramural translational research through set-asides. Instead, Klausner saw the uniquely collaborative environment of the NCI's intramural program as the ideal place to build much-needed translational infrastructure. Klausner's emphasis on multidisciplinary intramural collaboration played a central role in the evolving program for translational research in the NCI under his directorship.

From the beginning, Klausner focused on improving collaboration and long-term planning in the intramural program as the major issue surrounding translational research. Klausner saw the root of these problems in the "perverse incentives" built into a promotion system where leadership positions were distributed on the basis of the number of employees a scientist supervised rather than "the quality of your work and the importance of what you do."[106] His stated goal was to restore the NCI to an organization driven by scientific ideas rather than bureaucratic inertia.[107] To this end, Klausner sought to elevate high-ranking managers and administrators to the level of "folk heroes" whose actions were chiefly in service of scientific goals.[108] Throughout the NCI, Klausner strove to "de-bureaucratize" decision making by delegating authority as closely to the laboratory or clinic as possible.[109] Further, Klausner assembled groups of scientists and administrators from across different divisions to aid in collaboration and instituted several retreats where scientist-bureaucrats could contribute to programming decisions throughout the institute.[110] His goal in dashing hierarchy and distributing decision making was to instill a "culture of planning" in the NCI.[111] He hoped that interdisciplinary translational collaborations would emerge organically as scientists from different laboratories and clinics came into closer contact with one another.

Klausner's efforts toward a more open and transparent strategic planning process in the NCI was credited with helping to improve the "mood on the Hill" toward biomedical research funding, which disease advocates were also working hard to steer toward increased support for the NIH.[112] The mood soon grew so favorable that, in 1997, the Senate passed a nonbinding resolution to double funding for the entire NIH over the course of five years.[113] This resolution passed in the form of a budget amendment in 1998.

The new influx of funds into the NIH gave the NCI much-needed resources to continue building the "fundamental intellectual infrastructure" for translational research that Klausner perceived as sorely lacking.[114] While Broder's early efforts had been directed toward building translational infrastructure through small-scale extramural collaborations and focused cancer centers, Klausner was committed to building a parallel infrastructure in the intramural program. To accomplish this, he focused on making translational research a special emphasis of the new Division of Clinical Sciences (DCS).[115] Klausner's choice to head the DCS, Edison Liu, was brought in to secure this focus. Liu had acted as a principal investigator on a breast cancer SPORE at the University of North Carolina at

Chapel Hill and was determined to open up lines of communication between NCI clinicians and basic scientists that reflected his experiences in academia.[116] Learning from the SPORE model, Liu consolidated a number of laboratories in the DCS after taking office in an effort to generate a "critical mass" of investigators that would design innovative clinical trials around specific disease targets rather than disciplinary focus.[117] Additionally, Liu initiated a series of working groups, consortia, and awards to encourage collaboration, especially with scientists housed in the neighboring Division of Basic Sciences (DBS).

The NCI's renewed investment in intramural clinical research is particularly notable, both in light of complaints about bias against clinical research in the extramural granting process and in growing anxiety among clinicians that managed-care providers' reluctance to reimburse the cost of care associated with experimental treatments would jeopardize the entire academic clinical trial enterprise.[118] Compounded with a general lack of resources for funding clinical research, extramural trials seemed particularly threatened in the economic climate of the mid to late 1990s.[119] The NCI, on the other hand, was protected from the vagaries of managed care. Intramural clinicians received stable funding and were encouraged to pursue high-risk innovative research. Beginning in 1998, leadership in the DCS met with leadership in the DBS, the Division of Extramural Affairs, and the NCI director every two weeks to coordinate activities within and across NCI divisions.[120] Other programs designed to increase collaboration with industry, such as the Rapid Access to Intervention Development (RAID) program discussed in chapter 7, were also put into motion. Reforms like those implemented by Klausner and Liu made many projects in the DCS more closely resemble SPORE grants by emphasizing direct, multidisciplinary collaboration between laboratory and clinical scientists. In an interesting turn of events, Klausner's restructuring initiative reincorporated the institute's earlier efforts to encourage translational research in the extramural community as the basis for bureaucratic innovations in the intramural program.

Despite these ambitious restructuring efforts and Congress's promised doubling of the NIH budget, funding for the intramural program steadily shrank throughout Klausner's directorship. Between 1996 and 2000, intramural research dropped from 18 percent to 15.3 percent of the overall NCI budget.[121] In part, this reflected cost savings from Klausner's organizational restructuring; administrative streamlining initiatives alone saved more than $4 million by 1997.[122] However, by the close of the 1990s, it appeared that gains in bureaucratic efficiency won by downsizing the intramural program would come at the expense of scientific quality. Rather than fostering collaboration between intramural and extramural management, a review of the separation of intramural and extramural administration found that these 1995 reforms "disrupted communication" and created "redundant functions, confused business processes, and unhealthy competition between administrative units."[123] Management thus needed to be reconsolidated into a single office. Further bureaucratic restructuring had the potential to address a more urgent problem—the vanishing extramural management budget, which had dwindled to around 3 percent of the NCI's expenses.[124] Burdened by excessive workloads and low morale, workers in the extramural grants management units turned over at a rate of 25 percent; considering that 60 percent of the NCI's entire budget went toward extramural research grants, the lack of experience and resources in this unit threatened the basic mission of the NCI.[125]

Klausner was given an opportunity to retool his translational management vision when, as in 1995, a "leadership vacuum" allowed the institute to consider another reorganization of the intramural program. In March 2001, Edison Liu resigned from his post as director of the DCS. Liu's departure opened the door to another radical restructuring of the institute that combined the DCS and DBS into a single Center for Cancer Research (CCR).[126] The goal of the CCR, to be run by DBS director Carl Barrett, would be to develop a "new approach to integrated cancer research linking technology development, basic research, clinical research, and translational research."[127] Consolidation of the DBS and DCS was meant to facilitate translation "by providing a defined process for and support to researchers studying promising targeted treatments," including the creation of interdisciplinary "faculties" comprising both intramural and extramural scientists, new training programs in translational research, and adjunct appointments across laboratories that would enable scientists in different branches to collaborate with greater ease.[128]

Much thought went into the restructuring of the intramural program to better facilitate translational research in the new CCR. Nevertheless, some NCI scientists expressed continued reservations about collaborative and translational work. They felt that peer review still advantaged individual work and did not sufficiently reward translational research. In response to these concerns, Barrett pointed out that "he is seeking to change the way to evaluate investigators not only on their independent research, but also on their transdisciplinary efforts."[129] Beyond the intramural program, NCI leadership acknowledged that "conventional" approaches to research would need to be rethought to achieve effective translation, and that "NCI must help researchers create integrated research environments that foster the multidisciplinary collaborations needed to address the 'big picture' problems in cancer research."[130] The NCI's intramural researchers were in a position to lead the way in modeling translational research practices in the scientific community.

MAKING HPV VACCINES TRANSLATIONAL RESEARCH EXEMPLARS

Richard Klausner was an early and ardent supporter of the NCI's intramural HPV vaccine efforts. Like Broder before him, Klausner treated vaccine-oriented research on HPV as one of the institute's most significant translational undertakings. In September of 1996, less than a year after his appointment, Klausner convened an internal NCI meeting to discuss the institute's role in promoting HPV vaccine development.[131] Klausner would become particularly keen on the collaboration Schiller and Lowy were developing with other epidemiologists in the NCI and soon held up HPV vaccine efforts as exemplary of the kind of cross-divisional interactions he hoped his intramural reforms would encourage.[132]

By 1996, the NCI's phase I findings suggested the vaccine would be safe enough to test on a larger human population. Around this time, Schiller and Lowy initiated a series of collaborations with Mark Schiffman, an intramural NCI epidemiologist at the newly restructured Division for Cancer Epidemiology and Genetics. Schiffman was principal investigator on a study launched in 1993 that aimed to track the natural history of HPV infection in women in Guanacaste, Costa Rica, over seven years. Schiller and Lowy convinced Schiffman to collaborate on modified arms of the Guanacaste trial that would test an assay for HPV antibodies they had developed and, beginning in 1997, would serve as phase II and III trials for their L1 VLP vaccine.[133]

Despite Klausner's formal support of the project, the NCI lacked clear bureaucratic pathways for translating laboratory findings into vaccines. Klausner's enthusiasm for the HPV vaccine effort did not reflect the institute's dominant policy focus when it came to translational research. Instead, NCI leadership was banking on the potential of genomic information to yield new approaches to diagnostics and treatment.[134] As such, Lowy and Schiller continued to depend on their more experienced vaccinologist colleagues at NIAID to guide them through the bureaucratic process of interacting with the FDA to set up human trials.[135]

When it came to executing the trials in Guanacaste, Lowy and Schiller's relationship with Schiffman, as well as the relationship with NCI intramural scientist Allan Hildesheim that developed around their earlier collaborative phase I testing with NIAID, were also essential to their success. As Schiller recalls, these relationships "developed very naturally" in the NCI.[136] Schiller and Lowy were familiar with Schiffman and Hildesheim from routine bureaucratic tasks that involved joint meetings between their divisions in the NCI's extension at Shady Grove, Maryland. When the time came to initiate a scientific collaboration, they found that Klausner's focus on intramural translational research supported and rewarded such collaboration. In turn, NCI leadership would invoke the partnership between Schiller and Lowy's lab and Schiffman and Hildesheim's study as examples of successful translation encouraged by the organizational culture of the NCI.[137] In comparison to the phase I trial for which Schiller and Lowy depended on infrastructure located at Johns Hopkins, the NCI Guanacaste trials illustrate how Klausner's reforms created the means for collaborating to test innovations in-house more easily than in previous years. These reforms, which were done to increase the "intellectual infrastructure" for translating research, incentivized Schiller and Lowy to shift their vaccine efforts inward rather than seeking outside collaborators as they had for earlier testing.[138]

Though Schiller and Lowy could now collaborate with other NCI scientists to test their vaccine technology in human trials, they still relied on cooperation from private firms to develop the vaccine to scale. After promising phase I results, MedImmune transferred its license for the NCI's L1 VLP technology to GlaxoSmithKline (GSK), who would use it to develop Cervarix as a competitor to Merck's Gardasil.[139] Schiller and Lowy chose to use GSK's formulation in their own trials, as the pharmaceutical giant could provide sufficient material to meet their goal of vaccinating up to half of the Guanacaste study cohort of 10,000 women. As Lowy reported, GSK was happy to oblige.[140] Schiller announced the three- to four-year phase II/III Guanacaste trials to the NCAB in 1998, just as the phase I trials at Johns Hopkins were wrapping up.[141]

Collaborative efforts for HPV vaccine development in the NCI would also receive praise for their achievements in clinical trial diversity, a bureaucratic goal that was growing in importance throughout the NIH.[142] As Schiller noted in a 1998 NCAB meeting, the phase I trial at Johns Hopkins included "strong representation" of African American women, and the phase II/III Guanacaste trials enrolled a Latin American population whose circumstances more closely resembled those of the majority of poor women who would die from HPV-related cervical cancer around the globe than those of the enrollees in industry's U.S. or European trials.[143] Following on these trial successes, cervical cancer disparities in the United States, which are particularly striking among African Americans and Latinas, were singled out as the first target for the NCI's newly founded Center to Reduce Cancer Health Disparities in 2001. There was a sense among NCI scientist-bureaucrats that cervical cancer was a problem "we have an answer to" and that disparities among underserved populations were even more striking in the face of a promising prophylactic.[144]

Discussions of HPV vaccine research in the NCI's strategic planning process soon colligated around the issue of these cervical cancer disparities. In the Bypass Budget, the NCI directorate's major annual strategic planning document, the HPV vaccine was promoted as the best strategy for "comprehensively controlling" HPV infection and consequently eliminating health disparities in cervical cancer morbidity and mortality in the United States and abroad.[145] Similarly, the NCI-sponsored Gynecological Cancer Progress Review Group, convened in 2000, determined HPV vaccine development was of highest priority in the field because of its "high-impact" capacity to virtually eliminate cervical cancer worldwide.[146] In both his scientific and bureaucratic capacity, Lowy played a prominent role in the Gynecological Cancer Progress Review Group conferences and report and likely helped shape understandings of the HPV vaccine's public health potential. For NCI strategic planning purposes, the HPV vaccine was being reimagined as a technical innovation that would deliver real reductions in health disparities, both among racial and ethnic minorities and whites in the United States and among developing nations and the developed world.

Given Lowy's prominent role in strategic planning and his continued ascent through the NCI's bureaucratic apparatus, this shift in the language of strategic planning was likely influenced directly by the NCI's intramural vaccine development program. It had certainly been prefigured in the work of the NCI laboratory scientists and their epidemiological collaborators for at least five years prior. As Schiller and Lowy first noted in a 1996 publication, the majority of women who died of cervical cancer lived in developing nations. While Schiller and Lowy maintained that "an effective HPV vaccine may have a greater potential for reducing worldwide cancer burden than any other currently conceived anticancer program" such as routine Pap screening, lack of infrastructure made delivery of the vaccines being developed on the basis of the hepatitis B vaccine model (which utilized technology that required cold chain storage for three doses to be administered over 9–12 months) difficult to implement in these settings.[147] The solution to barriers against vaccination with an L1 VLP vaccine, according to NCI scientist-bureaucrats, was to explore alternative vaccine models more appropriate for resource-poor regions, including naked DNA vaccines, recombinant vaccines using live bacterial vectors, or transgenic plants that would allow VLPs to be ingested as food. However, as Schiller and Lowy noted, none of these different strategies was very well developed at the time. While they continued to discuss these approaches as alternatives better suited for developing nations for another ten years, they consistently cautioned that these technologies had not been demonstrated to be safe or efficacious.[148] Some of them, such as naked DNA vaccines, Schiller admitted to having little faith in as early as 1998.[149]

Yet since scientist-bureaucrats at the NCI had increasingly redefined the stakes of HPV vaccines in terms of *global* cervical cancer inequities, institute resources were put toward creating opportunities to fully explore low-cost vaccine alternatives that were not yet at an appropriate stage for development. These included efforts to develop second-generation vaccine technologies that NCI scientist-bureaucrats saw as extending or complementing ongoing work in the intramural program.[150] For example, the NCI awarded grants to academic collaborations with biotechnology firms exploring second-generation prophylactic HPV vaccines that promised to be "both economical and stable."[151] However, it is worth noting that these alternatives had not reached a stage of development where they could be considered viable until 2003. Even a 26 percent increase in the NCI's investments in novel HPV vaccine research between 2002 and 2003 left these alternative efforts at a major disadvantage vis-à-vis first-generation vaccines: by this time, NCI and industry phase III human trials on the first-generation L1 VLP vaccine were well under way, ensuring these vaccines would have a substantial first-mover advantage in the market.[152]

The results of the NCI's human trials, much like animal trials before them, were immediately very promising.[153] Congress broadly supported the institute's vaccine efforts, encouraging continued and accelerated collaboration within the NCI as well as between the NCI and industry toward the end of manufacturing an effective prophylactic vaccine.[154] With second-generation vaccines still in early development, NCI scientists saw special value in conducting parallel efficacy trials with industry that would test first-generation vaccines using protocols designed and controlled by the institute. Throughout the phase II and III Guanacaste trials, the NCI team continued to track women who had violated the three-shot protocol rather than dropping them from the study, which they assumed drug companies would do (in this case, Merck continued to follow protocol violators in at least one trial).[155] Schiller argued that only government trials could afford to follow protocol violators because they were not motivated by profit.[156] Though not strictly correct in this instance, such beliefs about the NCI's role as a supplementary force in vaccine research and development were important motivators for conducting follow-ups. The NCI's follow-ups showed that even women who failed to complete more than the first shot in the three-shot protocol showed antibody titers sufficient to suggest protection against the targeted HPV strains up to seven years after administration. Their findings led Schiller and Lowy to advocate for further research on a one-shot protocol for the first-generation vaccine as the most logistically practical and cost-effective alternative for vaccinating women in developing countries.[157] As the horizon for manufacturing generics for the vaccine in low-income countries became murkier around the World Trade Organization's 1994 Trade-Related Aspects of Intellectual Property (TRIPS) agreement, a reduced one-shot protocol allowed an alternative means of designing cost-effective HPV vaccination campaigns in developing nations that would address the global health stakes of the vaccine technology.[158]

By the time Merck's Gardasil was approved by the FDA in 2006, it had also become clear to administrators in the NCI, like then director John Niederhuber, that the purpose of continued vaccine development efforts was to extend coverage to underserved populations throughout the globe.[159] The vaccine was quickly held up by NCI scientist-bureaucrats as a "true example of translational research."[160] Testifying before Congress in 2006, Niederhuber insisted that the HPV vaccine could make a huge impact on cancer rates in the middle- and low-income countries that bear the greatest burden of HPV disease.[161] For NCI leadership, the story of HPV vaccine innovation illustrated how "basic discoveries arising from population studies, molecular biology, and immunology can be rapidly translated through public and private research efforts to solve significant public health problems, and in this case, perhaps the elimination of cervical cancer as a threat to women's health."[162]

CONCLUSION

One of the consistent sources of inspiration for the NCI's ongoing efforts at building a translational research infrastructure came from concomitant efforts by intramural scientists to develop and test a novel HPV vaccine. The distinctive approach to translational research emerging in the NCI's intramural research program allowed scientist-bureaucrats to interpret their efforts as offering countervailing or supplementary approaches to HPV vaccine development and testing as they imagined it to proceed in industry. It also allowed them to interpret the possibilities for developing HPV vaccines as serving the public good in accordance with the situational affordances of the technical, organizational, and institutional environments in which they conducted research.

Historians and sociologists of science have studied the complex political and cultural dimensions of HPV vaccination and associated cervical cancer prevention regimes.[163] However, few scholars have investigated the innovation processes that led to the technology that made the vaccines possible in the first place. This has left little room to combat suggestions that the design of the HPV vaccine primarily reflects the goals of a profit-oriented industry.[164] Yet this narrative conflates the process of initial development and the commercial product that emerged from necessary collaborations with private industry, which commands the nation's sole infrastructure for scalable vaccine production.

Though its investments in upstream research and testing are substantial, the United States has no federally funded production apparatus for manufacturing vaccines on an industrial scale.[165] As such, the government's ability to ensure scalable supplies of vaccines is dependent on the participation of private pharmaceutical companies. This configuration has been the status quo in vaccine research and development since the country began its first concerted vaccine R&D efforts; even during World War II, the military's capacity to produce sufficient supplies of vaccines and antibiotics was predicated upon the provision of contracts to private companies who worked at the behest of the nation. The pharmaceutical industry's willingness to produce vaccines primarily for consumption by the U.S.

government, once couched in the rhetoric of patriotic duty to the war effort, continued throughout the immediate postwar period as voluntarist contributions to national growth offered an economic policy counter to "communistic" state-directed research and development apparatus.[166]

But the 1990s followed on a period of precipitous decline in industry investment in vaccine research and development. Between 1967 and 1979, the number of pharmaceutical manufacturers in the United States halved; of the eighteen remaining American companies, only eight continued to produce vaccines.[167] Pharmaceutical manufacturers cited concerns over excessive federal regulation and liability litigation as major financial disincentives to continue producing vaccines, products with notoriously slender profit margins.[168] A consensus report issued by the Institute of Medicine and National Research Council in 1985 cautioned that "the availability of vaccines for public use depends entirely on the willingness of commercial manufacturers to undertake production. Numerous studies over the past two decades have raised the concern that our reliance on market incentives to ensure vaccine availability may lead to a failure to meet public health needs. Also, these incentives may not result in optimal levels of vaccine innovation."[169]

The prospect of market failure in vaccine production loomed large despite evidence that concerns over the profitability of vaccine products were overblown. In fact, Kendall Hoyt has shown that "traditional market-based formulas for innovation in industrial settings predict that greater economic incentives, technological opportunities, and firm capabilities in the latter half of the twentieth century should have led to a corresponding rise in innovations rates. Yet the data demonstrate a decline."[170] Declining vaccine innovation rates in industry suggest that many of the successful efforts the nation has seen in vaccine innovation may have instead been driven by nonmarket incentives—such as those enshrined in the scientific and bureaucratic culture of the NCI.

NCI scientists and clinicians consistently reported attention to the public health stakes of their research, first in relation to translation and, later, global disease reduction. The NCI's role in vaccine research and clinical testing shows the importance that government research played in determining the design of first-generation HPV vaccines. In addition to cross-licensing their patent through bureaucratic innovations that had been designed to foster market competition and drive down prices, NCI scientist-bureaucrats would continue their involvement in clinical testing on the basis of their assumption that only a government institute unconcerned with profit had the ability to collect more complete data on the vaccine. These interpretations of the NCI's mission reflect learning outcomes related to previous innovations such as nucleoside analogs and in turn would influence both the design of HPV vaccine research and the ongoing reconstruction of translational research in the intramural program. They would continue to inform the institute's conception of its role in public-health-relevant research and development as the political environment shifted in the new millennium.

CHAPTER 7

FROM ROADMAP TO MOONSHOT, 2002–2016

At the dawn of the new millennium, NCI scientist-bureaucrats had laid a solid foundation for developing translational research as a policy paradigm and a guide for cancer research practice. New models for funding innovative research, such as the Specialized Programs of Research Excellence (SPORE), offered many of the institute's most vocal public and political constituents a promising standard for realizing improvements in outcomes for the most deadly and intractable cancers in the United States. The doubling of the NIH budget coalesced with a seeming flood of emerging findings from across the life sciences, including the much-hyped Human Genome Project, to spur scientific and public optimism that new technologies for detecting, preventing, or treating cancer were just on the horizon.[1] Yet the NCI's political and scientific environment would shift quickly in the first years of the twenty-first century, as the administration of President George W. Bush brought a more austere fiscal attitude toward federal biomedical funding, driven by a desire to expand the role that private commercial entities played in executing the functions of government. The Bush administration installed a sympathetic cancer surgeon, Dr. Andrew von Eschenbach, as the new NCI director in service of this cause.

As NCI director, von Eschenbach would go against the scientific and bureaucratic grain of his predecessors in many respects, and his legacy as director would be marked by ignominy and failure. Though failure can often be overdetermined, this chapter explores von Eschenbach's legacy in light of his lack of familiarity with the organizational culture and practices of the NCI and his commitment to a conception of the organization's mission that was alien to the ways NCI scientist-bureaucrats and their principals defined the institute's dual mandate.

Scholars of scientific organizations have often attributed the success of scientific leaders to their effective socialization into the distinctive cultures of research as practiced in their organizations.[2] More recently, economists and historians have persuasively demonstrated that a similar socialization process among the cohort of scientists who became Public Health Service commissioned officers and served under intramural scientists as NIH associates during the Vietnam War led this cohort to experience long-lasting career advantages attributable to their early training in the NIH.[3] These scholars have argued that something distinctive to the environment for inquiry provided by the NIH enabled this cohort of "Yellow Berets" (so called because the position exempted them from the draft) to subsequently ascend to dominant positions in their scientific fields, as indicated by the unusual number who went on to earn Nobel Prizes.[4] Given that intramural scientists who spent their careers in the NCI have also been innovative, this outcome is more than a mere selection effect of talented scientists into the NIH associates program. The closeness with which scientific and bureaucratic tasks are bound for those intramural scientists who ascend to positions of leadership in the NCI enables the distinctive scientific environment found in the NIH's intramural programs and informs scientist-bureaucrats' distinctive and efficacious leadership styles, which may in turn exert an "influence effect" that helps explain the scientific and leadership success of even visiting associates such as the Yellow Berets.[5]

Throughout the history of the NCI, the majority of the institute's directors were practicing intramural scientist-bureaucrats in the NIH. This status would have socialized them into that distinct environment of intramural research they carried through into their bureaucratic practices. Past directors' successes in both intramural scientific and policy leadership stand out in stark contrast to von Eschenbach, an outsider who had spent his career in academic medicine and entered the directorship with an administrative vision inspired by corporate business literature. His plans to reshape the structure and culture of the NCI to reflect corporate management trends were at odds with the well-established interpretations of the institute's dual mission shared by other scientist-bureaucrats and even with the NCI's scientific and congressional advisors. The lack of fit between von Eschenbach's vision and the NCI's culture was attributable not only to philosophical differences between the presidentially appointed outsider and NCI scientist-bureaucrats but also to his apparent lack of recognizable managerial and scientific competence relative to the expectations cultivated by past institute leaders. Presidential patronage appointments to federal bureaucracies often invite concerns about the competence and effectiveness of appointees in comparison to that of career bureaucrats in the same agencies, and President George W. Bush famously confronted accusations of incompetence among many of his agency appointees.[6] What makes the von Eschenbach directorate stand out relative to prior NCI directorships is how important an interpretation of the scientific issues and stakes around the NCI's dual mission is to the performance of bureaucratic competence in this expert agency. In fundamental ways, the new director failed to formulate a vision for the NCI that was plausible in light of agency personnel's ongoing scientific and bureaucratic practices and their understandings of themselves as both scientists and public servants.

Analyzing the mismatch between von Eschenbach's pro-business policies and the NCI's culture also allows us to correct several misconceptions about the historical emergence of translational research. Though von Eschenbach was committed to opening more space for private commercial actors in the NCI, the coincidence of his leadership with the institute's role in helping craft important translational research policy, such the NIH Roadmap for Medical Research, should not be taken as evidence that these policies reflected a similar commitment to neoliberalism. Indeed, many of the key programs that served as blueprints for translational research policy during the NIH Roadmap era predate von Eschenbach's business-friendly directorship. Instead, these NCI programs emerged during the leadership of Directors Broder and Klausner, who were responding to perceived barriers to translational research in ways that addressed long-standing disconnects between the public capacity to produce innovations in government and university labs and the private infrastructure necessary for their commercial production. In particular, the Rapid Access to Intervention Development (RAID) program initiated during Klausner's directorship provided a model that inspired key programs in the NIH Roadmap for Medical Research. Thus, rather than advancing a coherent translational research policy subscribing to the neoliberal argument that market forces were superior to inefficient government agencies, the NIH Roadmap was informed by programs that were developed in part to address the limitations of the private sector in supporting successful translation.

Nor should the favorable attitude of the NCI director suggest that industry did in fact gain a foothold in the NCI during his administration. In several instances where von Eschenbach's market-friendly directorate attempted to incorporate special interests into policy decisions, actors on the National Cancer Advisory Board (NCAB) and NCI scientist-bureaucrats complained of a lack of information and communication from commercial interests about their preferences—which rules out the structural configuration obtaining in instances of regulatory capture where an agency "is overly responsive to the recommendations of regulated interests."[7] Instead, NCI scientist-bureaucrats' policy decisions remained largely informed by a combination of their experiences managing programs in the organization coupled with their understandings of how the NCI's mission gave the organization a distinctive position in the biomedical research economy.

ANDREW VON ESCHENBACH INHERITS AN ACCOUNTABILITY PROBLEM

NCI director Richard Klausner's reforms at the turn of the twenty-first century were explicitly aimed at achieving the goal of translational research in and through the institute. More so than in his first years at the helm, Klausner was working with a coherent understanding of what translational research entailed: collaborative, interdisciplinary efforts to rapidly move cutting-edge innovations into clinical testing.[8] Klausner fully embraced the oversight function of entities such as the NCAB, which he felt helped the NCI focus on its "top priority" of translational research.[9] Outside the NCI, however, calls for accountability were taking on an increasingly urgent tone. The extensive coalition of lobbyists and members of Congress who had succeeded in passing legislation to double the NIH budget in 1998 were also pushing for more translational research policies, with Congress explicitly urging the NCI to build better infrastructure and eliminate roadblocks to translation.[10] With the budget doubling well under way, such admonitions became more frequent, and calls for greater accountability in the use of government funds originated from more diverse sources. One surprising source was former NCI director Vincent DeVita. DeVita, backed by the American Cancer Society (ACS), argued that a sufficient knowledge base existed to begin delegating authority for developing intervention efforts outside the NCI (the Centers for Disease Control and Prevention was the favored competitor).[11] Klausner heartily disagreed, urging that the NCI's dual mission still necessitated further investment in and more careful stewardship of basic research.[12]

It was clear nonetheless that the influx of funds into the NCI consequent from the doubling of the NIH budget was creating a greater need to justify status quo expenditures on research. Early in 2001, the House Committee on Science warned of its expectation that the budget doubling would require the NIH to demonstrate "accountability" in its use of these taxpayer funds.[13] While Klausner saw the NCI's substantial investment in translational research as an indicator that the institute was doing its best to use government funds wisely, the recent election of conservative Republican president George W. Bush forecast fiscal retrenchment measures that could hobble high-risk federal investments in science. Fatefully, Klausner resigned on September 11, 2001, minutes before announcing to the NCAB that two planes had hit the World Trade Center in New York.[14]

President Bush would shortly thereafter appoint Andrew von Eschenbach (figure 7.1) as Klausner's replacement, and many would come to believe that the new director politicized the NCI in ways not seen since the War on Cancer first began. At von Eschenbach's swearing-in ceremony as director of the NCI, President's Cancer Panel chair Harold P. Freeman punctuated the mood

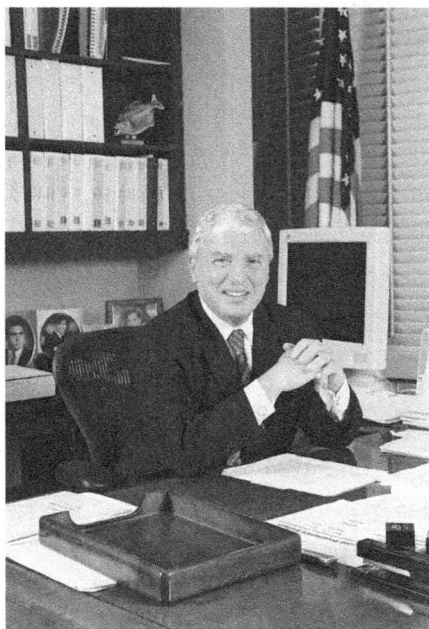

7.1 Andrew von Eschenbach in 2005.

Photo credit: Linda Bartlett, National Cancer Institute.

by drawing direct parallels between post-9/11 America and the setting during Nixon's presidency:

> President Bush declared a War against Terror about 30 days ago. President Nixon declared a War against Cancer about 30 years ago. The confluence of these events is something that I have thought about. We have made extraordinary advances in biomedical science over the last 30 years since the declaration of war against cancer, and America should be very proud of that progress. What we are facing now though, I think, is the need to expand that war, as we would in a military war, to cover all of the people of America. . . . Despite the great advances in science, we believe that there is a critical disconnect in America between what we discover and what we deliver to the American people. And that disconnect in itself is a cause of disparities. This is not just a medical and scientific issue, but in fact it is more than that. It is an ethical challenge for this great nation—a moral and ethical issue.[15]

Freeman concluded his speech by expressing his hope that von Eschenbach would prove the kind of leader who could leverage innovative research to address these cancer disparities. Freeman's focus had been then, as ever, on the disproportionate burden of cancer morbidity and mortality on America's marginalized racial and ethnic communities. It was not evident that most in NCI leadership shared such an overarching concern for equity. Nevertheless, they did share Freeman's optimism that translational research could serve as the mechanism for realizing important health gains in America.

Optimism that von Eschenbach would continue to nurture translational research at the NCI may have been high in part because the new director's prior academic research on biomarkers could be seen as leveraging discoveries to enable early detection of tumors.[16] Yet unlike his immediate predecessors, von Eschenbach was a complete outsider to the federal government. The surgeon came from a twenty-five-year career on the faculty of MD Anderson. More recently, he helped found the National Dialogue on Cancer, an organization that was overseen by former president George H. W. Bush and former first lady Barbara Bush. The National Dialogue on Cancer argued that enough research had been done on the biology of cancer and that it was time to ensure this science was put to use in developing new treatments. Von Eschenbach had also been president-elect of the increasingly oppositional American Cancer Society immediately preceding his selection as the new NCI director; this saw him leading the organization at a time when tensions between the ACS and NCI were high.

In a speech before the NCAB, the new director graciously promised to "build upon the programmatic infrastructure" of his predecessor Klausner, though he emphasized his own vision of translational research as one oriented toward application of extant cancer knowledge: "I will look forward to complementing what has gone on before by focusing specifically on the continued development of new knowledge and the translation of that knowledge into more effective interventions that will be directly applied to patients."[17] In an interview with *Cancer Letter*, he elaborated: "what I would like to add, is to help continue to promote the focus on not just nurturing the base and developing and promoting it, but also accentuating the complementary, translational piece, the creation of products, so to speak. To really enhance our portfolio of biologic-based interventions that have to do with prevention, treatment, as well as detection and diagnosis."[18] With the NIH budget doubling nearly complete, von Eschenbach envisioned such a turn toward corporate-style portfolio management as demanding a fresh approach to leadership that would "go beyond" the traditional budgeting and strategic planning mechanisms that had long formed the backbone of accountability and governance in the institute.[19]

Von Eschenbach's 2015 Goal

On the one-year anniversary of his first NCAB meeting, von Eschenbach reflected upon the recent statement by President George W. Bush that the War on Cancer was, for the first time in history, winnable. To this end, and in an effort to cement a new leadership role for the NCI in American cancer research under his directorship, von Eschenbach announced a "Challenge Goal" to "eliminate the suffering and death due to cancer, and to do it by 2015."[20]

The 2015 Challenge Goal was focused on what he called the "Three D's" of discovery, development, and delivery. Von Eschenbach proclaimed the Three D's would now "shape our mission and shape our vision" for long-term strategic planning in the NCI, which spurred innovation by targeting "aggressive, ambitious goals."[21] Von Eschenbach described a "roadmapping enterprise" that allowed the institute to identify areas of opportunity that could enable the ultimate fulfillment of the 2015 Challenge Goal. He noted how the NCI's efforts were also aimed at addressing ongoing NIH-wide roadmapping exercises and acknowledged that the NCI played a "critical leadership role" in reforms under way at the NIH and across the Department of Health and Human Services.

The reporting on this NCAB meeting by *Cancer Letter* was less than enthusiastic about von Eschenbach's 2015 Challenge Goal. Commentators noted that "von Eschenbach is taking a controversial step in a field that has a history of unrealistic promises."[22] The director's bold maneuver was met with a profound silence from the NCAB audience and the cancer community at large (including the ACS and "several oncologists and cancer activists" who declined to comment).[23] At the next NCAB meeting, this silence yielded to a flurry of pointed criticisms. Upon soliciting questions about the goal, von Eschenbach heard from distinguished NCAB members that the goal lacked: "realism," including viable metrics for the outcome of "eliminating suffering"; accountability for meeting benchmarks among NCI leadership; and potential to transform industry and regulatory practices to facilitate rapid approval of therapies. Scientific principals also critiqued the goal as inadequately articulated to public stakeholders and inattentive to the complexity of biological and political realities. The director's rejoinder, which largely entailed explaining the basic progression of cancer to a room full of distinguished oncologists and gesturing in a general way toward promising "strategic opportunities in the portfolio" at each point in this progression, may reasonably have been received as inadequate in addressing such serious concerns.[24]

When interviewed about the 2015 Challenge Goal after its announcement, the historian of science Robert Cook-Deegan commented that "eliminating cancer seems pretty out there, and unless the challenges are really well grounded in the science or technology, I fear that what it incites is regret in 2016."[25] He cautioned that, "to the degree that credibility matters—and I think it does—this is a dangerous game" von Eschenbach was playing.[26]

Von Eschenbach's credibility would in fact tarnish, though the unrealistic ambition of the 2015 Challenge Goal was rather a symptom than the underlying cause, which was a disconnect between von Eschenbach's vision and that of the NCI's scientist-bureaucrats and scientific principals. As it turned out, the 2015 Challenge Goal was "based on the agenda of the National Dialogue on Cancer," which von Eschenbach cofounded with George and Barbara Bush prior to being appointed head of the NCI by their son.[27] Throughout his tenure as NCI director, von Eschenbach maintained strong ties to the National Dialogue on Cancer that provoked concerns over conflict of interest and raised questions about his commitment to the NCI's standard policies and practices.[28] Not only did von Eschenbach substitute his own conception of the organization for the one shared by NCI career scientist-bureaucrats, he also insulated himself from their potential criticism by hiring a new team to populate the NCI Office of the Director. Many members of this team, such as Anna Barker and Mark Clanton, had personal connections with von Eschenbach or his former organizations, especially the National Dialogue on Cancer. The approaches cultivated in these organizations were distinct from, and often critical of, the NCI's typical approach to supporting cancer research and development. Thus, despite von Eschenbach's attempts to "overlay" his planning vision across extant administrative practices—and even numerous retreats oriented toward enlisting NCI leadership into his efforts to "synergize" and "streamline" the organization—the directorate's emerging management perspective sat in uneasy tension with scientist-bureaucrats' long-established conceptions of the NCI's mission.[29]

In one particularly consequential example, Anna Barker, whom von Eschenbach had brought in to serve in a new deputy directorship for strategic scientific initiatives position, announced the approval in March 2003 of a concept for the Academic Public-Private Partnership Program (AP4). The topic of industry collaboration had long been on the agenda of the research team Barker headed with von Eschenbach at the National Dialogue on Cancer, and there was some speculation that National Dialogue on Cancer agendas influenced AP4 much in the way they seemed to shape the 2015 Challenge Goal.[30] Though it may have reflected antecedent priorities of von Eschenbach and his cadre, AP4 was formally modeled after the National Science Foundation's Industrial/University Cooperative Research Centers, which provided funding and institutional support for collaborative translational research initiatives aimed at developing commercial cancer therapies for "underserved" cancers.[31] As Barker noted of the program, "these kinds of partnerships . . . can reduce the risk to the private sector"—effectively by shifting the risk of failed drugs from biotechnology and pharmaceutical companies to government and nonprofit academic and medical research facilities.[32] While the AP4 program was understood as a valuable tool for motivating the kinds of multi-institutional research and development collaborations necessary for successful drug development by many extramural scientists on the Board of Scientific Advisors (BSA) who approved the concept, Barker also presented it as a crucial initiative in meeting the 2015 Challenge Goal. The objective was to enable basic researchers working in government and academia to serve up targets for drug companies to develop. "Targeting has to pay off for us, actually, to hit our 2015 goals," she insisted.[33]

In shifting risk from private companies to public universities and government, AP4 exemplified the logic of neoliberal policies that were business friendly because they de-risked the research and development investments made by the private sector. Yet the ultimate approval of AP4 did not come without significant pushback from scientific principals on the BSA. Several BSA members raised significant concerns about the role private companies would play in such an enterprise. Reflecting upon an earlier report to the board by von Eschenbach on budget cuts that warned of looming fiscal constraints related to the mounting conflict with Iraq, BSA member Mack Roach argued that "when you have less money available . . . I feel a little uncomfortable being enthusiastic about an intellectual property nightmare and an underserved disease entity." Even if industry found such a program attractive enough to participate in and developed a successful commercial drug, Roach questioned, "what [would] the public get back out of" public-private ventures of the kind proposed?[34] Given their role in ensuring accountability to the NCI's dual mission, advisory board members such as Roach were skeptical that the possible outcomes of AP4 would best serve the public good. Scientific principals experienced in collaborating with industry were also skeptical of von Eschenbach's interpretation of the technical promise of AP4 in meeting his Challenge Goal. As BSA member William Kaelin asserted, "frankly, by historical standards, [the next generation of drug targets] should be on the blackboard now if we're going to have drugs to meet the 2015 deadline."[35] The contentious nature of these advisory board meetings offered early signs that von Eschenbach's approach was in misalignment with the practices that customarily characterized governance in the institute.

In a confrontational interview with Kirsten Boyd Goldberg and Paul Goldberg of *Cancer Letter*, von Eschenbach defended his 2015 Challenge Goal from what the periodical characterized as widespread skepticism among cancer researchers. The Goldbergs asserted that "the controversy comes in when you say 2015, because you are out on a limb. Your two predecessors in this office [Broder and Klausner] have specifically said, 'I am not making any predictions.' Other predecessors of yours have made predictions, with not the best outcomes for themselves."[36] Von Eschenbach defended the goal as necessary to "catalyze" collaborative research so the cancer research community could "rapidly accelerate the development of all of these opportunities and interventions" emerging from basic research.[37] In response to continued pushback that the 2015 Challenge Goal proposed to address "one of the greatest mysteries of the universe,"[38] von Eschenbach gestured obliquely to the need to "rapidly accelerate and catalyze" the existing science "in a collaborative and integrative way."[39] Such responses in turn elicited a query from the Goldbergs as to where von Eschenbach was getting his scientific advice.[40]

As became abundantly clear (due in no small part to *Cancer Letter's* investigative reporting), the National Dialogue on Cancer (renamed C-Change in 2004) was the source of many of von Eschenbach and his hand-picked office's controversial management strategies. The National Dialogue on Cancer, which deliberated behind closed doors and was the subject of ongoing concerns over transparency and illegal use of federal funds for government lobbying, was "together with the NCI . . . proposing fundamental changes" to American cancer research policy.[41] In addition to providing an external network from which von Eschenbach could hire loyal supporters into his administration, "the Dialogue set the stage for NCI Director Andrew von Eschenbach's controversial policies based on his 'challenge goal' to end suffering and death from cancer by the year 2015."[42]

Early in his directorship, von Eschenbach made clear through several actions that he was willing to commit the institute to various initiatives without consultation with intramural leaders or even advisory committees.[43] His Executive Committee filled out senior positions with external hires, even as he struggled to recruit personnel to major scientific management positions within the intramural program.[44] Indeed, von Eschenbach stated that he relied on long-standing intramural leadership to "[afford] me the opportunity of not having to immediately address organizational restructuring, but rather to really help focus more importantly on the future of the institution"—i.e., to develop the 2015 Challenge Goal.[45] By 2004, when private-sector outsourcing initiatives from the Office of Management and Budget were pressuring major downsizing of the NCI's full-time employees, von Eschenbach hired thirty-three new staff members to his Office of the Director, growing this unit to 25 percent of the institute's total employees.[46] In 2004, von Eschenbach created a new slate of deputy director positions that established "a new management structure between himself and the divisions," half of which positions he filled with his former National Dialogue on Cancer associates Barker and Clanton.[47] Von Eschenbach—who began referring to his position as the "CEO" of the NCI[48]—thus created a climate where he operated alongside a loyal executive team and remained relatively insulated from decision making among NCI scientist-bureaucrats employed in the institute's many laboratories and clinics.

Coupled with this structural insulation of von Eschenbach's Office of the Director and his continued refusal to abide by standard rules of propriety for government employees, von Eschenbach's leadership took on a cast of ignominy around the 2015 Challenge Goal. Though the tone of *Cancer Letter's* reporting on the 2015 Challenge Goal was always decidedly skeptical, this skepticism was reciprocated by members of the scientific community and NIH "insiders" who were "unable to point to any expression of support for von Eschenbach's goal" throughout the institutes.[49] Instead, the 2015 Challenge Goal came to embody von Eschenbach's failure to articulate his policy goals in accordance with reasonable and valid interpretations of the issues and stakes of the NCI's dual mission as enacted in the practices of institute scientist-bureaucrats.[50] Symbolic of his lack of integration into institute culture, von Eschenbach's statements on the 2015 Challenge Goal and his responses to criticisms changed very little over the duration of his directorship. He appeared to have developed a script around the Three D's and stuck closely to his "stump speech" in public engagements and in official communications and administrative planning and budgeting documents.[51] Tellingly, the director "who often resorts to imagery from books on business strategy" seemed to take away more from off-handed comments made by the likes of Bush-appointed NCAB member and conservative lobbyist David Koch than from interactions with institute staff.[52] Far from advancing the NCI's mission as intramural scientists understood it, "von Eschenbach's agenda has involved loosening regulations governing clinical research, lowering the bar for approval of cancer drugs, and privatizing tissue collection."[53]

Yet it was not the incredible hubris of the 2015 Challenge Goal in itself that led von Eschenbach to embody the failure of this new business-friendly NCI. His failure was a collective achievement that aggregated over time and across a series of performances by NCI staff and advisory bodies acting in opposition to the director's goals. This opposition had material consequences for scientific management in instances such as the BSA's refusal to fund a large proteomics initiative designed by von Eschenbach and his officers under the guise of meeting the 2015 goal. In "framing the focus" of the proteomics initiative in relation to rapidly developing a useful serum-screening test that could help meet the 2015 goal, the directorate made itself vulnerable to accusations like those of BSA member Tom Curran, who expressed reservations that the proposed initiative was "overpromising to the public" that revolutionary results would rapidly emerge "in a relatively short period of time" from a field that was itself in an early stage of development.[54] The NCI's scientific principals clearly disagreed with von Eschenbach's definition of what was at issue in proteomics research, just as they were at variance with his definitions of the stakes of cancer research expressed in the 2015 goal.

The policy issues offered to justify the program, which related to the need to build infrastructure that would unify a "cottage industry" in order to create the conditions from which proteomics innovations would later issue, were similar to the rationale NCI scientist-bureaucrats had successfully used to justify similar "big science" programs in the past. Such examples included the targeted virus programs discussed in chapters 2 and 3, which were approved at a time when there was no concrete evidence that a human cancer virus existed. Yet in this instance, the decision by von Eschenbach's Office of the Director to present the proteomics initiative as necessary to meeting the 2015 Challenge Goal proved fatal. Framed in relation to the stakes of the Challenge Goal, the inherent uncertainty of any such infrastructure-building enterprise was amplified by a hard deadline for yielding innovations. BSA member Jane Weeks pointedly criticized the proteomics initiative as underdeveloped in relation to its objective of leveraging patient specimens to develop early screening technologies—which Anna Barker acknowledged as one of the major achievements that would be necessary for meeting von Eschenbach's 2015 goal.[55] Von Eschenbach, who attended the meeting, was visibly perturbed and impatient to defend the strategic importance of this "infrastructure" project. He was forced instead to listen as a strong contingency of the board questioned the wisdom of using taxpayer monies to fund a "big science" project with vague goals. When one supportive member of the BSA, in an attempt to rescue the project, asked, "Can I make a motion to approve the concept in general," BSA chairman Robert Young responded with a vigorous head shake: "No. No, you cannot."[56]

At the same time the NCI's budget flattened under pressure from the Bush administration, von Eschenbach doubled down before congressional principals on his optimism that an end to suffering and death from cancer was imminent. Responding to a line of questioning from Senator Arlen Specter in May 2005, von Eschenbach suggested that an additional appropriation of $600 million per year would allow the NCI to meet its 2015 Challenge Goal in 2010.[57] While the Senate was finally swayed to provisionally endorse the goal (pending proof of sufficient progress since the War on Cancer in 1971), von Eschenbach's soaring rhetoric may have finally put too great a distance between his ambitions and the expectations of federal scientists.[58] Though von Eschenbach had excluded career NCI scientist-bureaucrats, including division directors in the intramural program, from informing budget proposals such as these, NIH advisors forced von Eschenbach to walk back his 2010 commitment in his official statement to Congress.[59] In the meantime, rumors continued to swirl that von Eschenbach's administration had created a "climate of fear among NCI staff and advisors."[60] NCI employees could not criticize the goal without risking accusations of "disloyalty," and a prevailing sense emerged among intramural scientists that they had to toe the party line on the 2015 Challenge Goal if they were to secure funding for any new proposals.[61] Morale understandably suffered: "'Some say, 'Let's hang in there and get the work done.' Most people here are dedicated," an NCI staff member said. "But there is a lot of worry about how NCI is going. You slide down too far, and it takes years to recover."[62]

The carefully cultivated culture of silence around frustration with von Eschenbach eventually broke out into "open resistance" shortly after President George W. Bush appointed him head of the FDA while he was still serving as NCI director.[63] The conflict of interest provoked concern from members of Congress and outrage from the media; von Eschenbach's timing involved him in serious scrutiny of Bush appointees following several accusations of cronyism on the part of those the president selected to occupy other federal positions.[64] In his capacity as chairman of the NCI Board of Scientific Advisors, Robert Young challenged von Eschenbach to clarify the nature of his dual appointment to the FDA and address the possibility of conflicts of interest and commitment.[65] Young's grilling came on the heels of a contentious retreat von Eschenbach held to discuss the NCI's cancer centers program, during which scientists lambasted the 2015 Challenge Goal as unrealistic.[66] The "ridicule" with which the 2015 Challenge Goal had long been greeted by extramural scientists was finally puncturing the bubble in which von Eschenbach had insulated his hand-picked directorate.[67]

Importantly, objections to the 2015 goal were both scientific and bureaucratic and implicated the NCI's competence on both fronts. As former NCI director Vincent DeVita would later remark, the 2015 Challenge Goal "sort of discredited [NCI] setting goals" because "it was so unclear what he actually meant, that it was clear to everybody that nothing of value . . . would ever come of it."[68] The opposition von Eschenbach faced from NCI bureaucrats and board members reflected fundamental disagreement about how the institute should be governed as a scientific agency. The 2015 goal was neither scientifically plausible nor bureaucratically sound in light of how these parties had customarily conceptualized the issues and stakes of translational research in the institute. Subsequent efforts to inform NIH-level planning, which proceeded under the auspices of NCI career scientist-bureaucrats, would better reflect interpretations of the issues and stakes of translational research that emerged from scientific conduct in the intramural program.

ORGANIZATIONAL REFORMS UNDER VON ESCHENBACH

The shift in organizational philosophy that accompanied von Eschenbach's leadership also motivated the director's efforts to restructure the NCI bureaucracy. Von Eschenbach was enamored with the business world and envisioned a leaner, more corporate model for the NCI. He was determined to integrate the institute's strategic planning "with a business plan to ensure a balanced portfolio in terms of opportunities and needs."[69] Fully embracing a portfolio-based approach to funding, which had been introduced in the NIH in the late 1990s as part of President Clinton's "Reinvention" initiatives but anemically implemented by management, von Eschenbach resolved to move strategic planning initiatives "from mechanism-based fund accounting to enterprise accounting."[70] In other words, the NCI would move away from models where specific programs, such as research project grants, were evaluated individually and toward a system that attempted to evaluate the overall performance of the entire agency. This approach reframed accountability in light of management techniques refined in private firms emphasizing increases in shareholder value, a stark departure from the way NCI scientist-bureaucrats and their principals had long interpreted accountability in terms of stewarding scientific investments to improve the health of the American populace. In accordance with this approach, von Eschenbach promised that funding for both intramural and extramural initiatives would be balanced in terms of value for taxpayer investments, with an emphasis on performance-based evaluation, and that the NCI would embrace more high-risk speculative initiatives with potentially larger payoffs.[71]

Despite a long history of collaborations with industry, von Eschenbach was the first NCI director to foreground public-private funding partnerships in management and pursue them aggressively as part of the institute's overall scientific strategy. He proposed private collaborations in the name of developing "synergy" and an "enabling culture" in the cancer community that would help scientists forge partnerships to more effectively bring drugs and diagnostic technologies to market.[72] Yet initiatives to shift expenses to the private sector also emanated from beyond the NCI and affected standard bureaucratic functions in addition to scientific strategy. In 2003, the Office of Management and Budget (OMB) Circular A-76 required institutes within the NIH to survey their administrative units to determine which functions could be put up for bids from private contracting firms.[73] Backlash against the OMB's initiative on the Hill was swift, with U.S. Rep. John Dingell lambasting the drive to outsource administrative labor as serving "right-wing privatization ideology" rather than the interests of science.[74] Alongside sympathetic congressional principals, NCI bureaucrats fought to retain in-house control over administrative functions and ultimately won the competition against private firms. Theirs was a pyrrhic victory—the NCI's winning bid proposed a radical consolidation of administrative functions that included dramatic cuts to full-time employee numbers.[75]

At the same time the NCI culled more than one-quarter of its administrative employees to comply with OMB requirements, von Eschenbach took the liberty of proliferating positions and initiatives that drew directly from the budget of the NCI Office of the Director (OD). He justified adding these new, highly paid administrators as supporting a new "shared governance" model in the OD, where decision making around organizational structure and resource management would be delegated through an enlarged executive committee.[76] The goal was "to broaden and increase the sphere of management of the entire enterprise" so that the goals of discovery, development, and delivery could be better integrated into the NCI's entire research portfolio.[77] In the ensuing years, NCI scientist-bureaucrats would take advantage of two opportunities to shift the institute's portfolio toward a greater emphasis on translational research as they defined it in relation to their routines of scientific research and organizational governance: intramurally, through efforts to "reengineer" the intramural program, and extramurally, through participation in the NIH Roadmap for Medical Research. Despite von Eschenbach's attempts to project a strong head office, these successful initiatives were designed and implemented by scientist-bureaucrats whose articulations of the NCI's mission differed from the director's.

Reengineering the Intramural Research Program

The need to "focus very intensely upon the NCI's internal, intramural program" was central to von Eschenbach's effort to "crystallize and define [the institute's] strategic opportunities . . . [to] add value to the rest of the enterprise." Throughout his announcement of the 2015 Challenge Goal, von Eschenbach gestured toward the role his new executive hires were playing in cementing this approach to strategic planning, enterprise accounting, and "value-added" intramural reforms. Despite the novel language imposed upon these reforms by the new director, their substance often had roots that predated von Eschenbach's entry into the organization. The intramural reforms of the early 2000s thus presented a meeting point between local understandings of translational research rooted in intramural scientific and bureaucratic practices and the novel perspective being cultivated in the OD. In response to criticism of his approach to long-term planning in the institute, von Eschenbach defended the idea that eliminating suffering and death from cancer was at least partially an "engineering problem."[78] It is thus unsurprising that his intense focus on the intramural program circulated around the issue of whether it was necessary to "reengineer" the intramural program to help meet the 2015 Challenge Goal.

In the spring of 2002, the NCI's Center for Cancer Research (CCR) director, Carl Barrett, formally began this reengineering process. Though much of the intramural program had been consolidated into the interdisciplinary CCR in 2000 as part of Klausner's effort to support translational research,[79] the goal of reengineering was to bring the intramural program closer in line with strategic initiatives emanating from the OD by encouraging existing tendencies toward interdisciplinary collaboration and translational research embodied in the CCR's organizational structure.[80] Reengineering was targeted toward accomplishing five goals: first, to maintain "value added" in the NCI by continuing to support high-risk and long-term projects; second, to encourage the development of new technologies; third, to support a unique clinical trial system; fourth, to provide interdisciplinary training for young researchers; and fifth, to ensure that peer review and reward systems encourage individual innovation as well as collaboration.[81]

The reengineering process was primarily informed by principal investigators in the NCI's intramural program, who participated through meetings, focus groups, and later through the various advisory channels to the OD located at or across the divisional level in the form of faculties, working groups, and steering committees. Barrett estimated that around 90 percent of the principal investigators in the intramural program were involved to some extent in faculties, working groups, and/or steering committees, which had organized "spontaneously" over the previous three years on the basis of the encouragement of then-director Klausner.[82] Barrett repeatedly marveled at the enthusiasm of intramural scientist-bureaucrats to participate in these collective efforts, particularly as they were unfunded and sustained purely by members' own initiative.

Based substantially upon input from these homegrown pockets of agency governance, which comprised almost 1,500 intramural employees, the reengineering committee established interdisciplinary Centers of Excellence within the CCR. In a similar fashion to the extramural SPORE program, these Centers of Excellence brought together interdisciplinary teams and created infrastructure to facilitate rapid translation of discoveries into clinical application.[83] The process of developing Centers of Excellence thus reflected an episode wherein earlier efforts to develop infrastructure for translational research in the extramural community fed back upon later efforts to shore up the intramural program's own capacity to expedite translational research in-house. Reflecting upon the accomplishments Barrett reported, von Eschenbach humbly assured he had "truly not done anything except preside, watching just unbelievably gifted people who care so very deeply and have such great gifts work together effectively as a team. And the progress that you're seeing . . . is progress that they are responsible for, they are making happening [sic] and I just have the privilege to preside over it."[84]

Barrett insisted that restructuring would be kept to a minimum during the reengineering process; the few changes that were made, such as renovations to Building 37 where many of the intramural laboratories were housed, were completed in order to improve "informal" communication and interaction among NCI scientists.[85] What emerged instead was a focus on changing the culture of the CCR to better support interdisciplinary, collaborative, and translational research. The spirit of these reforms harmonized with NCAB chairman John Niederhuber's interpretation of the Institute of Medicine's 2004 organizational report on the NIH, entitled "Enhancing the Vitality of the National Institutes of Health," which he argued encouraged changes to organizational strategy and administration rather than structure.[86] Spurred by the results of a recent survey on the culture of the NCI, von Eschenbach appointed NCI deputy director for management David Elizalde as head of a series of initiatives to improve the intramural program's training and reward structure. Central to Elizalde's implementation strategy was encouraging a culture of transdisciplinary research, which required sufficient balance across disciplines, as well as appropriate training and dedicated funding for team science.[87] On the development end, Elizalde's strategy also involved shoring up the clinical trials infrastructure at NCI and leveraging it as a resource in collaborations with academia and industry.[88]

With these intramural-extramural collaborations the NCI hoped to address concerns that the culture of biomedical research outside the NCI was antagonistic to interdisciplinary and translational research. In a 2004 conference sponsored by the President's Cancer Panel (PCP), experts puzzled over how to instill a "mission-oriented" focus in academia, where hiring and promotion decisions rewarded independent, investigator-initiated research.[89] The reports that issued from the PCP's deliberations emphasized the central role the NCI played as a source of funding, infrastructure, collaboration, and scientific as well as health leadership in cancer research.[90] More significantly, the NCAB's discussion of the PCP's analysis acknowledged the distinct environment for translational research in the NCI that could serve as a model for changing academic research cultures that in their judgment posed barriers to translation.[91] In presenting the panel's findings to the NCAB, PCP chair LaSalle Leffall, Jr., noted that a consistent theme had emerged around the perceived differences between how academia rewards investigator-initiated, discovery-oriented research and how the NCI's intramural program enables the development of such findings into medical interventions that address patient and community needs. Von Eschenbach argued that the NCI would leverage its intramural strengths to help foster an "enabling culture" of interdisciplinary and translational research in both the public and private sectors.[92] He presented the ongoing reengineering effort as offering opportunities for collaboration with extramural scientists and industry that could achieve this cultural change beyond the NCI itself.[93]

In February 2005, Barrett resigned as director of the CCR; in his stead, von Eschenbach appointed Robert Wiltrout, associate director of the government-owned, private-contractor-operated NCI-Frederick Cancer Center, as the new head of the CCR. Wiltrout's reengineering plan differed somewhat from what had evolved from Barrett and Elizalde's previous efforts. Initially, Wiltrout wanted to move CCR closer to a "hybrid" organizational model that would restructure existing labs and branches.[94] Given his former role in leadership at NCI-Frederick, the announcement of such an objective might forebode yet another effort to "overlay" exogenous models onto the local routines of intramural personnel. However, Wiltrout was convinced to keep Barrett's promise of only minimally restructuring the intramural program, and so he tested new models across existing structures or where planned consolidations of laboratories were taking place. Centers of Excellence provided the models as well as the resources for these cross-cutting initiatives, which Wiltrout attributed to the reengineering program's "changing the culture from what once was more of a silo-based mentality to actually a very interactive and cross-cutting organization."[95] The culmination of this cultural change was a shift in the evaluative criteria for intramural principal investigators, who were now formally rewarded for their participation in team-based collaborative science in addition to traditional investigator-initiated efforts as was typical in most academic environments.[96] Throughout his discussion of the reengineering program, Wiltrout and other leaders in the CCR upheld the HPV vaccine, discussed in chapter 6, as a prominent example of successful collaborations between NCI researchers within CCR Centers of Excellence, extramural scientists, and industry.[97] Wiltrout's efforts in reengineering the CCR thus hewed more closely to intramural scientists' routines than did the efforts of his counterparts in the OD.

As collaborations with academia and industry were increasingly integrated into strategic planning efforts in the CCR, the intramural program emphasized a vision of translational research more dependent upon partnerships with other government agencies, academia, and private industry. Partly as a result of the Translational Research Working Group's efforts, but also inchoate in these reengineering initiatives, was a more explicit distinction between "early translation," which they defined as the first interactions between basic and clinical research and considered to be within the NCI's purview, and "late translation," such as drug manufacture, which was assumed to be the purview of industry.[98] In 2006, Wiltrout presented evidence to the NCAB that the CCR's increasingly refined focus on early translation was indeed changing the culture of intramural research. Surveying the CCR, Wiltrout found that "70 percent of all publications from the CCR are based on collaborations, and half are collaborations with extramural investigators, many with universities and Cancer Centers."[99] In light of the extensive collaboration across laboratories, branches, and even the NIH, Wiltrout declared that distinctions between "basic" and "clinical" branches were merely matters of "convenience"; the intramural program was realizing a new era of integrated, translational cancer research from the ground up.[100]

THE NIH ROADMAP FOR MEDICAL RESEARCH

Von Eschenbach's agenda for reshaping the NCI unfolded contemporaneously with newly appointed NIH director Elias Zerhouni's early efforts to develop the NIH Roadmap for Medical Research. Zerhouni described the initial impetus for the roadmap as the outcome of pressure from Congress and the Bush administration to show the NIH was responsibly using the taxpayer funding that contributed to its recent budget doubling.[101] The earliest planning phases, which began in late 2002, specifically addressed ways to take advantage of emerging opportunities and eliminate barriers to translational research by reimagining the culture of scientific research and the structures available to realize discovery and translation. In 2002, roadmap planners identified four priorities, including investment in cutting-edge technologies such as nanotechnology and bioinformatics, novel and integrative approaches to studying biological systems, improvement of the nation's clinical research system to facilitate translation, and implementation of training programs and cultural changes that would enable large-scale interdisciplinary research to flourish.[102] By 2003, these priorities were whittled down to three more general goals: "(1) developing NIH competing strategy to follow in looking at new pathways to discovery; (2) developing a framework for adapting the new scientific teams to the changing model of how science is conducted; and (3) re-engineering the clinical research enterprise."[103]

According to von Eschenbach, many of the NCI's long-range planning initiatives helped Zerhouni develop the project in its early stages.[104] Many of the initiatives that ended up in the NIH Roadmap were "things that NCI has already been very actively and very aggressively engaged in."[105] As he pointed out, the NCI had already made progress on each of the NIH's roadmap priorities, particularly through efforts in the intramural CCR.[106] Though the roadmap integrated insights from each institute in the NIH, the NCI's previous success in committing resources to translational research initiatives and its prominent role in the roadmap planning process ensured that NIH Roadmap initiatives remained particularly relevant to the institute. In turn, von Eschenbach began referring to long-term strategic planning in the institute as a "roadmapping" exercise in itself.[107] He strove to make connections across institutes to maintain cohesion with NIH Roadmap goals and integrated the NCI's newly minted "roadmapping" strategies into both the long-standing strategic planning process and his own 2015 Challenge Goal.[108] Barrett ensured that the reengineering process in the CCR integrated roadmap goals, arguing that the NCI's intramural program was uniquely situated to conduct translational research.[109] Zerhouni's roadmap also closed in quickly on von Eschenbach's desire to collaborate with industry. Public-private partnerships, which Zerhouni downplayed in the earliest road-mapping priorities in favor of activities within the purview of the institutes, were more openly encouraged in September 2003 when Zerhouni officially unveiled the NIH Roadmap.[110]

During the initial roadmap implementation stage, which spanned the period 2003–2006, the NCI's role in shaping the translational research agenda continued to expand. At the outset, the NCI intramural program was presented as "a model for interdisciplinary and multidisciplinary research" of the kind the roadmap imagined comprising "research teams of the future."[111] Some of the special attributes of successful translational research conducted in the intramural program included having a "well-defined" sense of the "mission of the research team," which was built into the best practices of interdisciplinary translational research for the roadmap.[112]

Though the intramural program provided significant exemplars for envisioning successful translation that was based on federal collaborations, the NCI's extramural efforts—Cancer Centers, SPORE grants, and the RAID program in particular—were more influential in shaping the specific initiatives that emanated from the NIH roadmap. By 2004, NCI personnel spearheaded a number of roadmap projects, most notably the Translational Research Core Services project.[113] This project, led by the Division of Cancer Treatment and Diagnosis director James Doroshow, was one of the most crucial infrastructure-building programs in the roadmap. The format of the Translational Research Core Services program was modeled after the NCI's RAID program, by this time a popular extramural program that supported collaborations with academic scientists and small businesses.[114] Efforts to develop the Translational Research Core Services soon encouraged the NIH to adopt an NIH-wide RAID pilot program funded through the roadmap that promised to better facilitate translation.[115]

In colligating around a concept of translational drug development informed by the RAID program, these roadmap efforts were drawing upon an approach that had been substantially informed by NCI scientist-bureaucrats' understandings of the deficits of market-driven commercial drug development. RAID was first launched in 1998 as a "virtual drug company" that provided academic researchers access to the NCI's own contractual services at NCI-Frederick for preclinical drug testing of promising compounds. RAID explicitly selected compounds to develop on the basis of evaluations of the scientific merit of novel drugs, biologics, or vaccines rather than "pharmacoeconomics."[116] It is significant that RAID formed the basis for this foundational roadmap infrastructure project because, as Klausner and his colleagues in the NCI described it in its early years, much of the warrant for RAID was predicated upon an argument about market failure. NIH scientist-bureaucrats' adoption of a funding mechanism into the NIH Roadmap to support academic and small-business innovation because large pharmaceutical companies were overlooking valid compounds on the basis of economic considerations is a far cry from subsequent interpretations of the roadmap as a neoliberal gambit to enable further penetration of industry influence into academic science.[117] Indeed, nearly half of all RAID awards during the program's first five years were for biologics and vaccines—compounds that pharmaceutical companies were often reluctant to pursue because of the financial inefficiency of preclinical testing for these agents.[118]

The presumption that RAID should deliberately forego collaboration with big pharma to appropriately pursue the NCI's mission was revisited under von Eschenbach's directorship, as he hoped to involve private corporations in the program. However, the design of RAID dating back to Klausner (which only supported private collaboration on the condition that private collaborators were small businesses and thus categorically excluded partnerships with large private pharmaceutical and biotechnology companies), as well as concerns over conflict of interest, presented formal bureaucratic barriers to the program's co-optation by industry.[119] Additionally, RAID's administrators in the NCI pointed to continued lack of engagement by industry as limiting their ability to gain a better understanding of how the program *could* be used by these corporations. There was "some industry input, but very little" in the existing program, as NCI leadership "[had] not reached out to Big Pharma . . . because the goal is to try to avoid the necessary alliance or appearance of alliance with Big Pharma issues."[120]

In addition to programmatic concerns, commercial industry had historically shown little interest in RAID to begin with. NCI leadership identified a lack of clarity around intellectual property for the kinds of projects RAID typically sponsored as a disincentive to collaborate on the part of major pharmaceutical and biotechnology companies.[121] When scientific principals pressed the leadership in RAID and other industry-interfacing programs emerging in the NCI to solicit feedback on the actual concerns of Big Pharma and commercial biotechnology companies from their trade associations—Pharmaceutical Research and Manufacturers of America (PhRMA) and Biotechnology Innovation Organization (BIO)—the leadership found industry somewhat cagey. In attempting to account for its struggles in communicating with and recruiting the pharmaceutical industry to its advisory boards, NCI leadership interpreted industry as viewing the institute's new programs as either irrelevant to or in direct competition with their commercial efforts.[122] Industry's desire to obtain the most advantageous command over intellectual property rights for potential commercial products was identified as a point of contention; given the institute's focus on leveraging intellectual property rights to co-license NCI patents, it was unsurprising that industry was reluctant to cooperate.[123] In light of commercial industry's limited interest in the NCI, the RAID program remained focused on helping academics and small businesses partner for commercial development to enable "efficient translation from lead [discovery] to first-in-human clinical trial."[124] From here the NCI could but have faith that some larger opportunity to develop these compounds would follow from commercial industry's own initiative.[125]

RAID would go on to enhance the NCI's capacity to move promising drugs and biologics from early research into sufficient development to be of interest to private biotechnology and pharmaceutical concerns, but it would not serve as a means for industry to capture the institute's agenda. In this sense, RAID more closely mirrored the NCI's extant apparatus for enabling the patenting and licensing of intramural researchers' innovations. In fact, many NCI administrators touted its similarity to the intramural program's drug development approach as a positive attribute of the program.[126] As Doug Lowy would later point out, "the NCI receives more than three-quarters of royalties from all of NIH. We're one of the few institutes that has a positive cash flow. But while I say that, I want everyone to understand that public health is the principal purpose at the NIH for the licensing and patenting of our inventions."[127] By primarily serving those projects overlooked by industry, RAID provided a mechanism for realizing the NCI's dual mission at the interface of extramural research as well.

The inclusion of RAID and other translational research initiatives enabled the NIH Roadmap to realize its goal of catalyzing translation: 40 percent of all roadmap funds in 2005 went to translational research initiatives, compared to 25 percent in the NIH overall and 30 percent in the NCI.[128] In 2006, the NIH began its second phase of roadmap planning, which introduced two new priorities (one focused on the microbiome, the other on epigenetics).[129] However, "Roadmap 1.5" was quickly followed by the 2006 NIH Reform Act, which accompanied congressional reauthorization of the institutes. The NIH Reform Act ended the practice of culling funds from each institute to support roadmap projects, instead establishing a Common Fund in the NIH Office of the Director to be supported by separate appropriations.[130] The Common Fund took over all NIH Roadmap initiatives, continuing many of the projects until their projected termination but eliminating the roadmap nominally (at the time of this writing, the Common Fund continues to coordinate all trans-NIH initiatives descended from the roadmap).

Notably, in the implementation phase of the roadmap, each institute in the NIH was meant to "participate with their scientific communities in defining all components of the Roadmap" and "contribute equally and proportionately" to the planning process.[131] This made sense, given that the roadmap from 2003 to 2006 was funded primarily through money transferred from each institute's budget with supplements from the NIH. Over time, however, the NCI came to play a disproportionate role in trans-NIH agenda-setting and benefited more substantially from roadmap funding than the institute's monetary contributions might justify. During the initial phase of the roadmap, the NCI realized significantly greater returns in funding than the institute's contribution to the roadmap. Whereas the NCI contributed 13 percent of roadmap funds to the tune of $30.5 million, the institute was eventually awarded 18 percent of all roadmap funding, reaping roughly $42.1 million.[132] Reflecting upon the institute's success during this period, then NCI director John Niederhuber marveled at the institute's ability to "compete very effectively for Roadmap dollars."[133] But given that so many of the roadmap initiatives related to building infrastructure and resources for translational research were based on models developed at the NCI in the previous decade, the institute's success should be far from surprising.

Nevertheless, any windfall from the NCI's roadmap victory was offset by dwindling appropriations for the institute. In 2006, President George W. Bush slammed the NCI with the largest budget cut the institute had ever faced. Meager budgets meant the NCI failed to keep up with biomedical inflation; the institute's purchasing power had already plummeted 12 percent in just the past few years.[134] Von Eschenbach, whose overblown business rhetoric and fondness of alliteration *Cancer Letter* had long lampooned, was also under serious pressure as accusations of long-standing conflicts of interest came to a head when Bush appointed him director of the FDA while he was still serving as head of the NCI. The first director to face an atmosphere of "open resistance" from within the NCI as well as from extramural scientists,[135] in 2007 von Eschenbach stepped down from his post to direct the FDA full-time.

SHOOTING THE MOON—AGAIN

John Niederhuber had maintained a close collaborative relationship with von Eschenbach during the former's stint as chair of the NCAB, including moving into one of the controversial associate positions von Eschenbach created in the Office of the Director, before being appointed von Eschenbach's successor. After he formally assumed the directorship of the NCI in 2006, Niederhuber "stressed continuity of leadership at the Institute, pledging adherence to von Eschenbach's often-criticized" 2015 Challenge Goal.[136] Niederhuber continued to defend many of von Eschenbach's hires, including "the terrible witch of Bethesda," Anna Barker, who had inherited the extramural community's ire for her role in pushing von Eschenbach's expensive pro-business initiatives while R01 grant funding stagnated.[137] Though he did not criticize his predecessor publicly, in his first year Niederhuber reorganized the NCI Office of the Director to restore it to its structure before von Eschenbach's directorship and scrubbed all mention of the 2015 Challenge Goal from the NCI's official communications.[138]

Niederhuber spent the entirety of his tenure as NCI director presiding over an agency increasingly strapped for funding. When he parted ways with the NCI in 2010, he left behind an institute whose leadership of the preceding decade had "been marred by revelations of cronyism and conflicts of interest."[139] In this environment, as Paul Goldberg of *Cancer Letter* remarked, "applying the A-word—accountability—to NCI, [was] not a gratuitous dig."[140] When a young Obama administration, benefiting from a bipartisan effort by a group of moderate Republicans including longtime NIH advocate Arlen Specter, offered a handsome stimulus to the institutes in 2009 as part of the American Reinvestment and Recovery Act (ARRA), leaders from the extramural cancer community made clear their desire "to hold NIH accountable" for investing the money both quickly and wisely.[141] The ARRA influx marked the beginning of a funding rollercoaster at the NCI under the Obama administration, bookmarked on the opposite end by the "cancer moonshot" of 2016.

The lowest points of funding under the Obama administration were presided over by the newly appointed director of the NCI, Harold Varmus, a Nobel laureate who had previously served as head of the NIH from 1993 to 1999. More than a seasoned administrator, Varmus was an active researcher who enjoyed a broad reputation as one of the most significant living figures in cancer biology. During a town hall with NCI personnel after his official swearing-in on July 12, 2010, Varmus addressed a question about von Eschenbach's 2015 Challenge Goal by pledging to "make every effort to control cancer through science" without "mak[ing] promises that will be elusive."[142] His response was "drowned out by applause" from the NCI crowd.[143] Indeed, the excitement among NCI personnel in the town hall meeting was palpable, and Varmus's brief speech was peppered throughout with numerous spontaneous outbursts of laughter and applause.[144] Varmus's homecoming to federal science leadership (which he called "the most glorious manifestation I know of what government and democracy are capable of doing"[145]) thus marked a decisive shift in the NCI's leadership back to one of impactful scientist-bureaucrats with active stakes in ongoing research as well as institute management; in other words, Varmus slotted nicely into a culture based around the NCI's dual mission.

In moving into the directorship, Varmus's first act was to appoint Douglas Lowy to the position of deputy director, where he replaced the now-departing Anna Barker. In contrast with von Eschenbach's deputy, Doug Lowy (whom we met in chapter 6 as one of the inventors of the HPV vaccine) began his ascent through the NCI's leadership as one of the institute's native sons. Lowy acted as Varmus's "alter ego" and, upon Varmus's departure from the NCI in 2015, took over as acting director of the Institute.[146]

Though largely coincidental, the NCI's budget finally began to increase once again when Lowy was appointed acting director in March 2015. While "nice guy Lowy" began his stint by presiding over the first generous congressional appropriations for the institute in years, he would also shepherd a major influx of funds to the institute in the form of Vice President Joe Biden's "moonshot" initiative.[147] First announced by President Obama during the State of the Union address in January 2016, the new moonshot would honor Biden's son, Beau, who died of glioblastoma the previous year. The purpose of the moonshot was to accelerate progress in cancer research, with an emphasis on prevention and screening in addition to investments in cutting-edge basic research.[148] The NCI and its advisory bodies, evidently skittish about the language of a moonshot, initially reckoned this as the "Vice President's cancer initiative." In a March 2016 meeting of the BSA, Lowy acknowledged that the moonshot terminology carried with it some discomfiting baggage about engineering, cures, and "magic bullets."[149] He took care to point out, excerpting a speech Biden made during a recent visit to a cancer center in Pennsylvania, that the vice president did not expect the NCI to deliver on such lofty promises. *Cancer Letter* juxtaposed the moonshot's more reasonable interpretation of the issues and stakes of ongoing cancer research with the last attempt to set an ambitious goal for the NCI: "unlike Andrew von Eschenbach's unsuccessful plan to 'eliminate suffering and death due to cancer by 2015,' the Biden plan seeks to make 10 years' worth of progress in the next five years."[150]

Contrasting Lowy's leadership with von Eschenbach's helps put the striking differences in their style into perspective. Throughout his tenure as deputy and acting director of the NCI, Lowy's leadership was tightly coupled with his scientific projects. First, under the leadership of Varmus and Lowy, the NCI effected a decisive shift toward sustained focus on global health in 2010. This involved the creation of a Center for Global Cancer Research focused on addressing disparities in cancer morbidity and mortality between wealthy and developing nations. In introducing this new center, Director Varmus pointed to the importance of the NCI's work on the HPV vaccine in Latin America, which had demonstrated the efficacy and cost effectiveness of a single shot of the vaccine in preventing cervical cancer in low-income regions of the world.[151] Varmus indicated that the ongoing intramural HPV vaccine innovations, which now included attempts to develop cheaper next-generation vaccines in collaboration with pharmaceutical companies in middle-income nations, were a model for how to control this oncogenic virus into the future as well as a template for targeting other oncogenic pathogens such as Epstein-Barr virus (EBV).[152] The NCI's long-standing activities in Latin America, bolstered by these recent translational vaccine breakthroughs, would help form the basis for the institute's approach to global cancer research. Noting that "most deaths from cancer today occur in the poorest areas of the world . . . Dr. Varmus affirmed the NCI's responsibility to help address this."[153]

Lowy's commitment to HPV vaccine research would also inform how he interpreted priorities for the cancer moonshot early in its development. Presenting the concept to the BSA for the first time in March 2016, Lowy introduced the possibility of developing preventative vaccines as the first proposed priority for using these funds.[154] Along with NIH director Francis Collins, Lowy also published a perspectives piece in the *New England Journal of Medicine* announcing the cancer moonshot in May 2016.[155] As in his presentation to the BSA, Lowy listed the development of vaccines against cancer viruses, especially EBV, as a top priority for moonshot funding.[156] Though these specific efforts would fall further down the priority list as the moonshot's scientific agenda was subsequently refined through conversations with congressional and scientific principals, cancer vaccines retained a distinctive position in the program's prevention efforts throughout the planning phase.

The White House appointed a blue ribbon panel to develop a series of recommendations for how to distribute any funds allocated to the institute through the moonshot initiative. The timeline for producing a report was brisk; NCI leadership cautioned that it offered few opportunities for feedback from the public or broader cancer community on initiatives planned for the first fiscal year of funding in 2017. As such, the blue ribbon panel's final report, issued in September 2016, primarily reflected the priorities this group could develop and vet over the course of approximately 4 months.[157] Nevertheless, Lowy insisted that the major recommendations would allow the NCI to communicate to congressional principals "the scientific validity of what is being recommended as a really important way of augmenting what NCI is already doing."[158] The moonshot also won support from the NCI's principals on the NCAB and BSA in part because it avoided the pitfalls of promising on a "single achievable endpoint," instead seeking to accelerate research through investment such that what scientists projected they could achieve in ten years would be delivered in five.[159] As NCAB chair Tyler Jacks noted, even Biden seemed to understand "the fact that cancer is at least 200 diseases, and it is complex. So I think in his mind as well there's not a single planting of the flag."[160] For his part, Lowy was applauded for his ability to communicate specific research areas of promise to Congress, championing the moonshot by pointing to "ideas explaining circulating tumor cells, blood tests, biomarkers, early detection; things that are tangible to them."[161] His competence in advocating for the moonshot thus lay in his ability to interpret the issues and stakes of scientific and bureaucratic practices around promising initiatives at the NCI. In turn, moonshot goals were lauded by scientists and the trade press as "flexible enough to be realistic."[162]

Though funding for the moonshot was briefly jeopardized by Donald Trump's surprise election to the presidency in November 2016, it was funded with the passage of the 21st Century Cures Act that December. The Beau Biden Cancer

Moonshot allocated $1.8 billion for mandatory (as opposed to discretionary) activities in fiscal year 2017 related to the priorities of the blue ribbon panel's report. Though moonshot funding was set to expire in seven years, Joe Biden's 2020 election to the presidency reinvigorated the moonshot effort, which was reissued in 2022 with an explicit goal "to reduce the age-adjusted death rate from cancer by at least 50 percent within the next 25 years."[163]

CONCLUSION

Former NCI director Vincent DeVita once described the institute directorship as a "bully pulpit."[164] Yet the effectiveness of any given NCI director to shape national cancer policy depends crucially upon NCI scientist-bureaucrats and their principals to enact these policies through rule making, lawmaking, and changes in scientific organization and practice. As the model of environed social learning suggests, the durability of innovative science or policy change is won through its enactment in practices. To enact such policies in the laboratory and boardroom, scientist-bureaucrats at the NCI must interpret the issues and stakes of new policies as both plausible and broadly actionable in relation to their ongoing practices. In such instances, organizational innovations such as RAID are interpreted as compatible with the NCI's dual mission and find long life in the scientific and administrative programs of the organization. In other instances, less scientifically and organizationally plausible attempts at policy innovation, like the 2015 Challenge Goal, languish beyond the everyday scientific and bureaucratic life of the institute until administrative turnover allows them to be quietly banished.

Successful calibration of programmatic and operational goals in policy making is, like that of scientific and public health missions in experimentation, the outcome of a reiterative learning process. The acquisition of expert knowledge necessary for policy making is thus endogenous to bureaucratic organizations. Though analysis of endogenous bureaucratic competence tends to utilize informational models of expertise, this study indicates that practical competencies may be necessary to the formulation of policies that articulate plausible interpretations of the issues and stakes ingredient in complex scientific enterprises such as cancer research.[165] Though few NCI directors come from outside the NIH, those outsiders who do see policy success tend to establish research units in the

NIH that enable them opportunities to iteratively instantiate their policy visions into routines of scientific practice that unfold in the distinct local setting of the scientific bureaucracy. That Andrew von Eschenbach did not engage in research at the NCI during his tenure as director may not explain his failure, but it may help account for why his policies often lacked scientific and bureaucratic plausibility for NCI actors and advisors.

Despite the importance of scientist-bureaucrats' competency to policy success, the NCI remains dependent upon congressional principals to maintain adequate funding to make these policies relevant to the national community of cancer researchers. In the new millennium, the relationship between the NCI and Congress showed its first signs of systematic erosion. As the NCI's Office of Budget and Finance pointed out, the institute's purchasing power declined by 40 percent in the first fifteen years of the twenty-first century because of budget stagnation and real decline in appropriations.[166] Growing partisanship may also be to blame for the consistent failure to pass budgets on time in Congress. It has been the norm throughout the twenty-first century to rely on months of continuing resolutions every year before a spending bill makes it to the president's desk. The lack of timely appropriations has destabilized the regular functioning of the NCI as a federal bureaucracy. Opposition to Obama administration policies, including the Affordable Care Act, led to the ascent of Tea Party politics that pushed the Republican Congress further right. The funding crises that ensued—including federal sequestration and the 2013 government shutdown—caught a heretofore privileged realm of biomedical research funding in its wake. Comparing the 2013 shutdown to that of 1995, when he was at the helm of the entire NIH, Varmus noted a significant change in the political atmosphere. Given that conflicts over the Affordable Care Act were at the heart of the budget issues that led to the 2013 shutdown, Varmus likened the situation to a GOP-led Congress "hold[ing] the country hostage" in a manner "completely inconsistent with the better parts of our democracy."[167]

Yet it was not merely the changing tone of partisan politics that affected the NCI's standing in the nation's cancer enterprise. Since the dawn of the twenty-first century, the institute had begun to lose pride of place as the nation's leader in cancer research. Private pharmaceutical companies and the growing biotechnology industry increasingly commanded the power of global finance, which was changing the motives and means for conducting clinical trials. It is the broad political economic bent behind such financialization, coupled with austerity measures, that has led many STS scholars to suspect the NCI's fate reflects that of many other scientific organizations under neoliberalism.[168] That the historical realities of the NCI's changing approach to policy are more complex should not detract from the clear overall trend toward market-driven biomedicine. Nevertheless, the NCI's frequent role as a countervailing force in the neoliberalization of cancer research and development brings attention to the fragmented nature of federal government and to the significance of organizations as research sites where sociologists can study science governance in the making.

CONCLUSION

The history of cancer virus and vaccine research in the National Cancer Institute is a history of environed social learning. Confronted by reiterative problems of how to demonstrate the viral etiologies of cancers in an organization committed to improving health through both scientific and public policy innovation, NCI scientist-bureaucrats have been apt to pursue those projects that serve understandings of the public good built up through their experiences as both researchers and public servants. In the process, they often develop expertise in formulating popular and mission-relevant policies that thrust them into leadership positions in the institute. Whether they succeed or fail in achieving their stated scientific or policy goals, these scientist-bureaucrats' simultaneous service to science and the public good indelibly shapes the landscape of cancer research well beyond Bethesda.

When national cancer policy is the outcome of environed social learning, organizational outcomes in the NCI often precipitate changes throughout the broader biomedical ecology wherein the agency is situated. The infrastructure erected around virus cancer research contracts in the 1960s enabled the dramatic expansion of retrovirus expertise, giving birth to the "oncogene bandwagon" that drove molecular biology to prominence in cancer research in the final decades of the twentieth century.[1] In the process of attempting a targeted effort to develop cancer vaccines, the Virus Cancer Program's plans and infrastructure generated the scientific theories that led to its demise.[2] Subsequently, NCI policy shifted toward investigator-initiated basic research, in part as a response to criticisms from political principals in Congress and scientific principals on the National Cancer Advisory Board that vaccine programs had been inherently flawed.

Yet the problem of serving the institute's dual mission reemerged in the 1980s with the HIV/AIDS epidemic. The NCI's scientific investment in retrovirus research had equipped it with substantial resources to respond to the public health crisis, but the backlash against targeted research left scientist-bureaucrats to create informal collaborations from the ground up that would bring basic virology insights into the clinic for the development of effective AIDS treatments. These ad hoc interdisciplinary projects allowed bench scientists in the Laboratory of Tumor Cell Biology to rapidly identify a virus responsible for AIDS and to work closely with clinicians in the Clinical Oncology Program to test antiviral compounds that might be effective against the retrovirus. The NCI's intramural collaborative efforts not only led to the first major innovations in the epidemic—the creation of an HIV screening assay and the first generation of effective nucleoside analogs for treating AIDS—but also inspired new models of governing the transit of research findings from bench to bedside.

When the Clinical Oncology Program's Samuel Broder became NCI director in 1989, he worked to swing the policy pendulum back toward the institute's health mission. On the basis of his own experiences with HIV/AIDS innovation in the intramural program, he sought to establish the infrastructure necessary for effective translational research in extramural laboratories across the United States. Within the institute, the development of a human papillomavirus vaccine by intramural scientists provided a model for effective translation that responded to the changing legal, political, and economic environments for scientific innovation at the end of the twentieth century.

Yet it was the failure of a more market-friendly NCI director to enact policy reform that cemented NCI scientist-bureaucrats as experts on the scientific issues and stakes of translational research policy. By continuing to tailor their scientific and bureaucratic innovations to conceptions of the distinct ecology of scientific research and their place within it, NCI scientists preserved their conception of the dual mission in institute policy and prevented alternatives that defied it from being permanently incorporated into routine governance. In the process, NCI scientist-bureaucrats demonstrated the intimate and practical relationship between scientific and policy work in this government agency, whose outsized impact on the political economy of biomedicine makes it one of the most influential but overlooked bureaucracies in the U.S. federal government.

LESSONS FOR SOCIOLOGY AND STS

As a study in the growth of the U.S. administrative state, the NCI offers an illuminating case of a federal agency that effectively leverages taxpayer funding to produce new scientific and administrative capacities in addition to distributing funds to support scientific efforts outside the federal government.[3] Throughout the period examined here, the NCI applied this burgeoning scientific and administrative capacity to train researchers in fields of study underdeveloped elsewhere and to deliberately produce the material infrastructure, theoretical innovations, and novel products that drove cancer virus research and vaccine development forward in the United States and around the globe. The NCI can thus be examined as an important illustration of how expert bureaucrats construct the administrative capacity of federal agencies through long-term processes of policy change and organizational learning whereby bureaucrats creatively develop approaches to policy implementation that reshape the bureaucracy, the goals of political constituencies, and the role of the public in the innovation process.

Acknowledging that expert bureaucrats do not merely execute policies imposed by principals but rather play a role in generating innovations is important for sociologists looking to adapt insights from political science and economics to analyze processes of public policy and administration in action.[4] Principal-agent theories are used in these allied disciplines to emphasize problems of delegation and control from the perspective of principals, a perspective that treats the deviation of agents from the interests of principals as suspicious and indicative of undesirable practices such as shirking or corruption.[5] However, analyzing bureaucratic expertise and policy craft from the perspective of agents acting in their environments shows how innovation can emerge from creative responses to the constraints imposed by principals.[6] In closely examining the role that situated scientific and bureaucratic practices play in informing agents' interpretations of the issues and stakes of their policy work, this study joins others that aim to show the crucial role bureaucrats play in generating and maintaining administrative capacity.[7]

The story of the NCI's capacity as a productive instrument in the federal administrative apparatus is thus one illustration of how the "entrepreneurial state" has been realized in the United States.[8] The NIH, alongside other notable civilian science and technology agencies such as the Department of Energy and

NASA, has historically gone beyond merely incentivizing basic research with federal grants and contracts or supporting the private sector by seeding infrastructure; the agency has independently generated high-risk research that yielded some of the most important biomedical innovations of the past half-century. Examining governance at the NCI helps sociologists understand how this variety of "hidden industrial policy" stays hidden.[9] In addition to the structural configurations of a decentralized, cooperative, public-private innovation network that obscures the role of state support by disproportionately allocating credit and revenue to private entities, the hidden nature of the policy state ensures that little attention is drawn to the administrative activities supporting this structural configuration.[10] Much of the activity that proved consequential to shaping the policies affecting scientists at the NIH and throughout the academic community were forged in agency-level rule making and procedural interpretation, processes that frequently escape the attention of members of Congress, the scientific community, and lay citizens alike.[11]

To understand how these agencies successfully selected projects in the past, and how the state might better realize its potential for improving the public good through innovation in the future, requires us to couple theories of the entrepreneurial state with those of the policy state. As the NCI demonstrates, scientist-bureaucrats conceptualize themselves within an ecology structured by multiple principals and private commercial interests and formulate agency policies that enable them to address the gaps they interpret the government as best filling. From cancer virus infrastructure in the 1960s to 1970s to HIV/AIDS research in the 1980s and translational research in the 1990s to 2010s, the NCI's efforts have often involved creating infrastructure to assemble the disparate capacities of the nation's public and private researchers with an aim toward improving health for all. Appreciating how policy making unfolds within the NCI as an organization with a distinct structural configuration and organizational mission helps illustrate the environed social learning processes whereby interpretations of the political, economic, and scientific landscape are iteratively encoded into the policies and innovations NCI scientist-bureaucrats author.

Despite its successes in producing innovations for the public good, the NCI has consistently fallen short in its ability to fully realize its dual organizational mission through these innovations. As the cases of nucleoside analogs and HPV vaccines vividly illustrate, externalities related to the prospects of legislative action or executive branch inaction constrained the NIH's ability to exercise its own nominal intellectual property rights. Just as it is often difficult for NCI career scientists to anticipate the needs of commercial interests, these actors struggle to conceptualize dependency relations that are far removed from their standard governance practices. Issues surrounding the distribution or enforcement of their intellectual property rights in the United States and abroad thwarted the visions of intramural researchers who helped innovate nucleoside analogs and HPV vaccines. These scientist-bureaucrats, whose science and policy innovations were carefully crafted to serve their conceptions of the public good, did not reckon the logic of patent law or international trade disputes that would ultimately stymie their efforts.[12]

Appreciating the importance and complexity of such dependencies requires a shift away from common conceptions of state policies as mitigating market failure and toward acknowledgment of more complex dynamics than those commonly postulated in models of neoliberal science. Far from a story of either regulatory capture or market failure, these examples of innovation at the NCI help illustrate how a far more systemic problem of *network failure* limits the institute's ability to effectively distribute its own innovations to the (increasingly global) public. Whereas market failure encourages scholars to look for places for the state to intervene where market incentives are insufficient to encourage the private sector to produce public goods, the theory of network failure draws our attention to how the distributed structure of research, development, and distribution builds complex webs of interdependencies between private and public entities with numerous interconnected points of possible failure. Whitford and Schrank note that network failure is particularly likely in situations where sophisticated production demands coordination between public and private organizations with different resources and competencies, but where some of these organizations either lack the requisite competence to succeed in creating an innovation or are prone to opportunistic behavior that intentionally co-opts innovation for purposes that serve their interests rather than sustaining the network.[13] In the case of both nucleoside analogs and HPV vaccines, the near-total control of U.S. drug manufacture by private industry created the conditions for opportunistic pharmaceutical companies to price drugs beyond the reach of low-income Americans and patients in developing nations, while the lack of coordination or will on the part of Congress and the White House ensured that NCI inventors were unable to overcome these structural limitations to maximize the public health impact of their innovations.

Network failures help explain why risks remain concentrated in the public sector while rewards are reaped primarily by private interests, *even in agencies that have not been captured by those interests*.[14] The NIH, like most federal institutions that administer billions of dollars in taxpayer funds, is sometimes suspected of creating policies that serve special interests over the public good. But "regulatory capture is very commonly misdiagnosed and mistreated" by social scientists and public commentators alike[15]—and not least in this instance because the NIH is not a regulatory agency by any traditional means. As I have shown throughout this study, policy making at the NCI is influenced by career scientists' interpretation of the institute's statutory obligations as expressed in its dual-mission charter and informed by the interests of congressional and scientific principals. The need for NCI scientist-bureaucrats to learn policy by doing, and their tendency to make policy meaningful in relation to their own scientific practices, has created a culture where the institute's mission remains salient in everyday organizational practices. The lack of information about industry desires among NCI scientist-bureaucrats, strikingly illustrated in the attempt to modify the RAID program discussed in chapter 7, demonstrates the low level of industry penetration in NCI policy. This low industry penetration exists even where advisory boards offer a mechanism for limited representation of special interests in NCI governance. By unpacking the structures of governance and routines of agency-level policy craft at the NCI, this study helps us understand how the NIH retains remarkable control over its internal scientific agenda, and why it remains curiously impervious to special interest lobbying.[16] In the process of challenging claims of industry capture, network failure redirects attention to the interconnected dynamics of the innovation ecosystem, where the behavior of commercial pharmaceutical and biotechnology firms that outsource vaccine research and development capacity in service of short-term financial performance can, in the long run, undermine the capacity to scale up the production of effective medicines discovered by government or academic scientists working in service of nonmonetary incentives.[17]

This discussion of the NCI's role in building state capacity for biomedical innovation also has clear implications for how scholars in science and technology studies (STS) approach the relationship between states and markets. Much as Mazzucato and Block and Somers chided economists and sociologists for presuming the kind of market fundamentalism that Karl Polanyi long ago debunked as an ideology of state erasure, STS scholars can similarly be taken to task for assuming that state action is perennially corrupted by neoliberalism.[18] STS writings on the political economy of cancer research often presume market dominance over a captured state, such that commercial interests' profit motives control the shape and trajectory of biomedical innovations. As I have shown in the case of the HPV vaccine, assuming neoliberal motives behind commercialized innovations can lead scholars to erroneous historical conclusions.[19] Yet these assumptions also limit the extent to which STS can properly theorize the emergence of translational research as a new biomedical paradigm.[20]

Critics of translational research in STS have rightly commented that policy discussions focus primarily on the promissory nature of medical innovations to the detriment of theorizing how the prevailing structural conditions of research, development, and medical delivery in the United States present their own impediments to improvement of health outcomes.[21] This study tracks the development, dating back to the 1940s, of a dual mission in the NCI that has transmitted the spirit of cancer melioration through biomedical innovation into present-day attempts to improve the nation's health through translational research. While the governance structures and social learning processes characteristic of policy making at the NCI have ensured that translational research hews closely to scientists' understandings of how innovation and public health can complement one another, it is unclear whether the paradigm of translational research—or any prior paradigm that has embodied the "biomedical settlement" of the 1940s[22]—can address the systemic issues affecting cancer patients today. In the continued absence of universal health care, U.S. cancer patients continue to confront a highly fragmented and unequal system of care. As intramural researchers at the NCI's Center for Cancer Research continue to pioneer potentially lifesaving innovations, from Dr. Steven Rosenberg's cancer immunotherapies to Dr. Genoveffa Franchini's prospective HIV vaccines, ordinary Americans and citizens around the globe struggle to access even basic care. Despite the NCI's transformative track record of innovation and its capacity for repeated comprehensive reconstitution of the nation's biomedical infrastructure over the past seventy years, it should be abundantly clear to policy makers that the institute's mission to improve health will remain limited without dramatic changes to the way the American health care system allocates resources to the public.

Despite these systemic limitations to realizing its dual mission, the NCI provides a particularly noteworthy case for examining how institutional change can emerge gradually from the iterative process of interpreting rules in ordinary practice, offering a compelling counterpoint to punctuated models of path dependence that typically rely on exogenous shocks to explain change.[23] Unlike the dominant sociological frameworks of new institutionalism and field theory, the approach used here does not assume inertia or reproduction as the governing dynamic of organizational life at the NCI.[24] Instead, NCI scientist-bureaucrats engage organizational practices within an environment that makes their dual normativity particularly evident. In sorting through the coupled issues and stakes that motivate their scientific and policy work, NCI scientists iteratively and often creatively reconstruct the mission of the organization in ways that encourage innovation. Appreciating how the full ecological environments toward which NCI scientist-bureaucrats act when solving problems that are simultaneously relevant to their scientific and policy ends affect their experimental and bureaucratic trajectories offers a powerful illustration of how social learning occurs in technically sophisticated bureaucracies.

LESSONS FOR THE FUTURE OF BIOMEDICAL RESEARCH POLICY

Though this study demonstrates how the NCI was able to maintain a distinct position of autonomy and authority vis-à-vis other federal agencies even as the political and economic environment changed dramatically over the century, there is reason to suspect the NIH's privileged position may be eroding. Growing political polarization at the turn of the twenty-first century has empowered political agendas that seek to undermine the legitimacy and function of the administrative state.[25] Nowhere was this more evident than during the COVID-19 pandemic, when noted scientist-bureaucrat and NIAID director Anthony Fauci became a prominent target of right-wing politicians and pundits. As conservative trust in scientific expertise continues to decline, the autonomy the NIH has enjoyed due in part to the complexity of the scientific expertise necessary to execute the agency's mandate may dissipate as politicians propose alternative forms of knowing to counter scientist-bureaucrats' expertise.[26] Such a change would fundamentally alter the NCI's existing relationship with its congressional principals into a more adversarial one subject to increased and potentially unpredictable forms of monitoring.

Concerns about the ultimate utility of biomedical innovation to health outcomes and accountability of NCI policy to democratic sentiments should continue to be addressed. Yet the success of the NCI in contributing to some of the most significant innovations in cancer research since the mid-twentieth century should also clarify the stakes of hasty institutional reform. This study goes beyond merely supporting the argument that the state plays an entrepreneurial role in innovation. Indeed, it would not be far-fetched to suggest that the NIH has been the single most significant force in driving biomedical innovation in the United States throughout the twentieth century. Its overwhelming support of upstream academic and government research helped yield the material innovations and train the innovators who maintained American dominance in global R&D throughout this period. In its heyday, the intramural NIH associates program nurtured young scientists who would go on to compose "more than a third of all physician winners of the Nobel Prize in Physiology or Medicine" in the past quarter-century.[27] Yet many alumni of the NIH express concern about the institute's continuing capacity to conduct innovative and boundary-expanding research. Many of these observers remark that the shift toward lucrative oncology practices in large hospitals has overwhelmed physicians' incentives to conduct groundbreaking and curiosity-driven research in favor of patient care and clinical trials.[28] More concerningly, former NCI director Samuel Broder lamented that the "administrative flexibility" of the institutes has so degraded that "the NIH of today might find it difficult or impossible to respond to the AIDS epidemic in the same way that it did in the early 1980s."[29]

The very success of federal science in contributing to innovation has made the NIH's potential decline a matter of concern for the entire innovation ecosystem, particularly when it comes to public-health-relevant innovations such as vaccines. Since the 1970s, private investment in basic vaccine research has declined precipitously. As most major pharmaceutical manufacturers disinvested from in-house vaccine research and development, the production of novel vaccine candidates became concentrated in academic and government laboratories. The NIH has become increasingly relevant in vaccine innovation as other public players, such as the Walter Reed Army Institute of Research, lost much of their capacity for vaccine innovation when the military transitioned to a system that contracted for services from the lowest bidder in the private sphere in the 1990s.[30] The importance of concentrated competencies for vaccine innovation within the NIH was again illustrated when a team led by Dr. Barney Graham,

NIAID intramural scientist and deputy director of the NIH Vaccine Research Center, developed the enabling technology used in Moderna's mRNA vaccine against COVID-19.[31] In this instance, the continued vulnerabilities created by network failures related to pharmaceutical companies' high pricing and aggressive intellectual property protection manifested in the continued emergence of deadly variants of COVID-19 in regions of the globe with low vaccination rates. With another mRNA vaccine on the horizon—this time against Epstein-Barr virus, an agent that has been under study at the NCI for some fifty years and was a focus of vaccine development in planning for the 2016 Cancer Moonshot—issues of how the NIH will manage its intellectual property in service to its public mission remain urgent.

Acknowledging the importance of the NIH to innovation should also lead us to reevaluate what is sometimes called the social contract of science.[32] What do we expect science to deliver to society, and who shall be its champions? For decades, a system based on allocating federal grants to scientists conducting fundamental health research has been seen as wise industrial policy, encouraging the flow of knowledge that can form the basis for new innovations. Yet fully acknowledging the role government scientists play in directly producing many of the innovations later licensed by commercial companies also raises the question whether taxpayer monies truly benefit the public or are simply being plundered by private interests. Recognizing the processes whereby NCI scientists govern will enable more considered and efficacious approaches to resolving problems that entangle macro-level questions of political economy with micro-level dramas of scientific innovation.

METHODOLOGICAL APPENDIX

The conclusions drawn in this study are based on extensive historical sociological research into the scientific and bureaucratic activities of NCI intramural researchers spanning the period 1948–2018. The bulk of the evidence I draw upon is derived from the annual reports generated by administrative and intramural research units in the NCI throughout this period. Annual reports were obtained from the National Archives and Records Administration in College Park, Maryland, and the NIH Intramural Database (https://intramural.nih.gov/search/index.taf). Between July 2014 and June 2015, I conducted on-site research at the National Archives and Records Administration in College Park, Maryland; the National Library of Medicine in Bethesda, Maryland; and the Library of Congress in Washington, D.C. I also consulted digital sources from the National Cancer Institute Division of Extramural Affairs Advisory Board meeting archives; the National Institutes of Health Office of NIH History archives; the National Cancer Institute intranet; the Food and Drug Administration; and the U.S. Government Printing Office. Additionally, I analyzed forty-four oral history interviews from the National Institutes of Health Oral History Project; these interviews were conducted primarily with NCI scientist-bureaucrats who are no longer living. I collected two additional oral histories to contribute to the Oral History Project archive; these interviews are of living subjects and were conducted in 2015 and 2017. This results in a total of forty-six oral history interviews used in this study (see table A.1).

In addition to archival and oral history sources, I consulted published scientific articles and technical reports produced by the historical figures I study. Some scientist-bureaucrats produced memoirs or clinician histories of the major scientific and bureaucratic events in which they took part; I analyzed these as retrospectives that could complement or supplement information corroborated by

TABLE A.1 Oral History Interviews Analyzed

Carl G. Baker	Edward Gelmann	Ira Pastan
Calvin Baldwin	Michael Gottesman	Alan Rabson
J. Carl Barrett	Christine Grady	John Schiller*
Edward Beeman	Janet Hartley	Edward Scolnick
William Blattner	John Heller	James Shannon
Samuel Broder	James Holland	Michael Shimkin
Bruce Chabner	Harriet Huebner	Arthur Upton
Robert Chanock	Gary Kelloff	Harold Varmus
Albert Dalton	Ruth Kirchstein	Thomas Waldmann
Vincent DeVita	Paul Kotin	Flossie Wong-Staal
Anthony Fauci	Lloyd Law	James Wyngaarden
Donald Fredrickson	Arthur Levine	Robert Yarchoan
Emil Frei	Douglas Lowy*	John Ziegler
Emil Freireich	Robert Manaker	Gordon Zubrod
Robert Gallo	Paul Marks	
William Gay	John Moloney	

Interviews conducted by the author are indicated with an asterisk (*); all others were gathered from the archives of the National Institutes of Health Oral History Project (https://history.nih.gov/display/history /NIH+Oral+Histories).

archival or oral history sources. A number of historians of science and medicine have produced secondary analyses of the programs and projects discussed here, which I also make use of where appropriate. To maintain focus on the relations between NCI scientist-bureaucrats and scientific and congressional principals, I drew upon journalistic reporting primarily from venues that serve these specialized audiences, such as *Science, Nature, Cancer Letter,* and the *Federal Register.* I used reporting from these journalistic sources to contextualize major scientific and bureaucratic events as they unfolded in real historical time. While I necessarily exclude some of the discourse around the NCI reported in the popular press given my theoretical focus, they did not escape my notice. Controversies around Gallo, the cause of AIDS, and the HPV vaccine, for example, appeared in the popular press throughout the period I study but are beyond the scope of my analysis.

A NOTE ON SOURCES

As the evidence that forms the basis of the argument in this book is historical, it is necessary to appreciate the rhetorical and memorial function of the various media I draw upon in constructing my interpretations. The documents that populate archives are structured by curatorial decisions made by scientists, secretaries, administrators, archivists, and others about which documents are or are not worth preserving. Similarly, interview and oral history responses are narratives motivated by the interviewers' and interviewees' desires to tell particular kinds of stories for reasons that may sometimes be difficult to reconstruct. The selectivity of organizational documents and actor standpoints is often a matter of methodological concern in history, sociology, and science and technology studies (STS), and I take these concerns about data production seriously. Further, I appreciate that the organizational tasks that lead these evidentiary sources to be produced in the form we confront them is of central theoretical importance to the study of scientist-bureaucrats' practices. The materiality of documents and the meanings encoded in narratives comprise features of the environment that actors can elide or make salient, reproduce or transform, in light of the problems they confront at any given time.

As a historical sociologist, I am obligated to make a good faith effort to situate these artifacts in relation to the immediate context of their production. I have done my best to fulfill this scholarly mandate but admit that there may be omissions, elisions, and errors of which I am unaware that open different perspectives on the events under discussion. To ensure the integrity of my analysis, I developed a strategy for triangulating my interpretations among the different sources available for analysis. Official NCI documents, scientific publications, and a mixture of contemporaneous reporting in professional presses and/or post hoc oral or written recollections of scientists were carefully compared to ensure the relationships between practices and innovation outcomes were not discursively artifactual. Major discrepancies between information reported in different sources were uncommon and almost exclusively involved minor variations in how events were reported in journalistic outlets, oral histories, or personal memoirs. Where these discrepancies exist, I default to the most authoritative source as determined by structures of public accountability—for example, official documents subject to editorial oversight or publications subject to peer review—in guiding my interpretation.

CASE SELECTION

From extensive archival evidence I constructed a theoretical sample of cancer virus and vaccine projects that took place in the NCI intramural research program throughout the seventy-year period of study. This sampling strategy was driven by a desire to discover (1) why the NCI was so innovative in the areas of virus and vaccine studies despite their counterintuitive relationship to cancer, which is popularly conceived as a heritable or degenerative disease; and (2) why so many in the NCI's bureaucratic leadership corps seemed to be drawn from among the ranks of virus and vaccine research units. After months of inductive research in the archives, I abductively hypothesized that virus and vaccine research, because of its promissory capacity to improve the health of the greatest number of Americans through public health interventions, was unusually complementary to the institute's dual mission. The decision to study cancer virus and vaccine efforts was thus not the outcome of randomly sampling a representative pool of projects from across the NCI intramural program but was instead driven by theoretical concerns involving precisely these projects' *non*-representativeness. Innovation is a rare event; consistently innovative research units perhaps more so. Cancer virus and vaccine efforts in the NCI intramural program are striking outliers in their scientific success and their organizational impact. The goal of the study is to understand how these two dimensions of the institute may be related.

To construct a within-case temporal comparison of cancer virus and vaccine efforts in the NCI, I sampled to include a range of projects that were both successful and unsuccessful, oriented toward a wide selection of human and animal viruses, and conducted by principal investigators with varying career lengths in the institute. I summarize the sample in table A.2.

While I took care to analyze a range of cases across the whole history of cancer virus and vaccine research in the NCI, limiting my study to these fields of inquiry necessarily limits the possible patterns that could manifest in my data. Even within the field of cancer virus and vaccine research, some work of great historical importance included in this sample had to be excluded or minimized for the sake of forming a coherent narrative of appropriate length and focus for a book. For instance, the work of Marjorie Robert-Guroff and of Genoveffa Franchini on HIV vaccines, which builds upon work that each began in the Laboratory of Tumor Cell Biology under Robert Gallo, has been innovative and significant to virology and vaccinology for decades. I excluded these projects because, bureaucratically, HIV vaccine efforts were no longer centralized in the NCI and, scientifically, HIV had long ago shed its direct association with cancer by the time these principal investigators began their independent lines of

TABLE A.2 Theoretical Sample of Intramural Cancer Virus and
Vaccine Projects in the NCI from 1948 to 2018

Principal Investigator Name	Project Range	Principal Investigator Name	Project Range
Sarah Stewart	1954–1970	Berge Hampar	1969–1982
Lloyd Law	1954–1989	Stuart Aaronson	1970–1993
W. Ray Bryan	1954–1960	Dharam Ablashi	1970–1991
Clyde Dawe	1955–1982	Edward Scolnick	1971–1982
Alan Rabson/Jose Costa	1958–1983	Wade Parks	1971–1977
John Moloney	1958–1968	Raoul Benveniste	1973–2004
Robert Manaker	1958–1966	Doug Lowy	1976–2018
Mary Fink	1959–1970	David Klein	1976–1979
Joseph DiPaolo	1966–1999	Meir Kende	1976–1979
Robert Huebner	1966–1982	Samuel Broder	1977–1988
Janet Hartley	1967–1975	Peter Howley	1978–1993
Robert Gallo	1968–1996	Jay Berzofsky	1978–2018
George Todaro	1968–1982	Johng Rhim	1980–2000
Paul Levine	1969–1982	Dean Mann	1983–1996
Paul Arnstein	1969–1993	C. Richard Schlegel	1983–1993
Padman Sarma	1969–1981	Marjorie Robert-Guroff	1987–2018
Wilna Woods	1969–1975	Peter Nara	1989–1997
Gary Kelloff	1969–1982	Genoveffa Franchini	1990–2018

inquiry. Nevertheless, these projects remain exemplary of the broader trends that manifest in the main narrative of the book.

There is more yet to be done in exploring the vast scientific and bureaucratic history of the NCI. I hope that this study, in its strengths as well as its limitations, may compel future scholars to continue investigating this complex and fascinating federal agency.

NOTES

INTRODUCTION

1. Siddhartha Mukherjee, *The Emperor of All Maladies: A Biography of Cancer* (New York: Scribner, 2010).

2. "Lifetime Risk of Developing or Dying from Cancer," American Cancer Society, https://www.cancer.org/cancer/cancer-basics/lifetime-probability-of-developing-or-dying -from-cancer.html. Lifetime risk calculation is based on the NCI's Surveillance Epidemiology and End Results (SEER) data for 2014–2016, which records cancer incidence and death rates throughout the United States.

3. Susan Sontag, *Illness as Metaphor* (New York: Farrar, Straus and Giroux, 1978); S. Lochlann Jain, *Malignant: How Cancer Becomes Us* (Berkeley: University of California Press, 2013).

4. Roderik F. Viergever and Thom C. C. Hendriks, "The 10 Largest Public and Philanthropic Funders of Health Research in the World," *Health Research Policy and Systems* 14, no. 12 (2016): 1–15.

5. The National Cancer Act of 1937, S. 2067, 75th Congress, 1st session (1937). Text of Public Law 244 provided by the National Cancer Institute, "National Cancer Act of 1937," posted February 16, 2016, https://www.cancer.gov/about-nci/overview/history /national-cancer-act-1937.

6. "Mission and Goals," National Institutes of Health, https://www.nih.gov/about-nih/what -we-do/mission-goals.

7. Jean-Paul Gaudillière and Ilana Löwy, eds., *Heredity and Infection: The History of Disease Transmission* (New York: Routledge, 2012).

8. For a review, see Edgar Kiser, "Comparing Varieties of Agency Theory in Economics, Political Science, and Sociology: An Illustration from State Policy Implementation," *Sociological Theory* 17, no. 2 (1999): 146–70.

9. Elisabeth Clemens and James M. Cook, "Politics and Institutionalism: Explaining Durability and Change," *Annual Review of Sociology* 25, no. 1 (1999): 441–66; George Steinmetz, ed., *State/Culture: State Formation After the Cultural Turn* (Ithaca, NY: Cornell University Press, 1999); Kimberly J. Morgan and Ann Shola Orloff, eds., *The Many Hands of the State: Theorizing Political Authority and Social Control* (New York: Cambridge University Press,

2017); Erin Metz McDonnell, *Patchwork Leviathan: Pockets of Bureaucratic Effectiveness in Developing States* (Princeton, NJ: Princeton University Press, 2020).

10.   Charles Tilly, *Coercion, Capital, and European States, AD 990–1992* (Cambridge, MA: Blackwell, 1992).

11.   Chandra Mukerji, *Territorial Ambitions and the Gardens of Versailles* (New York: Cambridge University Press, 1997); Patrick Carroll, *Science, Culture, and Modern State Formation* (Berkeley: University of California Press, 2006).

12.   Robin W. Scheffler and Natalie B. Aviles, "State Planning, Cancer Vaccine Infrastructure, and the Origins of the Oncogene Theory," *Social Studies of Science* 52, no. 2 (2022): 174–98.

13.   Mariana Mazzucato, *The Entrepreneurial State: Debunking Public vs. Private Sector Myths* (New York: Public Affairs, 2015); Fred Block and Matthew R. Keller, eds., *State of Innovation: The U.S. Government's Role in Technology Development* (Boulder, CO: Paradigm, 2011); Suzanne Mettler, *The Submerged State: How Invisible Government Policies Undermine American Democracy* (Chicago: University of Chicago Press, 2011).

14.   The centrality of the NIH is most strikingly demonstrated in network analyses, where it forms a well-connected yet entirely unexplored node in dense networks of academic and industry innovation; see John F. Padgett and Walter W. Powell, *The Emergence of Organizations and Markets* (Princeton, NJ: Princeton University Press, 2012). For a similar critique of how sociologists elide the role of the government in establishing biomedical markets, see Steven P. Vallas, Daniel Lee Kleinman, and Dina Biscotti, "Political Structures and the Making of U.S. Biotechnology," in *State of Innovation: The U.S. Government's Role in Technology Development*, ed. Fred Block and Matthew R. Keller (Boulder, CO: Paradigm, 2011), 57–76.

15.   Mettler, *The Submerged State*, 6.

16.   Touchstone perspectives on neoliberalism in biomedicine include Kaushik Sunder Rajan, *Biocapital: The Constitution of Postgenomic Life* (Durham, NC: Duke University Press, 2006); Nikolas Rose, *The Politics of Life Itself: Biomedicine, Power, and Subjectivity in the Twenty-First Century* (Princeton, NJ: Princeton University Press, 2007). For a critique of this interpretation of science and technology policy from STS, see Elizabeth Popp Berman, "Not Just Neoliberalism: Economization in US Science and Technology Policy," *Science, Technology, & Human Values* 39 no. 3 (2014): 397–431.

17.   Classic studies include Yaron Ezrahi, *The Descent of Icarus: Science and the Transformation of Contemporary Democracy* (Cambridge, MA: Harvard University Press, 1990); David Guston, *Between Politics and Science: Assuring the Integrity and Productivity of Research* (Cambridge: Cambridge University Press, 2000); Sheila Jasanoff, *Designs on Nature: Science and Democracy in Europe and the United States* (Princeton, NJ: Princeton University Press, 2011); Daniel Lee Kleinman, *Politics on the Endless Frontier: Postwar Research Policy in the United States* (Durham, NC: Duke University Press, 1995); Chandra Mukerji, *A Fragile Power: Scientists and the State* (Princeton, NJ: Princeton University Press, 1989); and Theodore M. Porter, *Trust in Numbers: The Pursuit of Objectivity in Science and Public Life* (Princeton, NJ: Princeton University Press, 1996).

18.   Karen Orren and Stephen Skowronek, *The Policy State: An American Predicament* (Cambridge, MA: Harvard University Press, 2017), 110.

19. Joan Fujimura, *Crafting Science: A Sociohistory of the Quest for the Genetics of Cancer* (Cambridge, MA: Harvard University Press, 1996); Monica J. Casper and Adele E. Clarke, "Making the Pap Smear Into the 'Right Tool' for the Job: Cervical Cancer Screening in the USA, Circa 1940–95." *Social Studies of Science* 28, no. 2 (1998): 255–90.

20. Steven Epstein, *Impure Science: AIDS, Activism, and the Politics of Knowledge* (Berkeley: University of California Press, 1996); Steven Epstein, *Inclusion: The Politics of Difference in Medical Research* (Chicago: University of Chicago Press, 2007).

21. Scott Frickel and Kelly Moore, eds., *The New Political Sociology of Science: Institutions, Networks, and Power* (Madison: University of Wisconsin Press, 2006).

22. In STS, David Guston has applied principal-agent theory to conceptualize some policy dynamics in agencies such as the NIH; see Guston, *Between Politics and Science*.

23. As Guston notes, this general observation of the "uncheckability" of science by its patrons was also made in Stephen P. Turner, "Forms of Patronage," in *Theories of Science in Society*, ed. Susan E. Cozzens and Thomas F. Gieryn (Bloomington: Indiana University Press, 1990), 185–211.

24. The first formulation of information asymmetry as a source of bureaucratic agency autonomy vis-à-vis political principals is attributed to Max Weber, "Bureaucracy," in *From Max Weber: Essays in Sociology*, ed. H. H. Girth and C. Wright Mills (Oxford: Oxford University Press, 1958), 196–244.

25. Sean Gailmard and John W. Patty. *Learning While Governing: Expertise and Accountability in the Executive Branch* (Chicago: University of Chicago Press, 2012), 25.

26. Gailmard and Patty, *Learning While Governing*, 39.

27. David H. Guston, "Stabilizing the Boundary Between US Politics and Science: The Role of the Office of Technology Transfer as a Boundary Organization," *Social Studies of Science* 29, no. 1 (1999): 91.

28. Guston, "Stabilizing the Boundary," 104.

29. In taking the extramural grantee's perspective as primary, Guston notes that this creates an "iterated" principal-agent structure between the NCI and grantee scientists where it is interpreted as an intermediary bureaucratic organization that enforces implicit contracts between the government and grant recipients. Guston, "Stabilizing the Boundary," 105. For a similar perspective, see Dietmar Braun, "Who Governs Intermediary Agencies? Principal-Agent Relations in Research Policy-Making," *Journal of Public Policy* 13, no. 2 (1993): 135–62.

30. For an overview of multiple-principal models across the social sciences, see Bart Voorn, Marieke van Genugten, and Sandra van Thiel, "Multiple Principals, Multiple Problems: Implications for Effective Governance and a Research Agenda for Joint Service Delivery," *Public Administration* 97, no. 3 (2019): 671–85.

31. Daniel Carpenter, *The Forging of Bureaucratic Autonomy* (Princeton, NJ: Princeton University Press, 2001); Daniel Carpenter, *Reputation and Power* (Princeton, NJ: Princeton University Press, 2014). For a more general model of why this outcome is common, see Thomas H. Hammond and Jack H. Knott, "Who Controls the Bureaucracy? Presidential Power, Congressional Dominance, Legal Constraints, and Bureaucratic Autonomy in a Model of Multi-institutional Policy-Making," *Journal of Law, Economics, and Organization* 12, no. 1 (1996): 119–66.

32. Sheila Jasanoff, *The Fifth Branch: Science Advisers as Policymakers* (Cambridge, MA: Harvard University Press, 1998).

33. Voorn et al., "Multiple Principals, Multiple Problems," 680–82. Braun comments on the similarity in training between federal scientist-bureaucrats and the scientists they fund as creating closeness between these parties; see Braun, "Who Governs Intermediary Agencies?," 153–54. Though I refer here to scientists on advisory boards of the NCI, a similar closeness to what Braun describes should be imagined to exist for similar reasons.

34. Sean Gailmard, "Multiple Principals and Oversight of Bureaucratic Policy-Making," *Journal of Theoretical Politics* 21, no. 2 (2009): 178. Though Gailmard's model assumes legislative oversight and the NCAB is an executive committee, the basic principle vis-à-vis collective action problems in multiple-principal situations should extend to an intermediary modeled after those discussed in Voorn et al., "Multiple Principals, Multiple Problems."

35. Chris Caswill, "Principals, Agents and Contracts," *Science and Public Policy* 30, no. 5 (2003): 337–46.

36. Gailmard and Patty, *Learning While Governing.*

37. Kiser notes that sociologists commonly sacrifice the parsimony of formal agency models in favor of theoretical perspectives that allow them to better capture multiscalar social forces, such as organizational and institutional relationships, that traditionally motivate sociological analysis; see Kiser, "Comparing Varieties of Agency Theory." While I hope political scientists and economists would find the discussion of how innovation is possible among motivated agents in a context where multiple principals vie to enforce their interests through shifting strategies of monitoring and oversight illuminating, my more primary goal of understanding how science is shaped in ways that reflect particular organizationally specific interpretations of mission and public good is intended to resonate with sociologists and STS scholars.

38. For a discussion of the legacy of pragmatism in STS, see Natalie B. Aviles, "Scientific Innovation as Environed Social Learning," in *Inquiry, Agency, and Democracy: The New Pragmatist Sociology*, ed. Neil Gross, Isaac Ariail Reed, and Christopher Winship (New York: Columbia University Press, 2022), 231–55. For the classic sociological treatment of principal-agent theory built upon rational actor assumptions, see James Coleman, *Foundations of Social Theory* (Cambridge, MA: Harvard University Press, 1990), 145–62.

39. Josh Whitford, "Pragmatism and the Untenable Dualism of Means and Ends: Why Rational Choice Theory Does Not Deserve Paradigmatic Privilege," *Theory and Society* 31, no. 3 (2002): 325–63.

40. In reviewing many empirical and experimental applications of principal-agent theory, Miller finds ample evidence that "irrational" cultural assumptions, such as those around reciprocity and gift exchange, may account for a sizable proportion of the outcomes that principal-agent models presume to emanate from rational calculation instead; see Gary J. Miller, "The Political Evolution of Principal-Agent Models," *Annual Review of Political Science* 8, no. 1 (2005): 217.

41. For a review of the STS literature on expertise, see Harry Collins and Robert Evans, *Rethinking Expertise* (Chicago: University of Chicago Press, 2008).

42. For programmatic statements of practice theories of organization, see Theodore R. Schatzki, "On Organizations as They Happen," *Organization Studies* 27, no. 12 (2006): 1863–73; Martha S. Feldman and Wanda J. Orlikowski, "Theorizing Practice and Practicing Theory," *Organization Science* 22, no. 5 (2011): 1240–53.

43. Timothy Besley and Maitreesh Ghatak, "Competition and Incentives with Motivated Agents," *American Economic Review* 95, no. 3 (2005): 616.

44. Gailmard and Patty, *Learning While Governing*, 28.

45. Mariusz Finkielsztein and Izabela Wagner, "The Sense of Meaninglessness in Bureaucratized Science," *Social Studies of Science* 53, no. 2 (2022): 271–86.

46. These findings are consistent with those that find increased productivity of workers in mission-oriented government and nonprofit organizations, as described in Besley and Ghatak, "Competition and Incentives with Motivated Agents." Additional support in the sociological literature can be found in McDonnell, *Patchwork Leviathan*.

47. McDonnell, *Patchwork Leviathan*, 6.

48. A similar dual mission was observed among public servants in the National Weather Service; see Phaedra Daipha, *Masters of Uncertainty: Weather Forecasters and the Quest for Ground Truth* (Chicago: University of Chicago Press, 2015).

49. Diane Vaughan, *The Challenger Launch Decision: Risky Technology, Culture, and Deviance at NASA* (Chicago: University of Chicago Press, 1996); Diane Vaughan, "The Role of the Organization in the Production of Techno-Scientific Knowledge," *Social Studies of Science* 29, no. 6 (1999): 913–43; Janet Vertesi, *Shaping Science: Organizations, Decisions, and Culture on NASA's Teams* (Chicago: University of Chicago Press, 2020).

50. Adele Clarke and Susan Leigh Star, "The Social Worlds Framework: A Theory/Methods Package," in *The Handbook of Science and Technology Studies*, 3rd ed., ed. Edward J. Hackett et al. (Cambridge, MA: MIT Press, 2008), 113–37. For exemplary illustrations of the social worlds analytic in STS, see Susan Leigh Star and James R. Griesemer, "Institutional Ecology, 'Translations' and Boundary Objects: Amateurs and Professionals in Berkeley's Museum of Vertebrate Zoology, 1907–39," *Social Studies of Science* 19, no. 3 (August 1, 1989): 387–420; Fujimura, *Crafting Science*.

51. Joseph Rouse, *Articulating the World* (Chicago: University of Chicago Press, 2015). I have more fully specified the connection between social worlds and Rouse's pragmatism in Aviles, "Scientific Innovation as Environed Social Learning."

52. My use of social learning builds upon a substantial literature in organizational sociology; see Chris Argyris and Donald A. Schön, *Organizational Learning: A Theory of Action Perspective* (Reading, MA: Addison-Wesley, 1978); Mark Easterby-Smith, Mary Crossan, and Davide Nicolini, "Organizational Learning: Debates Past, Present and Future," *Journal of Management Studies* 37, no. 6 (September 1, 2000): 783–96; Barbara Levitt and James G. March, "Organizational Learning," *Annual Review of Sociology* 14 (1988): 319–40. A fuller discussion of how the model of environed social learning fits into these debates in organizational sociology can be found in Aviles, "Scientific Innovation as Environed Social Learning."

53. Richard Swedberg, "Colligation," in *Concepts in Action: Conceptual Constructionism*, ed. Håkon Leiulfsrud and Peter Sohlberg (Leiden: Brill, 2017), 64.

54. Rouse, *Articulating the World*.

55.   Andrew Abbott, *Processual Sociology* (Chicago: University of Chicago Press, 2016), 33.

56.   R. Keith Sawyer, *Explaining Creativity: The Science of Human Innovation* (Oxford: Oxford University Press, 2011), 8.

57.   Jeffrey Haydu, "Making Use of the Past: Time Periods as Cases to Compare and as Sequences of Problem Solving," *American Journal of Sociology* 104, no. 2 (1998): 339–71.

58.   Readers interested in studies of how organized science can lead to failure are directed toward Vaughan, *The Challenger Launch Decision*; Daipha, *Masters of Uncertainty*.

59.   Other significant organizations involved in cancer virus and vaccine innovation in the United States besides the NCI are analyzed in Gregory J. Morgan, *Cancer Virus Hunters: A History of Tumor Virology* (Baltimore, MD: Johns Hopkins University Press, 2022), which examines research conducted at the Rockefeller Institute for Medical Research and Cold Spring Harbor Laboratory; and Louis Galambos and Jane Eliot Sewell, *Networks of Innovation: Vaccine Development at Merck, Sharp and Dohme, and Mulford, 1895–1995* (Cambridge: Cambridge University Press, 1997), which looks at work done in Merck & Company's internal laboratories.

60.   Frank J. Rauscher Jr. and Michael B. Shimkin, "Viral Oncology," in *NIH: An Account of Research in Its Laboratories and Clinics*, ed. DeWitt Stetten and W. T. Carrigan (Orlando, FL: Academic Press, 1984), 350–67.

61.   Kristen Intemann and Inmaculada de Melo-Martín, "Social Values and Scientific Evidence: The Case of the HPV Vaccines," *Biology and Philosophy* 25 no. 2 (2010): 203–13; Kaushik Sunder Rajan and Sabina Leonelli, "Introduction: Biomedical Trans-Actions, Postgenomics, and Knowledge/Value," *Public Culture* 25 no. 3 (2013): 463–75. For discussions of how market logic has infiltrated academic science, see Elizabeth Popp Berman, *Creating the Market University: How Academic Science Became an Economic Engine* (Princeton, NJ: Princeton University Press, 2011); Philip Mirowski, *Science-Mart: Privatizing American Science* (Cambridge, MA: Harvard University Press, 2011); Daniel Lee Kleinman, *Impure Cultures: University Biology and the World of Commerce* (Madison: University of Wisconsin Press, 2003); Mark Dennis Robinson, *The Market in Mind: How Financialization Is Shaping Neuroscience, Translational Medicine, and Innovation in Biotechnology* (Cambridge, MA: MIT Press, 2019).

62.   Galambos and Sewell, *Networks of Innovation*; Kendall Hoyt, *Long Shot: Vaccines for National Defense* (Cambridge, MA: Harvard University Press, 2012); Edward Shorter, *The Health Century* (New York: Doubleday, 1987).

63.   For a review of historical changes to the vaccine industry in the United States and Europe in the latter half of the twentieth century, see Stuart Blume, "Towards a History of 'the Vaccine Innovation System,' 1950–2000," in *Biomedicine in the Twentieth Century: Practices, Policies, and Politics*, ed. Caroline Hannaway, 255–86 (Washington, DC: IOS Press, 2008).

64.   September 1, 1994, memo from NIH Legal Advisor to Robert H. Purcell, NIAID, "The $100,000 Cap on Royalties to Inventors in the Federal Technology Transfer Act," Harold Varmus papers, Box 7, Folder 1 (Bethesda, MD: National Library of Medicine, 1994). This cap was recently raised to $150,000, though this remains slight compared to the compensation nongovernment inventors receive when they retain personal intellectual property rights.

65. Guston, "Stabilizing the Boundary," 102.

66. The concepts of "basic" and "applied" research have their own variable legacy across this period of study and can be subject to contestation; see Jane Calvert, "The Idea of 'Basic Research' in Language and Practice," *Minerva* 42 no. 3 (2004): 251–68.

67. See Galambos and Sewell, *Networks of Innovation.*

68. Peter Keating and Alberto Cambrosio, *Cancer on Trial: Oncology as a New Style of Practice* (Chicago: University of Chicago Press, 2011); Robin Wolfe Scheffler, *A Contagious Cause: The American Hunt for Cancer Viruses and the Rise of Molecular Medicine* (Chicago: University of Chicago Press, 2019); Fujimura, *Crafting Science.*

1. MEDICINE, MELIORISM, AND THE MAKING OF A MODERN NCI

1. Victoria A. Harden, *Inventing the NIH: Federal Biomedical Research Policy, 1887–1937* (Baltimore, MD: Johns Hopkins University Press, 1986).

2. Stephen P. Strickland, *Politics, Science, and Dread Disease: A Short History of United States Medical Research Policy* (Cambridge, MA: Harvard University Press, 1972), 235.

3. Richard Rettig, *Cancer Crusade: The Story of the National Cancer Act of 1971* (Lincoln, NE: iUniverse, 2005), 46.

4. Richard Mandel, *A Half-Century of Peer Review: 1946–1996* (Bethesda, MD: Division of Research Grants, National Institutes of Health, 1996), 5.

5. Text of bill quoted in Ludwig Hektoen, "The National Cancer Institute Act," *California and Western Medicine* 49, no. 6 (December 1938): 499–500.

6. Sheila Jasanoff, *The Fifth Branch: Science Advisers as Policymakers* (Cambridge, MA: Harvard University Press, 1998).

7. Rachel Kahn Best, *Common Enemies: Disease Campaigns in America* (New York: Oxford University Press, 2019).

8. Bhaven N. Sampat, "Mission-Oriented Biomedical Research at the NIH," *Research Policy* 41, no. 10 (2012): 1730.

9. Sampat, "Mission-Oriented Biomedical Research at the NIH," 1732. Congressional ethics reforms in 2007 also had a chilling effect on hard earmarks.

10. Deepak Hegde and Bhaven Sampat, "Can Private Money Buy Public Science? Disease Group Lobbying and Federal Funding for Biomedical Research," *Management Science* 61, no. 10 (2015): 2281–98.

11. Hegde and Sampat, "Can Private Money Buy Public Science," 2293.

12. Colin Koopman, *Pragmatism as Transition: Historicity and Hope in James, Dewey, and Rorty* (New York: Columbia University Press, 2009), 167.

13. Robin Wolfe Scheffler, *A Contagious Cause: The American Hunt for Cancer Viruses and the Rise of Molecular Medicine* (Chicago: University of Chicago Press, 2019), 4.

14. Strickland, *Politics, Science, and Dread Disease,* 233.

15. See Daniel Lee Kleinman, *Politics on the Endless Frontier: Postwar Research Policy in the United States* (Durham, NC: Duke University Press, 1995).

16. Strickland, *Politics, Science, and Dread Disease,* 16.

17. Strickland, *Politics, Science, and Dread Disease,* 18–19.

18. Mandel, *A Half-Century of Peer Review,* 12.

19. Beatrix Hoffman, *Health Care for Some: Rights and Rationing in the United States Since 1930* (Chicago: University of Chicago Press, 2012), 41.

20. Strickland, *Politics, Science, and Dread Disease*, 19.

21. The influence of McIntyre's opposition to a national health care bill on Roosevelt's decision to exclude health care from Social Security legislation is documented in Hoffman, *Health Care for Some*, 25.

22. Strickland, *Politics, Science, and Dread Disease*, 22–23.

23. Strickland, *Politics, Science, and Dread Disease*, 23; see also Paul Starr, *The Social Transformation of American Medicine: The Rise of a Sovereign Profession and the Making of a Vast Industry* (New York: Basic Books, 1982).

24. Kleinman, *Politics on the Endless Frontier*, 150.

25. Strickland, *Politics, Science, and Dread Disease*, 29.

26. Strickland, *Politics, Science, and Dread Disease*, 30.

27. Daniel Sledge, *Health Divided: Public Health and Individual Medicine in the Making of the Modern American State* (Lawrence: University Press of Kansas, 2017), 9.

28. Sledge, *Health Divided*, 10.

29. AMA spokesperson Dr. Olin West, 1937, quoted in Strickland, *Politics, Science, and Dread Disease*, 14.

30. Strickland, *Politics, Science, and Dread Disease*, 55; see also Starr, *The Social Transformation of American Medicine*.

31. Sledge, *Health Divided*, 111.

32. Sledge, *Health Divided*, 111–112.

33. Sledge, *Health Divided*.

34. The AMA's vociferous and highly successful opposition to Truman's national health care proposals are well documented in Starr, *The Social Transformation of American Medicine*.

35. Starr, *The Social Transformation of American Medicine*, 289.

36. Starr, *The Social Transformation of American Medicine*, 336. Indeed, a major objection to many of the modest proposals for health care reform or expansion were scuttled by Southern Democrats if they posed even a minor threat of social reorganization, i.e., by enabling or enforcing racial integration; see Strickland, *Politics, Science, and Dread Disease*; and Hoffman, *Health Care for Some*.

37. Starr, *The Social Transformation of American Medicine*, 337.

38. Starr, *The Social Transformation of American Medicine*, 343.

39. Starr, *The Social Transformation of American Medicine*, 347.

40. Angela N. H. Creager. "Mobilizing Biomedicine: Virus Research Between Lay Health Organizations and the U.S. Federal Government, 1935–1955," in *Biomedicine in the Twentieth Century: Practices, Policies, and Politics*, ed. Caroline Hannaway (Amsterdam: IOS Press, 2008), 171–201.

41. Rettig, *Cancer Crusade*, 19.

42. Rettig, *Cancer Crusade*, 34.

43. Rettig, *Cancer Crusade*, 35.

44. Starr, *The Social Transformation of American Medicine*, 343.

45. Strickland's history of postwar cancer research policy benefits from interviews with both Lasker and Mahoney, who shared their motivations for building the cancer lobby extensively with that author.

46. Strickland, *Politics, Science, and Dread Disease*, 33.
47. Strickland, *Politics, Science, and Dread Disease*, 33.
48. Strickland, *Politics, Science, and Dread Disease*, 34.
49. Scheffler, *A Contagious Cause*, 85.
50. Scheffler, *A Contagious Cause*, 85.
51. Scheffler, *A Contagious Cause*, 86.
52. Scheffler, *A Contagious Cause*, 87.
53. Scheffler, *A Contagious Cause*, 87.
54. Scheffler, *A Contagious Cause*, 94.
55. Strickland, *Politics, Science, and Dread Disease*, 39–40.
56. See Best, *Common Enemies*.
57. Strickland, *Politics, Science, and Dread Disease*, 48.
58. Strickland, *Politics, Science, and Dread Disease*, 50.
59. Strickland, *Politics, Science, and Dread Disease*, 49.
60. Strickland, *Politics, Science, and Dread Disease*, 175.
61. Mandel, *A Half-Century of Peer Review*, 62.
62. Mandel, *A Half-Century of Peer Review*, 66.
63. Starr, *The Social Transformation of American Medicine*, 347.
64. Mandel, *A Half-Century of Peer Review*, 68.
65. Mandel, *A Half-Century of Peer Review*, 74. The use of radiation in cancer research and therapy was a particularly noteworthy example of coupling material infrastructure with styles of laboratory and clinical practice, and the use of extramural cooperative groups anticipates the circulation of protocols in clinical oncology described in Peter Keating and Alberto Cambrosio, *Cancer on Trial: Oncology as a New Style of Practice* (Chicago: University of Chicago Press, 2011).
66. Scheffler, *A Contagious Cause*, 81.
67. Starr, *The Social Transformation of American Medicine*, 370.
68. Strickland, *Politics, Science, and Dread Disease*, 259.
69. Starr, *The Social Transformation of American Medicine*, 343.
70. The surgeon general formalized these decentralized relationships among institutes and the NIH, and between the NIH and PHS, in 1951; see Mandel, *A Half-Century of Peer Review*, 57.
71. Rettig, *Cancer Crusade*, 53.
72. Buhm Soon Park, "Disease Categories and Scientific Disciplines: Reorganizing the NIH Intramural Program, 1945–1960," in *Biomedicine in the Twentieth Century: Practices, Policies, and Politics*, ed. Caroline Hannaway (Amsterdam: IOS Press, 2008), 27–58.
73. Rettig, *Cancer Crusade*, 50.
74. David Cantor. "Radium and the Origins of the National Cancer Institute," in *Biomedicine in the Twentieth Century: Practices, Policies, and Politics*, ed. Caroline Hannaway (Amsterdam: IOS Press, 2008), 95–146.
75. Rettig, *Cancer Crusade*, 50–51.
76. Scheffler, *A Contagious Cause*, 94.
77. Rettig, *Cancer Crusade*, 58; and Scheffler, *A Contagious Cause*, 94.
78. Rettig, *Cancer Crusade*, 61.
79. Rettig, *Cancer Crusade*, 61.

80. Rettig, *Cancer Crusade*, 10.

81. Scheffler, *A Contagious Cause*, 96.

82. Strickland, *Politics, Science, and Dread Disease*, 75.

83. Strickland, *Politics, Science, and Dread Disease*, 185.

84. Strickland, *Politics, Science, and Dread Disease*, 186.

85. Strickland, *Politics, Science, and Dread Disease*, 195.

86. John F. Kennedy, text of speech at the Little White House, Warm Springs, Georgia (October 10, 1960). Papers of John F. Kennedy, Pre-Presidential Papers. Senate Files. Speeches and the Press. Speech Files, 1953–1960 (JFKSEN-0912-068, John F. Kennedy Presidential Library and Museum). Digitized copy available at https://www.jfklibrary .org/asset-viewer/archives/JFKSEN/0912/JFKSEN-0912-068.

87. Strickland, *Politics, Science, and Dread Disease*, 132.

88. Strickland, *Politics, Science, and Dread Disease*, 131–32.

89. Rettig, *Cancer Crusade*, 10.

2. CANCER VIRUSES AND THE PROMISE OF A VACCINE, 1958–1968

1. "Introduction," Intramural Research Program (Non-Clinical Programs). National Cancer Institute, *Annual Report 1962* (National Archives and Records Administration II, College Park, MD [hereafter NARA II], Record Group 443, UD-WW Entry 4, Box 3), 908.

2. For a history of Ludwik Gross's tumor virus studies and their relationship to early cancer virus efforts in the NCI led by Sarah Stewart, see Gregory J. Morgan, "Ludwik Gross, Sarah Stewart, and the 1950s Discoveries of Gross Murine Leukemia Virus and Polyoma Virus," *Studies in History and Philosophy of Science Part C: Studies in History and Philosophy of Biological and Biomedical Sciences* 48, part B (2014): 200–209.

3. National Cancer Institute, *Analysis of Program Activities 1954, Volume II* (Bethesda, MD: U.S. Department of Health, Education, and Welfare, 1954), 2–3.

4. Doogab Yi, "Governing, Financing, and Planning Cancer Virus Research: The Emergence of Organized Science at the U.S. National Cancer Institute in the 1950s and 1960s," *Korean Journal for the History of Science* 38, no. 2 (2016): 321–49; and Robin Wolfe Scheffler, *A Contagious Cause: The American Hunt for Cancer Viruses and the Rise of Molecular Medicine* (Chicago: University of Chicago Press, 2019).

5. This discussion is elaborated in greater detail in Robin Wolfe Scheffler and Natalie B. Aviles, "State Planning, Cancer Vaccine Infrastructure, and the Origins of the Oncogene Theory," *Social Studies of Science* 52, no. 2 (2022): 174–98.

6. Edward Shorter, *The Health Century* (New York: Doubleday, 1987), 197.

7. "Project Report 427," National Cancer Institute, *Analysis of Program Activities 1954, Volume II* (Bethesda, MD: U.S. Department of Health, Education, and Welfare, 1954), 3.

8. See Ton van Helvoort, "A Century of Research Into the Cause of Cancer: Is the New Oncogene Paradigm Revolutionary?" *History and Philosophy of the Life Sciences* 21, no. 3 (1999): 293–330.

9. "Project Report 427," National Cancer Institute, *Analysis of Program Activities 1954, Volume II*, 6.

10. "Project Report 433," National Cancer Institute, *Analysis of Program Activities 1956, Volume II* (Bethesda, MD: U.S. Department of Health, Education, and Welfare, 1956), 281.

11. Morgan, "Ludwik Gross, Sarah Stewart, and the 1950s Discoveries of Gross Murine Leukemia Virus and Polyoma Virus," 204.

12. "Bernice Eddy, Ph.D. (1903–1989)," National Institutes of Health, https://history.nih.gov /display/history/Eddy%2C+Bernice.

13. Priority over the discovery of the SE polyomavirus was contested, as Gross himself would claim to have detected the virus first; see Morgan, "Ludwik Gross, Sarah Stewart, and the 1950s Discoveries of Gross Murine Leukemia Virus and Polyoma Virus."

14. "Project Report 524," National Cancer Institute, *Annual Report of Program Activities 1958, Volume II* (Bethesda, MD: U.S. Department of Health, Education, and Welfare, 1958), 1031.

15. Many women who made early contributions to cancer virology and vaccinology saw their careers limited by sexism as described in Morgan, *Cancer Virus Hunters: A History of Tumor Virology* (Baltimore, MD: Johns Hopkins University Press, 2022).

16. Shorter, *The Health Century*, 198.

17. "Project Report 433," National Cancer Institute, *Annual Report of Program Activities 1958, Volume II* (Bethesda, MD: U.S. Department of Health, Education, and Welfare, 1958), 637–40.

18. "Project Report 416a," National Cancer Institute, *Annual Report of Program Activities 1958, Volume II* (Bethesda, MD: U.S. Department of Health, Education, and Welfare, 1958), 601.

19. "Project Report 416b," National Cancer Institute, *Annual Report of Program Activities 1958, Volume II* (Bethesda, MD: U.S. Department of Health, Education, and Welfare, 1958), 672.

20. This situation was frequently discussed in meetings of advisory boards. Researchers also reported that limitations of space and personnel prevented them from pursuing experiments planned for a given fiscal year; see, e.g., "Project Report 427d," National Cancer Institute, *Annual Report of Program Activities 1959, Volume II* (Bethesda, MD: U.S. Department of Health, Education, and Welfare, 1959), 632.

21. Carl G. Baker, "Administrative History of the National Cancer Institute's Viruses and Cancer Programs, 1950–1972," 9. National Institutes of Health, https://history.nih.gov /research/downloads/SpecialVirusCaPrgm.pdf.

22. "Virology Research Resources Branch," National Cancer Institute, *Annual Report 1962* (NARA II, Record Group 443, UD-WW Entry 4, Box 3), 178.

23. "Virology Research Resources Branch," National Cancer Institute, *Annual Report 1962*, 179.

24. Baker, "Administrative History of the National Cancer Institute's Viruses and Cancer Programs," 14.

25. Scheffler, *A Contagious Cause*, 102.

26. For an extensive history of the CCNSC, see Peter Keating and Alberto Cambrosio, *Cancer on Trial: Oncology as a New Style of Practice* (Chicago: University of Chicago Press, 2011).

27. Baker, "Administrative History of the National Cancer Institute's Viruses and Cancer Programs," 23 (emphasis in original).

28. Baker, "Administrative History of the National Cancer Institute's Viruses and Cancer Programs," 23.

29. Richard Rettig, *Cancer Crusade: The Story of the National Cancer Act of 1971* (Lincoln, NE: iUniverse, 2005), 64.

30. Baker, "Administrative History of the National Cancer Institute's Viruses and Cancer Programs," 44.

31. Baker, "Administrative History of the National Cancer Institute's Viruses and Cancer Programs," 35. The so-called Fountain Committee, headed by U.S. Rep. Lawrence Fountain, launched a series of investigations beginning in 1959 into alleged misappropriations of NIH funds that led to accusations the NIH lacked the administrative capacity to properly oversee its large budgets. Though embarrassing for NIH director James Shannon, the effects on the NIH budget were confined to a mild and short-lived downward adjustment to the NIH budget in 1963–1965, which did not affect the steady growth in cancer virus research in the NCI. See Stephen P. Strickland, *Politics, Science, and Dread Disease: A Short History of United States Medical Research Policy* (Cambridge, MA: Harvard University Press, 1972), 170–78.

32. Rettig, *Cancer Crusade*, 65.

33. Baker, "Administrative History of the National Cancer Institute's Viruses and Cancer Programs, 35.

34. Baker, "Administrative History of the National Cancer Institute's Viruses and Cancer Programs, 49–50.

35. Baker, "Administrative History of the National Cancer Institute's Viruses and Cancer Programs, 31.

36. Scheffler, *A Contagious Cause*, 70.

37. Baker, "Administrative History of the National Cancer Institute's Viruses and Cancer Programs," 35.

38. Baker, "Administrative History of the National Cancer Institute's Viruses and Cancer Programs," 35, 49.

39. Baker, "Administrative History of the National Cancer Institute's Viruses and Cancer Programs," 49.

40. Daryl E. Chubin and Kenneth E. Studer, "The Politics of Cancer," *Theory and Society* 6, no. 1 (1978): 55–74; and Scheffler, *A Contagious Cause*, 177–80.

41. Strickland, *Politics, Science, and Dread Disease*, 203.

42. Strickland, *Politics, Science, and Dread Disease*, 204–5.

43. U.S. Department of Health, Education and Welfare, Office of the Secretary, Office of the Assistant Secretary of Health and Scientific Affairs, *Report of the Secretary's Advisory Committee on the Management of National Institutes of Health Research Contracts and Grants* (Washington, D.C.: Government Printing Office, 1966); and Rettig, *Cancer Crusade*, 64.

44. Scheffler, *A Contagious Cause*, 122.

45. "Collaborative Research, Operations Branch," National Cancer Institute, *Annual Report 1962* (NARA II, Record Group 443, UD-WW Entry 4, Box 3), 16.

46. Baker, "Administrative History of the National Cancer Institute's Viruses and Cancer Programs," 111.

47. I use the actor's category "scientist-manager" to refer to this subset of scientist-bureaucrats working in the virus cancer programs wherever relevant. Readers should be advised that scientist-managers are a subset of the more general scientist-bureaucrats specific to

this historical period who supervised contract researchers in addition to fulfilling their usual bureaucratic functions.

48. Baker, "Administrative History of the National Cancer Institute's Viruses and Cancer Programs," 37.

49. "Office of the Director," National Cancer Institute, *Annual Report 1962* (NARA II, Record Group 443, UD-WW Entry 4, Box 3), 1.

50. "Project Report 3011c," National Cancer Institute, *Annual Report 1962* (NARA II, Record Group 443, UD-WW Entry 4, Box 3), 1569.

51. Scheffler and Aviles, "State Planning, Cancer Vaccine Infrastructure, and the Origins of the Oncogene Theory."

52. "Office of the Director," National Cancer Institute, *Annual Report 1962* (NARA II, Record Group 443, UD-WW Entry 4, Box 3), 1.

53. Baker, "Administrative History of the National Cancer Institute's Viruses and Cancer Programs," 40.

54. "Virology Research Resources Branch," National Cancer Institute, *Annual Report 1965* (NARA II, Record Group 443, UD-WW Entry 4, Box 4), 649.

55. "Virology Research Resources Branch," National Cancer Institute, *Annual Report 1965*, 649.

56. "Virology Research Resources Branch," National Cancer Institute, *Annual Report 1965*, 649.

57. "Virology Research Resources Branch," National Cancer Institute, *Annual Report 1962* (NARA II, Record Group 443, UD-WW Entry 4, Box 3), 181.

58. "Virology Research Resources Branch," National Cancer Institute, *Annual Report 1965*, 651.

59. "Virology Research Resources Branch," National Cancer Institute, *Annual Report 1965*, 651.

60. "Office of the Director," National Cancer Institute, *Annual Report 1962*, 1–2.

61. "Virology Research Resources Branch," National Cancer Institute, *Annual Report 1962*, 183.

62. "Director of Intramural Research, Summary Report," National Cancer Institute, *Annual Report 1962* (NARA II, Record Group 443, UD-WW Entry 4, Box 3), 910.

63. Though the "C-type" virus designation was decommissioned as viruses were identified and classified into other virus families in the 1970s, it was used throughout the 1960s to refer to a group of RNA viruses that share certain morphological similarities and whose particles are often recovered from cell cytoplasmic channels or bone marrow.

64. Baker, "Administrative History of the National Cancer Institute's Viruses and Cancer Programs," 47.

65. Huebner's fortunes at NIAID were waning at the time, and NCI provided a significant source of funding that enabled him to pursue his interests in tumor viruses; see Edward A. Beeman. "Robert J. Huebner, M.D.: A Virologist's Journey," 340 and 361–62. National Institutes of Health, https://history.nih.gov/research/downloads/HuebnerBiography.pdf. Huebner would officially join the NCI in 1967, though his transfer to the NCI was initiated in 1962 (Baker, "Administrative History of the National Cancer Institute's Viruses and Cancer Programs," 47). Baker would later call Huebner one of the great

"generals" in the War on Cancer (Baker, "Administrative History of the National Cancer Institute's Viruses and Cancer Programs," 338).

66. Baker, "Administrative History of the National Cancer Institute's Viruses and Cancer Programs," 69–70.

67. Ray Bryan, Laboratory of Viral Oncology, NCI, February 5, 1963. Status report of the Human Cancer Virus Task Force. Memorandum to Scientific Directorate, NCI. Reproduced in Baker, "Administrative History of the National Cancer Institute's Viruses and Cancer Programs," 78–79.

68. Baker, "Administrative History of the National Cancer Institute's Viruses and Cancer Programs," 80.

69. Beeman, "Robert J. Huebner, M.D.," 344.

70. Bryan memorandum from Baker, "Administrative History of the National Cancer Institute's Viruses and Cancer Programs," 80.

71. Baker, "Administrative History of the National Cancer Institute's Viruses and Cancer Programs," 80.

72. For descriptions of the NIH Research Administration Discussion Group, see Yi, "Governing, Financing, and Planning Cancer Virus Research"; and Scheffler, *A Contagious Cause*, 106–8.

73. Yi, "Governing, Financing, and Planning Cancer Virus Research," 331.

74. Scheffler, *A Contagious Cause*, 108.

75. Rettig, *Cancer Crusade*, 66–67.

76. Scheffler, *A Contagious Cause*, 120.

77. The assumption that the impetus for funding virus cancer research in the NCI came from outside undergirds the argument of Doogab Yi; see Yi, "Governing, Financing, and Planning Cancer Virus Research."

78. Frank Rauscher and Robert Reisinger, *Special Virus Leukemia Program Progress Report #4* (Bethesda, MD: U.S. Department of Health, Education and Welfare, 1964).

79. Discussion materials, NIH Group for Discussion of Research Administration Meeting, January 23, 1957, 1; quoted in Scheffler, *A Contagious Cause*, 107. The personal papers of Carl G. Baker, which included this and other important memoranda, were once housed in the National Library of Medicine but were lost in the late 2010s.

80. "Special Report: Virus Cancer Program" (for Director, NCI), January 1962. Baker Papers, Virus and Cancer Programs, Backup Memoranda 1950–1962, 1962; quoted in Scheffler and Aviles, "State Planning, Cancer Vaccine Infrastructure, and the Origins of the Oncogene Theory," 180.

81. "Office of the Director, Introduction," National Cancer Institute, *Annual Report 1965* (NARA II, Record Group 443, UD-WW Entry 4, Box 4), 2.

82. Scheffler, *A Contagious Cause*, 135.

83. Scheffler, *A Contagious Cause*, 135.

84. Scheffler argues that this dual life of prospective human cancer viruses was effected by transforming them into "administrative objects; see Scheffler, *A Contagious Cause*, 126. In subsequent work, Scheffler and Aviles add to this focus an emphasis on the materiality of cancer virus infrastructure over their administrative performance; see Scheffler and Aviles, "State Planning, Cancer Vaccine Infrastructure, and the Origins

of the Oncogene Theory." Both perspectives remain relevant to this interpretation of the SVLP.

85.   Scheffler and Aviles, "State Planning, Cancer Vaccine Infrastructure, and the Origins of the Oncogene Theory."

86.   Working groups were formed for development; testing and monitoring; epidemiology; resources and logistics; production; biohazards control and containment; special animal leukemia ecology studies; and human leukemia therapy (Baker, "Administrative History of the National Cancer Institute's Viruses and Cancer Programs," 136).

87.   "Office of the Director, Introduction," National Cancer Institute, *Annual Report 1965*, 1.

88.   Louis M. Carrese and Carl G. Baker, "The Convergence Technique: A Method for the Planning and Programming of Research Efforts," *Management Science* 13, no. 8 (1967): B420–B438.

89.   Scheffler and Aviles, "State Planning, Cancer Vaccine Infrastructure, and the Origins of the Oncogene Theory," 181.

90.   "Office of the Director, Introduction," National Cancer Institute, *Annual Report 1965*, 1–2.

91.   Beeman, "Robert J. Huebner, M.D.," 352.

92.   "Office of the Director, Introduction," National Cancer Institute, *Annual Report 1965*, 1.

93.   Baker, "Administrative History of the National Cancer Institute's Viruses and Cancer Programs," 145.

94.   Morgan, "Ludwik Gross, Sarah Stewart, and the 1950s Discoveries of Gross Murine Leukemia Virus and Polyoma Virus."

95.   See Nicholas Wade, "Special Virus Cancer Program: Travails of a Biological Moonshot," *Science* 174, no. 4016 (1971): 1311. Sociologists of science were not immune to this utilitarian interpretation, as evidenced by Studer and Chubin's argument that the program's continued focus on C-type RNA viruses in no small part reflected its constituent scientists' career stakes; see Chubin and Studer, "The Politics of Cancer."

96.   Baker, "Administrative History of the National Cancer Institute's Viruses and Cancer Programs," 114.

97.   "Office of the Director, Introduction," National Cancer Institute, *Annual Report 1966* (NARA II, Record Group 443, UD-WW Entry 4, Box 5), 5–6.

98.   "Scientific Director for Etiology Summary Report," National Cancer Institute, *Annual Report 1966* (NARA II, Record Group 443, UD-WW Entry 4, Box 5), 498.

99.   "Virus Leukemia & Lymphoma Branch Summary Report," National Cancer Institute, *Annual Report 1966* (NARA II, Record Group 443, UD-WW Entry 4, Box 5), 1005.

100. "Project Report 4823," National Cancer Institute, *Annual Report 1966* (NARA II, Record Group 443, UD-WW Entry 4, Box 5), 1028.

101. "Project Report 4823," National Cancer Institute, *Annual Report 1966* (NARA II, Record Group 443, UD-WW Entry 4, Box 5), 1034.

102. "Project Report 4823," National Cancer Institute, *Annual Report 1966* (NARA II, Record Group 443, UD-WW Entry 4, Box 5), 1034.

103. Morgan, *Cancer Virus Hunters*, 115–16.

104. Farah Huzair and Steve Sturdy, "Biotechnology and the Transformation of Vaccine Innovation: The Case of the Hepatitis B Vaccines 1968–2000," *Studies in History and*

Philosophy of Science Part C: Studies in History and Philosophy of Biological and Biomedical Sciences 64 (2017): 12–13. Ironically, former SVCP researcher Edward Scolnick would go on to spearhead Merck's subsequent effort to develop a second-generation hepatitis B vaccine using recombinant subunit proteins instead of the human plasma system first developed by Blumberg. These projects unfolded in the 1980s, well after the SVCP was shuttered. For analysis of Merck's efforts to develop the recombinant subunit hepatitis B vaccine, see Huzair and Sturdy, "Biotechnology and the Transformation of Vaccine Innovation," 14–16; and Louis Galambos and Jane Eliot Sewell, *Networks of Innovation: Vaccine Development at Merck, Sharp and Dohme, and Mulford, 1895–1995* (New York: Cambridge University Press, 1997), 172–76.

105.   "Virus Leukemia & Lymphoma Branch Summary Report," National Cancer Institute, *Annual Report 1966* (NARA II, Record Group 443, UD-WW Entry 4, Box 5), 998.

106.   "Virus Leukemia & Lymphoma Branch Summary Report," National Cancer Institute, *Annual Report 1966*, 1010.

107.   Scheffler and Aviles, "State Planning, Cancer Vaccine Infrastructure, and the Origins of the Oncogene Theory."

108.   Baker, "Administrative History of the National Cancer Institute's Viruses and Cancer Programs," 125.

109.   The convergence technique was also implemented in the Chemotherapy Program, whose participants maintained a similar distance from industry techniques as SVLP scientists did from NASA. For more on convergence in the CCNSC, see Keating and Cambrosio, *Cancer on Trial*, 171–74.

110.   Beeman, "Robert J. Huebner, M.D.," 364.

111.   Beeman, "Robert J. Huebner, M.D.," 374.

112.   Scheffler, *A Contagious Cause*, 131–35.

113.   Kenneth Endicott, "Reorganization of the National Cancer Institute," Memo to James Shannon, Director, NIH (June 25, 1965). National Institutes of Health Office of the Director Central Files (NARA II, Record Group 443, UD-06D Entry 1, Box 49, Folder 12), 3.

114.   "Scientific Director for Etiology Summary Report," National Cancer Institute, *Annual Report 1966* (NARA II, Record Group 443, UD-WW Entry 4, Box 5), 494.

115.   Baker, "Administrative History of the National Cancer Institute's Viruses and Cancer Programs," 145.

116.   Gretchen Case, "Carl Baker Oral History Interview Transcript," part I (November 20, 1996), 17. Office of NIH History Oral History Archive, https://history.n12ih.gov/archives/downloads/Bakerinterview1996.pdf.

117.   Wade, "Special Virus Cancer Program," 1311.

118.   For example, SVLP scientists failed to route meeting minutes to project officers and sometimes did not inform project officers when or where section meetings would be held. February 2, 1967 meeting minutes of the Special Virus Leukemia Program. Cancer Chemotherapy Program, 1969–81 (NARA II, Record Group 443, UD-UP Entry 7, Box 3, Folder 5), 1–2.

119.   June 1, 1967, meeting minutes of the Special Virus Leukemia Program. Cancer Chemotherapy Program, 1969–81 (NARA II, Record Group 443, UD-UP Entry 7, Box 3, Folder 5), 3.

120. Wade, "Special Virus Cancer Program," 1307.

121. Thus the earliest programs to examine cancers beyond leukemia in the SVLP targeted sarcomas associated with C-type leukemia virus strains that NCI researchers Moloney and Bryan had previously discovered; see Beeman, "Robert J. Huebner, M.D.," 375–76.

122. "Special Virus-Leukemia Program Summary," National Cancer Institute, *Annual Report of Program Activities, 1967* (NARA II, Record Group 443, UD-WW Entry 4, Box 5), 1049.

123. "Special Virus-Leukemia Program Summary," National Cancer Institute, *Annual Report of Program Activities, 1967*, 1049.

124. John H. Kelso, Executive Officer, PHS, July 14, 1967, "Reorganization of the Office of the Associate Director for Program, National Cancer Institute." Memo to William H. Stewart, Attorney General. National Institutes of Health Office of the Director Central Files (NARA II, Record Group 443, UD-06D Entry 1, Box 49, Folder 12).

125. Carrese and Baker, "The Convergence Technique," B436.

126. Jane Calvert, "The Idea of 'Basic Research' in Language and Practice," *Minerva* 42, no. 3 (2004): 251–68; but see Philip Mirowski, *Science-Mart: Privatizing American Science* (Cambridge, MA: Harvard University Press, 2011), 47–56, for an analysis of its roots in interwar debates over the economics of science.

127. Rettig, *Cancer Crusade*, 79.

128. Baker, "Administrative History of the National Cancer Institute's Viruses and Cancer Programs," 276.

129. Baker, "Administrative History of the National Cancer Institute's Viruses and Cancer Programs," 280.

130. Scheffler, *A Contagious Cause*, 119.

131. Rettig, *Cancer Crusade*, 66–67.

132. Department of Health, Education, and Welfare, *Biomedical Science and Its Administration: A Study of the National Institutes of Health (Wooldrige Report)* (Washington, D.C.: White House, 1965), 39. Quoted in Rettig, *Cancer Crusade*, 66.

133. Scheffler, *A Contagious Cause*, 121.

134. Scheffler, *A Contagious Cause*, 122. Though Scheffler presents this exchange as one between the Lasker-controlled American Cancer Society and the NCI, it is more accurate to position Lasker's sallies against contracting in the NACC where she had some measure of statutory oversight vis-à-vis the NCI. Appreciating the NACC's authority in advising the NCI's scientific and policy agenda makes the stakes of her objections to NCI-controlled contracting for bureaucrats such as Baker and Endicott more apparent.

135. September 7, 1967, meeting minutes of the Special Virus Leukemia Program. Cancer Chemotherapy Program, 1969–81 (NARA II, Record Group 443, UD-UP Entry 7, Box 3, Folder 5), 3.

136. "Viral Carcinogenesis Branch Summary Report," National Cancer Institute, *Annual Report of Program Activities, 1967*, 921–22.

137. "Viral Carcinogenesis Branch Summary Report," National Cancer Institute, *Annual Report of Program Activities, 1967*, 921.

138. See January 5, 1967, meeting minutes of the Special Virus Leukemia Program. Cancer Chemotherapy Program, 1969–81 (NARA II, Record Group 443, UD-UP Entry 7, Box 3, Folder 5), 3.

139. These "Joint Working Conferences" became an annual tradition where virus-cancer researchers shared unpublished research and brainstormed. See Baker, "Administrative History of the National Cancer Institute's Viruses and Cancer Programs," 204, 209.

140. See Beeman, "Robert J. Huebner, M.D.," 344–45.

141. See Natalie B. Aviles, "The Little Death: Rigoni-Stern and the Problem of Sex and Cancer in 20th-Century Biomedical Research," *Social Studies of Science* 45, no. 3 (2015): 394–415.

142. Beeman, "Robert J. Huebner, M.D.," 375–76.

143. "Associate Scientific Director for Viral Oncology Summary Report," National Cancer Institute, *Annual Report of Program Activities, 1968* (NARA II, Record Group 443, UD-WW Entry 4, Box 5), 894.

144. "Associate Scientific Director for Viral Oncology Summary Report," National Cancer Institute, *Annual Report of Program Activities, 1968,* 895.

145. "Associate Scientific Director for Viral Oncology Summary Report," National Cancer Institute, *Annual Report of Program Activities, 1968,* 895.

146. "Associate Scientific Director for Viral Oncology Summary Report," National Cancer Institute, *Annual Report of Program Activities, 1968,* 895.

147. "Associate Scientific Director for Viral Oncology Summary Report," National Cancer Institute, *Annual Report of Program Activities, 1968,* 913.

148. "Associate Scientific Director for Viral Oncology Summary Report," National Cancer Institute, *Annual Report of Program Activities, 1968,* 934 (emphasis in original).

149. "Associate Scientific Director for Viral Oncology Summary Report," National Cancer Institute, *Annual Report of Program Activities, 1968,* 935.

150. "Associate Scientific Director for Viral Oncology Summary Report," National Cancer Institute, *Annual Report of Program Activities, 1968,* 935.

3. MOVING TARGETS IN THE WAR ON CANCER, 1969–1979

1. "Associate Scientific Director for Viral Oncology Summary Report," National Cancer Institute, *Annual Report of Program Activities, 1968* (National Archives and Records Administration II, College Park, MD [hereafter NARA II], Record Group 443, UD-WW Entry 4, Box 5), 904.

2. "Associate Scientific Director for Viral Oncology Summary Report," National Cancer Institute, *Annual Report of Program Activities, 1968,* 906.

3. "Associate Scientific Director for Viral Oncology Summary Report," National Cancer Institute, *Annual Report of Program Activities, 1968,* 905–6.

4. For a summary of work on mouse mammary tumor virus originated by Jackson Laboratory researcher John Bittner, see Gregory J. Morgan, *Cancer Virus Hunters: A History of Tumor Virology* (Baltimore, MD: Johns Hopkins University Press, 2022), 23–29.

5. "Associate Scientific Director for Viral Oncology Summary Report," National Cancer Institute, *Annual Report of Program Activities, 1969, Part II* (NARA II, Record Group 443, UD-WW Entry 4, Box 6), 1050.

6. Robin Wolfe Scheffler and Natalie B. Aviles, "State Planning, Cancer Vaccine Infrastructure, and the Origins of the Oncogene Theory," *Social Studies of Science* 52, no. 2 (2022): 185.

7.   Quoted in Kenneth E. Studer and Daryl E. Chubin, *The Cancer Mission: Social Contexts of Biomedical Research* (Beverly Hills, CA: Sage, 1980), 99.

8.   Scheffler and Aviles, "State Planning, Cancer Vaccine Infrastructure, and the Origins of the Oncogene Theory," 185.

9.   "Scientific Director for Etiology Summary Report," National Cancer Institute, *Annual Report 1970, Part II* (NARA II, Record Group 443, UD-WW Entry 4, Box 6), 688.

10.   "Scientific Director for Etiology Summary Report," National Cancer Institute, *Annual Report 1970, Part II*, 689 (emphasis in original).

11.   "Viral Carcinogenesis Branch Summary Report," National Cancer Institute, *Annual Report of Program Activities, 1969, Part II*, 1139.

12.   Carl G. Baker, "Administrative History of the National Cancer Institute's Viruses and Cancer Programs, 1950–1972," 245. National Institutes of Health, https://history.nih.gov /research/downloads/SpecialVirusCaPrgm.pdf.

13.   Statement reproduced in "Etiology Area Summary Report," National Cancer Institute, *Annual Report of Program Activities, 1969, Part II*, 657 (emphasis in original).

14.   Baker, "Administrative History of the National Cancer Institute's Viruses and Cancer Programs," 251–52.

15.   Baker, "Administrative History of the National Cancer Institute's Viruses and Cancer Programs," 259 (emphasis in original).

16.   Richard Rettig, *Cancer Crusade: The Story of the National Cancer Act of 1971* (Lincoln, NE: iUniverse, 2005), *Cancer Crusade*, 10.

17.   Rettig, *Cancer Crusade*, 79.

18.   Rettig, *Cancer Crusade*, 93–94.

19.   This goal was almost universally regarded as dubious by cancer scientists in the NCI. See Edward A. Beeman. "Robert J. Huebner, M.D.: A Virologist's Journey," 423. National Institutes of Health, https://history.nih.gov/research/downloads/HuebnerBiography.pdf.

20.   Baker, "Administrative History of the National Cancer Institute's Viruses and Cancer Programs," 304–5.

21.   Internal memo, "Justification for Mounting an Expanded Cancer Research Program Within NIH Rather than Establishing a Separate Cancer Authority Reporting to the President" (February 2, 1971). National Institutes of Health Office of the Director Central Files (NARA II, Record Group 443, UD-06D Entry 1, Box 94, Folder 2).

22.   Baker, "Administrative History of the National Cancer Institute's Viruses and Cancer Programs," 304–5.

23.   Robin Wolfe Scheffler, *A Contagious Cause: The American Hunt for Cancer Viruses and the Rise of Molecular Medicine*. Chicago: University of Chicago Press, 2019, 155.

24.   Council of the NCI Assembly of Scientists to NCI Director, "Analysis of S.4564 by the Council of the NCI Assembly of Scientists." Memo to Carl Baker, Director, NCI (March 5, 1971). National Institutes of Health Office of the Director Central Files (NARA II, Record Group 443, UD-06D Entry 1, Box 29, Folder 13), 1.

25.   Council of the NCI Assembly of Scientists to NCI Director, "Analysis of S.4564," 3 (emphasis in original).

26.   Testimony of members of the National Panel of Consultants on the Conquest of Cancer before the Senate Health Subcommittee (March 10, 1971). National Institutes of Health

Office of the Director Central Files (NARA II, Record Group 443, UD-06D Entry 1, Box 14, Folder 3), 12–13 (emphasis in original).

27. Robert Huebner, "Cancer Conquest Program." Memo to Edward David, Leonard Laster, Robert Marston, Carl Baker, and James Shannon (September 15, 1971). National Institutes of Health Office of the Director Central Files (NARA II, Record Group 443, UD-06D Entry 1, Box 93, Folder 6).

28. Rettig, *Cancer Crusade*, 291.

29. Rettig, *Cancer Crusade*, 297.

30. Baker, "Administrative History of the National Cancer Institute's Viruses and Cancer Programs," 296.

31. Rettig, *Cancer Crusade*, 297.

32. Rettig, *Cancer Crusade*, 298.

33. Baker, "Administrative History of the National Cancer Institute's Viruses and Cancer Programs," 361–62.

34. Rettig, *Cancer Crusade*, 311.

35. "Office of the Director, Introduction," National Cancer Institute, *Annual Report of Program Activities Fiscal Year 1971, Part III* (Bethesda, MD: U.S. Department of Health, Education and Welfare, 1971), b.

36. Scheffler, *A Contagious Cause*, 164.

37. Baker, "Administrative History of the National Cancer Institute's Viruses and Cancer Programs," 311–14.

38. Carl Baker, Director, NCI, "An Expanded Research and Development Program on Cancer," Draft Report (February 2, 1971). National Institutes of Health Office of the Director Central Files (NARA II, Record Group 443, UD-06D Entry 1, Box 14, Folder 3).

39. National Cancer Institute, "National Cancer Plan Approaches Session: Guidance Material." First planning session, Arlie Conference Center, Warrenton, Virginia (October 24–29, 1971). National Institutes of Health Office of the Director Central Files (NARA II, Record Group 443, UD-06D Entry 1, Box 93, Folder 6).

40. John H. Schneider, Scientific and Technical Information Officer, NCI, "Summary of Project Areas Proposed for the National Cancer Plan" (September 1972). National Institutes of Health Office of the Director Central Files (NARA II, Record Group 443, UD-06D Entry 1, Box 94, Folder 7), A-3.

41. Baker, "Administrative History of the National Cancer Institute's Viruses and Cancer Programs," 344.

42. NCI Planning and Analysis staff collected information from scientists during the planning conferences at Arlie House as well as from a follow-up survey conducted by JRB Associates, Inc., that reflected variation in how scientists ranked many approaches, especially those more distant from basic research (e.g., cancer control efforts). See Baker, "Administrative History of the National Cancer Institute's Viruses and Cancer Programs," 354–55.

43. Baker, "Administrative History of the National Cancer Institute's Viruses and Cancer Programs," 317–18.

44. Baker, "Administrative History of the National Cancer Institute's Viruses and Cancer Programs," 321.

45. Baker, "Administrative History of the National Cancer Institute's Viruses and Cancer Programs," 360.

46. Transcript of Vincent T. DeVita, Jr., oral history, conducted by Gretchen A. Case, June 5, 1997, 14 (National Cancer Institute Oral History Project, Office of NIH History, Bethesda, MD) [hereafter DeVita oral history]. https://history.nih.gov/display/history /NIH+Oral+Histories.

47. DeVita oral history, 13.

48. Vincent T. DeVita, Jr., and Elizabeth DeVita-Raeburn, *The Death of Cancer: After Fifty Years on the Front Lines of Medicine, a Pioneering Oncologist Reveals Why the War on Cancer Is Winnable—and How We Can Get There* (New York: Sarah Crichton Books, 2015), 133.

49. DeVita, Jr., and DeVita-Raeburn, *The Death of Cancer*, 145.

50. DeVita, Jr., and DeVita-Raeburn, *The Death of Cancer*, 147–48.

51. DeVita oral history, 26–27.

52. The Sisco Report was initiated on the basis of grievances arising from within NIH. Combined with long-standing external critiques of expensive contract initiatives in both NCI and the National Heart Institute, the secretary of the Department of Health, Education and Welfare found that these complaints warranted the largest-scale investigation of NIH contracting to date. See "Review of Research Contract Management at National Institutes of Health (Sisco Report)" (April 1969). National Institutes of Health Office of the Director Central Files (NARA II, Record Group 443, UD-06D Entry 1, Box 127, Folder 9).

53. James W. Schriver, Chief, Management Survey and Review Branch, "Research Contract Management at National Institutes of Health." Memo to Associate Director for Administration, NIH (May 8, 1969). National Institutes of Health Office of the Director Central Files (NARA II, Record Group 443, UD-06D Entry 1, Box 127, Folder 9).

54. Carl Baker, Director, NCI, "Status Report #6: National Cancer Program." Memo to Robert Marston, Director, NIH (January 13, 1972). National Institutes of Health Office of the Director Central Files (NARA II, Record Group 443, UD-06D Entry 1, Box 94, Folder 7).

55. "Summary Report, Office of the Associate Scientific Director for Viral Oncology." National Cancer Institute, *Annual Report of Program Activities Fiscal Year 1973, Part III* (Bethesda, MD: U.S. Department of Health, Education and Welfare, 1973), 782.

56. Baker, "Administrative History of the National Cancer Institute's Viruses and Cancer Programs," 360.

57. One study by the comptroller general found that centralized contracting administration utilizing traditional line channels through the NCI and NIH caused unnecessary delays of 1-1/2 months, primarily because of duplication of administrative efforts. See Comptroller General, "Administration of Contracts and Grants for Cancer Research," Report to the Committee on Labor and Public Welfare, United States Senate (March 5, 1971). National Institutes of Health Office of the Director Central Files (NARA II, Record Group 443, UD-06D Entry 1, Box 96, Folder 11).

58. "Proposed Report: President's Review of the Administrative Processes of the National Cancer Program" (April 1973). National Institutes of Health Office of the Director Central Files (NARA II, Record Group 443, UD-06D Entry 1, Box 95, Folder 1).

59. Surveys and Investigations Staff, House Appropriations Committee, "A Report to the Committee on Appropriations, U.S. House of Representatives, on Research Programs Funded Through Contracts Rather than Grants, National Institutes of Health, U.S. Department of Health, Education, and Welfare" (January 1973). National Institutes of Health Office of the Director Central Files (NARA II, Record Group 443, UD-06D Entry 1, Box 128, Folder 2).

60. "Report of the NIH Program Mechanisms Committee" (February 14, 1973). National Institutes of Health Office of the Director Central Files (NARA II, Record Group 443, UD-06D Entry 1, Box 20, Folder 1).

61. Surveys and Investigations Staff, "A Report to the Committee on Appropriations," 29–30.

62. National Cancer Program, "Operational Plan FY 1977–1981" (August 1974). National Institutes of Health Office of the Director Central Files (NARA II, Record Group 443, UD-06D Entry 1, Box 95, Folder 2), II-12.

63. "Office of the Director, Introduction," National Cancer Institute, *Annual Report of Program Activities Fiscal Year 1971, Part III* (Bethesda, MD: U.S. Department of Health, Education and Welfare, 1971), g-h.

64. "Office of the Director, Introduction," National Cancer Institute, *Annual Report of Program Activities Fiscal Year 1971, Part III* (Bethesda, MD: U.S. Department of Health, Education and Welfare, 1971), h.

65. "Office of the Associate Director for Program Planning and Analysis," National Cancer Institute, *Annual Report of Program Activities Fiscal Year 1971, Part III* (Bethesda, MD: U.S. Department of Health, Education and Welfare, 1971), 7.

66. Harold Varmus, *The Art and Politics of Science* (New York: Norton, 2009), 79.

67. Scheffler and Aviles, "State Planning, Cancer Vaccine Infrastructure, and the Origins of the Oncogene Theory," 187.

68. Scheffler and Aviles, "State Planning, Cancer Vaccine Infrastructure, and the Origins of the Oncogene Theory," 187.

69. "Virus Cancer Program Report on Scientific Activities Continues," *Cancer Letter* 1, no. 31 (August 1, 1975): 3–4.

70. "Virus Cancer Program Report on Scientific Activities Continues," *Cancer Letter*, 6.

71. "Virus Cancer Program Includes 'Some of the Best Basic Research Anywhere,' Moloney says," *Cancer Letter* 2, no. 2 (January 9, 1976): 3.

72. Scheffler, *A Contagious Cause*, 199.

73. Varmus, *The Art and Politics of Science*, 80.

74. Detailed accounts of these experiments can be found in Scheffler and Aviles, "State Planning, Cancer Vaccine Infrastructure, and the Origins of the Oncogene Theory"; and in Scheffler, *A Contagious Cause*, 192–202.

75. "NCI Virus Program Has 'Important Extension of Virology' as New Approach To Etiology," *Cancer Letter* 2, no. 17 (April 23, 1976): 4.

76. Transcript of Edward Scolnick oral history, conducted by Gretchen A. Case, June 24, 1998. Office of NIH History, Oral History Archive. https://history.nih.gov/display/history/Scolnick%2C+Edward+1998.

77. For histories detailing the ascent of the cellular oncogene hypothesis in molecular cancer research, see Michel Morange, *A History of Molecular Biology*, trans. Matthew Cobb

(Cambridge, MA: Harvard University Press, 1998); and Ton van Helvoort, "A Century of Research Into the Cause of Cancer: Is the New Oncogene Paradigm Revolutionary?" *History and Philosophy of the Life Sciences* 21, no. 3 (1999).

78. Joan Fujimura, *Crafting Science: A Sociohistory of the Quest for the Genetics of Cancer* (Cambridge, MA: Harvard University Press, 1996).

79. For extensive discussion of the arguments extramural scientists made about investigator-initiated research in opposition to targeted research, see Studer and Chubin, *The Cancer Mission*; and Scheffler, *A Contagious Cause*.

80. Nicholas Wade, "Special Virus Cancer Program: Travails of a Biological Moonshot," *Science* 174, no. 4016 (1971): 1306.

81. Wade, "Special Virus Cancer Program," 1307.

82. Wade, "Special Virus Cancer Program," 1308.

83. Scheffler, *A Contagious Cause*, 157.

84. Scheffler, *A Contagious Cause*, 148.

85. Matthew D. McCubbins and Thomas Schwartz, "Congressional Oversight Overlooked: Police Patrols versus Fire Alarms," *American Journal of Political Science* 28, no. 1 (1984): 166.

86. Nicholas Wade, "Cancer Politics: NIH Backers Mount Late Defense in House," *Science* 174, no. 4005 (1971): 127–31.

87. Scheffler, *A Contagious Cause*, 171–72.

88. Scheffler, *A Contagious Cause*, 168.

89. Scheffler, *A Contagious Cause*, 173.

90. Scheffler, *A Contagious Cause*, 172.

91. Scheffler, *A Contagious Cause*, 174.

92. Scheffler, *A Contagious Cause*, 174–76.

93. The SVCP changed its name to the VCP in the midst of the Zinder Committee's investigation, but the report uses the acronym SVCP to refer to the program.

94. Quoted in "Zinder Report Asks SVCP to Switch Most Research to Grants, Spread Work Among More Scientists, Change Review Groups," *Cancer Letter* 1, no. 7 (March 22, 1974): 2.

95. "Zinder Report," *Cancer Letter*, 2.

96. "Report of the Ad Hoc Review Committee of the SVCP (Zinder Report)" (October 31, 1973). National Institutes of Health Office of the Director Central Files (NARA II, Record Group 443, UD-06D Entry 1, Box 96, Folder 6), 9.

97. "Report of the Ad Hoc Review Committee of the SVCP," National Institutes of Health Office of the Director Central Files, 15.

98. "Report of the Ad Hoc Review Committee of the SVCP," National Institutes of Health Office of the Director Central Files, 29.

99. Barbara Culliton, "Cancer: Select Committee Calls Virus Program a Closed Shop," *Science* 182, no. 4117 (1973): 1111.

100. "Office of the Associate Scientific Director for Viral Oncology Summary Report," National Cancer Institute, *Annual Report of Program Activities Fiscal Year 1973, Part III* (Bethesda, MD: U.S. Department of Health, Education and Welfare, 1973), 778.

101. Beeman, "Robert J. Huebner, M.D.," 458.

102. "NCAB to Monitor Virus Program; NCI Answers Zinder Report Criticisms," *Cancer Letter* 1, no. 21 (June 28, 1974): 3.

103. "NCAB to Monitor Virus Program," *Cancer Letter*, 3.

104. Scheffler, *A Contagious Cause*, 177.

105. "National TV Attack on Cancer Program Gets Response from Schmidt; Some NCAB Members Side with Kornberg," *Cancer Letter* 1, no. 21 (June 28, 1974).

106. Scheffler, *A Contagious Cause*, 179.

107. National Cancer Program, "1975 Annual Plan for FY 1977–1981." National Institutes of Health Office of the Director Central Files (NARA II, Record Group 443, UD-06D Entry 1, Box 95, Folder 3), lv.

108. "Office of the Director Division of Cancer Research Resources and Centers," National Cancer Institute, *Annual Report 1975–1976, Part V* (Bethesda, MD: U.S. Department of Health, Education and Welfare, 1976), 4.

109. "Research Contracts Branch," National Cancer Institute, *Annual Report 1975–1976, Part I* (Bethesda, MD: U.S. Department of Health, Education and Welfare, 1976), 59.

110. "The Congressional Committee System: Historical Overview," in *Final Report of the Joint Committee on the Organization of Congress* (December 1993). Archives of the U.S. House of Representatives Committee on Rules. https://archives-democrats-rules.house.gov /Archives/jcoc2.htm.

111. Stephen P. Strickland, *Politics, Science, and Dread Disease: A Short History of United States Medical Research Policy* (Cambridge, MA: Harvard University Press, 1972), 217.

112. "Schmidt's Influence in for Another Test; Shingleton Nominated to Panel," *Cancer Letter* 3, no. 23 (June 10, 1977): 3.

113. "Lasker Pushes NCI to Get Research Results Quicker, Into Practice Sooner," *Cancer Letter* 1, no. 17 (May 31, 1974): 3.

114. Beeman, "Robert J. Huebner, M.D.," 483.

115. Robert Manaker, Louis Sibal, and John Moloney, "Scientific Activities at the National Cancer Institute: Virology," *Journal of the National Cancer Institute* 59, no. 2 (1977): 631.

116. "In Brief," *Cancer Letter* 2, no. 14 (April 2, 1976): 1.

117. "Rauscher Tells Flood EC Support Percentage 'Good'; Obey Unfriendly," *Cancer Letter* 2, no. 10 (March 5, 1976): 2–3.

118. For a discussion of the political ascent of environmental carcinogen research, see Scheffler, *A Contagious Cause*, 206–13.

119. Scheffler, *A Contagious Cause*, 210.

120. "Obey Attacks Eppley, Shubik, NCI, Asks for Complete GAO Report," *Cancer Letter* 3, no. 23 (June 10, 1977): 3. Though Shubik was a long-standing target of the young congressman, his criticisms of NCI-contracted work conducted by the Shubik-run Epley Institute spilled over into an indictment of the NCI's contracting operations generally.

121. June 6, 1978, meeting minutes of the Bureau-Institute-Division Directors, National Institutes of Health. National Institutes of Health Office of the Director Central Files (NARA II, Record Group 443, UD-06D Entry 1, Box 40, Folder 5), 3–4.

122. Arthur C. Upton, Director, NCI, "Report by the Inspector General—NCI Contracting Operations." Memo to Office of Inspector General (April 10, 1978). National Institutes of Health Office of the Director Central Files (NARA II, Record Group 443, UD-06D Entry 1, Box 129, Folder 2).

123. "Summary Report, Division of Cancer Cause and Prevention," National Cancer Institute, *Annual Report 1975–1976, Part III-A* (Bethesda, MD: U.S. Department of Health, Education and Welfare, 1976), 40.

124. A Laboratory of DNA Tumor Viruses was founded in the VOP in 1976 "to recognize the increased emphasis on molecular-genetic approach [*sic*] to cancer-virus studies and the role of DNA viruses in cancer." "Summary Report, Office of the Associate Director, Viral Oncology Program," National Cancer Institute, *Annual Report 1975–1976, Part III-B* (Bethesda, MD: U.S. Department of Health, Education and Welfare, 1976), 1124.

125. Studer and Chubin, *Cancer Mission*, 54. For a discussion of zur Hausen's emerging research agenda on HPV and human cancer, see Natalie B. Aviles, "The Little Death: Rigoni-Stern and the Problem of Sex and Cancer in 20th-Century Biomedical Research," *Social Studies of Science* 45, no. 3 (2015): 394–415.

126. Scheffler, *A Contagious Cause*, 219–22.

127. Studer and Chubin, *Cancer Mission*, 211–12.

128. Studer and Chubin, *Cancer Mission*, 228.

129. Studer and Chubin, *Cancer Mission*, 57; for a discussion of how Baltimore quickly acquired large supplies of murine retrovirus from Todaro and the SVCP, see Scheffler, *A Contagious Cause*, 142.

130. Fujimura, *Crafting Science*; and Peter Keating and Alberto Cambrosio, *Cancer on Trial: Oncology as a New Style of Practice* (Chicago: University of Chicago Press, 2011).

131. Several examples of this approach can be found in John F. Padgett and Walter W. Powell, *The Emergence of Organizations and Markets* (Princeton, NJ: Princeton University Press, 2012).

4. BACK TO BASICS: HUMAN CANCER
RETROVIRUS RESEARCH, 1980–1984

1. Transcript of Robert Gallo oral history, conducted by Victoria Harden and Dennis Rodrigues, August 24, 1994, 26 (In Their Own Words: NIH Researchers Recall the Early Years of AIDS, Office of NIH History and Stetten Museum, Bethesda, MD) [hereafter Gallo oral history 1]. https://history.nih.gov/display/history/Transcripts.

2. Vincent T. DeVita, "The Governance of Science at the National Cancer Institute: A Perspective on Misperceptions," *Cancer Research* 43, no. 8 (1983): 3970.

3. Transcript of Vincent T. DeVita, Jr., oral history, conducted by Gretchen A. Case, June 5, 1997, 39; 47–48 (National Cancer Institute Oral History Project, Office of NIH History, Bethesda, MD) [hereafter DeVita oral history]. https://history.nih.gov/display/history/NIH+Oral+Histories.

4. DeVita oral history, 19.

5. Voncent T. DeVita, Jr., and Elizabeth DeVita-Raeburn, *The Death of Cancer: After Fifty Years on the Front Lines of Medicine, a Pioneering Oncologist Reveals Why the War on Cancer is Winnable—and How We Can Get There* (New York: Sarah Crichton Books, 2015), 62–63.

6. DeVita oral history, 47.

7. DeVita oral history, 49.

8. DeVita oral history, 41.

9.   Robin Wolfe Scheffler, *A Contagious Cause: The American Hunt for Cancer Viruses and the Rise of Molecular Medicine* (Chicago: University of Chicago Press, 2019), 226–27.

10.   DeVita, "The Governance of Science at the National Cancer Institute," 3969.

11.   DeVita, "The Governance of Science at the National Cancer Institute," 3969.

12.   DeVita, "The Governance of Science at the National Cancer Institute," 3971.

13.   Vincent T. DeVita, "On Special Initiatives, Critics, and the National Cancer Program," *Cancer Treatment Reports* 68, no. 1 (1984): 2.

14.   DeVita, "On Special Initiatives, Critics, and the National Cancer Program," 3.

15.   DeVita, "On Special Initiatives, Critics, and the National Cancer Program," 2.

16.   DeVita, "On Special Initiatives, Critics, and the National Cancer Program," 4.

17.   DeVita, "The Governance of Science at the National Cancer Institute," 3969.

18.   DeVita, "On Special Initiatives, Critics, and the National Cancer Program," 2.

19.   DeVita, "The Governance of Science at the National Cancer Institute," 3969.

20.   Marjorie Sun, "Hatch Batters NCI with Straus Case," *Science* 212, no. 4501 (1981): 1366.

21.   Chiefs of Laboratories and Clinics, "Support for DeVita," *Science* 213, no. 4503 (1981): 9.

22.   DeVita, "The Governance of Science at the National Cancer Institute," 3971.

23.   DeVita, "The Governance of Science at the National Cancer Institute," 3970.

24.   DeVita oral history, 11–12. DeVita also recounts several such episodes in chapters 5 and 6 of his memoir; see DeVita and DeVita-Raeburn, *The Death of Cancer.*

25.   DeVita oral history, 14.

26.   DeVita oral history, 14.

27.   DeVita and DeVita-Raeburn, *The Death of Cancer*, 153.

28.   DeVita and DeVita-Raeburn, *The Death of Cancer*, 154.

29.   DeVita and DeVita-Raeburn, *The Death of Cancer*, 154.

30.   DeVita and DeVita-Raeburn, *The Death of Cancer*, 155.

31.   Peter Keating and Alberto Cambrosio, *Cancer on Trial: Oncology as a New Style of Practice* (Chicago: University of Chicago Press, 2011), 196 (emphasis in original).

32.   DeVita and DeVita-Raeburn, *The Death of Cancer*, 157.

33.   DeVita and DeVita-Raeburn, *The Death of Cancer*, 154.

34.   DeVita and DeVita-Raeburn, *The Death of Cancer*, 161.

35.   DeVita and DeVita-Raeburn, *The Death of Cancer*, 153.

36.   DeVita and DeVita-Raeburn, *The Death of Cancer*, 165.

37.   DeVita and DeVita-Raeburn, *The Death of Cancer*, 167.

38.   DeVita and DeVita-Raeburn, *The Death of Cancer*, 174.

39.   DeVita and DeVita-Raeburn, *The Death of Cancer*, 168.

40.   "New NCAB: Weak (for Now) in Grant Reviewing, Confused Over Issues," *Cancer Letter* 8, no. 48 (December 10, 1982): 5.

41.   "New NCAB," *Cancer Letter*, 5.

42.   Between 1982 and 1984, Rowley wrote several letters to *Science* "urging the appointment of highly qualified scientists to the Board and criticizing the last round of Reagan appointees"; see "In Brief," *Cancer Letter* 10, no. 3 (January 20, 1984): 1. Though this deficiency was addressed in the 1984 appointments to the NCAB, until this time the board was generally inclined to accept the NCI's recommendations on most policy issues until David Korn became NCAB chairman in late 1984. The lack of major pushback from the

NCAB to this point allowed the NCI to play an outsized role in shaping the direction of institute governance throughout the first four-and-a-half years of the decade.

43. DeVita, "The Governance of Science at the National Cancer Institute," 3971.

44. DeVita, "The Governance of Science at the National Cancer Institute," 3971.

45. Testimony before the Subcommittee on Investigations and Oversight of the Committee on Science and Technology, U.S. House of Representatives, reported in Peter J. Fischinger and Vincent T. DeVita, "Governance of Science at the National Cancer Institute: Perceptions and Opportunities in Oncogene Research," *Cancer Research* 44, no. 10 (1984): 4693–96.

46. Fischinger and DeVita, "Governance of Science at the National Cancer Institute," 4693.

47. Fischinger and DeVita, "Governance of Science at the National Cancer Institute," 4693.

48. DeVita, "The Governance of Science at the National Cancer Institute," 3973.

49. DeVita, "The Governance of Science at the National Cancer Institute," 3973.

50. DeVita, "The Governance of Science at the National Cancer Institute," 3973.

51. National Cancer Advisory Board, "Summary of Meeting, January 30–February 1, 1984," 2–3 (National Cancer Institute Division of Extramural Activities, NCAB digital archive). https://deainfo.nci.nih.gov/advisory/ncab/archive/index.htm.

52. This goal was developed by the NCI during an Executive Staff retreat in January 1984; National Cancer Advisory Board, "Summary of Meeting, January 30–February 1, 1984," 4.

53. DeVita, "The Governance of Science at the National Cancer Institute," 3973.

54. DeVita, "The Governance of Science at the National Cancer Institute," 3973.

55. DeVita, "The Governance of Science at the National Cancer Institute," 3973.

56. Gallo oral history 1, 4

57. Gallo oral history 1, 8.

58. Saul Shepartz, "Annual Report, Division of Cancer Treatment," *Annual Report of Program Activities, National Cancer Institute, Fiscal Year 1980, Part VI-A* (Bethesda, MD: U.S. Department of Health and Human Services, 1980), 2.

59. Robert C. Gallo, "Project CM Z01-CM-06117-08," *Annual Report of Program Activities, National Cancer Institute, Fiscal Year 1980, Part VI-A* (Bethesda, MD: U.S. Department of Health and Human Services, 1980), 652.

60. Robert Gallo, *Virus Hunting: AIDS, Cancer, and the Human Retrovirus* (New York: Basic Books, 1991), 64–67.

61. Gallo, *Virus Hunting*, 92.

62. Gallo oral history 1, 30; and Gallo, *Virus Hunting*, 38.

63. Gallo oral history 1, 26.

64. Gallo oral history 1, 9.

65. Gallo oral history 1, 10.

66. Gallo oral history 1, 10. Rosenberg would use these and other materials from NCI bench scientists to develop the first immunotherapeutic protocols in the institute.

67. Gallo oral history 1, 24.

68. Gallo oral history 1, 24.

69. Gallo, *Virus Hunting*, 42.

70. Gallo, *Virus Hunting*, 42.

71. Gallo, *Virus Hunting*, 43.

72. Gallo, *Virus Hunting*, 42.

73. Gallo, *Virus Hunting*, 43.

74. Gallo oral history 1, 15.

75. Gallo oral history 1, 15.

76. Gallo, *Virus Hunting*, 85.

77. Gallo, *Virus Hunting*, 68.

78. For accounts of these uses in the STS literature, see Joan Fujimura, *Crafting Science: A Sociohistory of the Quest for the Genetics of Cancer* (Cambridge, MA: Harvard University Press, 1996); and Hans-Jörg Rheinberger, *Toward a History of Epistemic Things: Synthesizing Proteins in the Test Tube* (Stanford, CA: Stanford University Press, 1997).

79. Gallo, *Virus Hunting*, 68.

80. Gallo, *Virus Hunting*, 71.

81. Gallo, *Virus Hunting*, 71–75.

82. Gallo oral history 1, 21.

83. Gallo, *Virus Hunting*, 76–77.

84. Gallo, *Virus Hunting*, 84–86.

85. Gallo, *Virus Hunting*, 93.

86. Gallo's recollection of the responsible parties in this episode were thin nearly twenty years on, but he suggests another MD on the project, Dr. Robert Gallagher, may have sent the samples to Dr. Ethan Shevach in the Clinical Center for analysis. Gallo oral history 1, 21.

87. Gallo oral history 1, 21.

88. Gallo, *Virus Hunting*, 77–79.

89. Gallo oral history 1, 21.

90. Gallo, *Virus Hunting*, 93.

91. Gallo, *Virus Hunting*, 100–101.

92. Gallo, *Virus Hunting*, 102–3.

93. Gallo, *Virus Hunting*, 104–5.

94. Gallo, *Virus Hunting*, 110–13.

95. The infamy of the MO cell line comes from the patent protection extended to this early biotechnology product. Subsequent debates over ownership and royalty rights ensued between Golde, his various employers, and the donor himself.

96. "Annual Report of the Laboratory of Tumor Cell Biology," *Annual Report of Program Activities, National Cancer Institute, Fiscal Year 1982, Part VI-A* (Bethesda, MD: U.S. Department of Health and Human Services, 1982), 604.

97. These findings were published in V. S. Kalyanaraman et al., "A New Subtype of Human T-cell Leukemia Virus (HTLV-II) Associated with a T-cell Variant of Hairy Cell Leukemia," *Science* 218, no. 4572 (1982): 571–73.

98. In 1985, genetic analysis showed that HTLV-3, LAV, and ARV were subvariants of the same virus, which came to be known as HIV.

99. Steven Epstein, *Impure Science: AIDS, Activism, and the Politics of Knowledge* (Berkeley: University of California Press, 1996), 80–97.

100. The NCI's Richard Adamson told the Board of Scientific Counselors that the NCI would work with NIAID to issue a request for applications to stimulate interest because the "NCI has been expecting traditional R01 to study the relationship of viruses to AIDS, 'but they have not come in.'" Quoted in "DCCP Board Approves Concepts of New Grants Totaling $1.4 Million a Year," *Cancer Letter* 9, no. 7 (February 18, 1983): 4.

101. Gallo, *Virus Hunting*, 134–35.

102. Transcript of Robert Gallo oral history, conducted by Victoria Harden and Dennis Rodrigues, November 4, 1994, 8 (In Their Own Words: NIH Researchers Recall the Early Years of AIDS, Office of NIH History and Stetten Museum, Bethesda, MD) [hereafter Gallo oral history 2]. https://history.nih.gov/display/history/Transcripts.

103. Gallo, *Virus Hunting*, 13–16.

104. Gallo oral history 1, 35.

105. "Annual Report, Division of Cancer Treatment," *Annual Report of Program Activities, National Cancer Institute, Fiscal Year 1983, Part VI-A* (Bethesda, MD: U.S. Department of Health and Human Services, 1983), 3.

106. Transcript of Samuel Broder oral history, conducted by Victoria Harden and Caroline Hannaway, February 2, 1997, 18 (Oral History Archive, Office of NIH History) [hereafter Broder oral history]. https://history.nih.gov/archives/downloads/broderfeb97.pdf.

107. Gallo, *Virus Hunting*, 142.

108. In May 1982, panic over AIDS contamination among researchers and clinicians had triggered reactive prohibitions on AIDS research in some institutions, while many scientists and physicians simply refused to work with AIDS patients or their materials. Gallo is quick to note that this makes these two female technicians "among the first researchers to culture cells from AIDS patients regularly" (Gallo, *Virus Hunting*, 140). Because of annual reporting standards at the NCI as well as scientific publication conventions, technicians are rarely acknowledged for their contributions to research. In an attempt to remedy the historical omissions created by this professional disenfranchisement, I note the names, roles, and contributions of technicians where credited scientists report them. As such disclosures are not normative, I can only acknowledge the systematic omission of these perspectives from the historical record in those cases where credited scientists have not named technicians specifically.

109. Gallo oral history 1, 35; and Gallo, *Virus Hunting*, 141.

110. Gallo oral history 1, 34.

111. Gallo, *Virus Hunting*, 140–41.

112. Gallo, *Virus Hunting*, 143.

113. Gallo, *Virus Hunting*, 143.

114. Gallo, *Virus Hunting*, 150–53.

115. Genoveffa Franchini, quoted in Gallo, *Virus Hunting*, 155–56.

116. Gallo oral history 2, 11–12.

117. Gallo oral history 2, 12–13; and Gallo, *Virus Hunting*, 159–60.

118. Gallo, *Virus Hunting*, 178.

119. Gallo, *Virus Hunting*, 173.

120. Gallo, *Virus Hunting*, 173.

121. Gallo, *Virus Hunting*, 175.

122. Gallo, *Virus Hunting*, 178–79. Popovic's actions in this experiment led to accusations, later discredited, that the lab had intentionally stolen LAV from Montagnier's lab.

123. Gallo, *Virus Hunting*, 178.

124. Gallo, *Virus Hunting*, 179.

125. Gallo, *Virus Hunting*, 180.

126. "Summary Report, Associate Director for Developmental Therapeutics Program," *Annual Report of Program Activities, National Cancer Institute, Fiscal Year 1982, Part VI-A* (Bethesda, MD: U.S. Department of Health and Human Services, 1982), 180–81.

127. Gallo, *Virus Hunting*, 183.

128. Gallo, *Virus Hunting*, 181.

129. Gallo, *Virus Hunting*, 186.

130. Gallo, *Virus Hunting*, 185.

131. Gallo, *Virus Hunting*, 185.

132. Gallo, *Virus Hunting*, 185.

133. Gallo, *Virus Hunting*, 195–97.

134. Gallo, *Virus Hunting*, 186.

135. Gallo, *Virus Hunting*, 192.

136. "Gallo's Finding: HTLV-III Is the Cause of AIDS; Blood Test Soon," *Cancer Letter* 10, no. 17 (April 27, 1984): 6.

137. Victoria Harden, *AIDS at 30: A History* (Washington, D.C.: Potomac Books, 2012), 63–64.

138. For the perspectives of the main interlocutors, see Gallo, *Virus Hunting*; Luc Montagnier, *Virus: The Co-Discoverer of HIV Tracks Its Rampage and Charts the Future* (New York: Norton, 2000). The journalist John Crewdson's infamous series of exposés on alleged wrongdoings by Gallo published in the *Chicago Tribune*, of which Gallo was subsequently cleared by the NIH Office of Scientific Integrity, are collected in John Crewdson, *Science Fictions: A Scientific Mystery, a Massive Cover-up, and the Dark Legacy of Robert Gallo* (New York: Little, Brown, 2002). Crewdson's reporting has long been discredited in the scientific community (see, e.g., Martin Delaney, "Double Jeopardy for Gallo," *Science* 296, no. 5573 [2002]: 1615–17) and even triggered an exculpatory response in Nikolas Kontaratos's dissertation, self-published as *Dissecting a Discovery* (Bloomington, IN: Xlibris Corporation, 2006). Scholarly accounts include those by the sociologist Steven Epstein in *Impure Science* and by the historian Victoria Harden in *AIDS at 30*.

139. Gallo, *Virus Hunting*, 208.

140. Robert C. Gallo and Luc Montagnier, "The Chronology of AIDS Research," *Nature* 326, no. 6112 (1987): 435–36.

141. Gallo, *Virus Hunting*, 202–3.

142. "Project Z01-CM-07201-01," *Annual Report of Program Activities, National Cancer Institute, Fiscal Year 1984, Part VI* (Bethesda, MD: U.S. Department of Health and Human Services, 1984), 507.

143. "NIH Restructures AIDS Effort; New Research Thrusts Okayed by Advisors," *Cancer Letter* 10, no. 38 (October 5, 1984): 6.

5. HIV RESEARCH AND DRUG DEVELOPMENT, 1985–1989

1. Quoted in Sandra Panem, *The AIDS Bureaucracy: Why Society Failed to Meet the AIDS Crisis and How We Might Improve Our Response* (Cambridge, MA: Harvard University Press, 1988), 95.

2. "NCI Gets $1.258 Billion in Final Appropriations for Fiscal '86," *Cancer Letter* 11, no. 46 (November 29, 1985): 4.

3. This concern was reiterated in NCAB meetings throughout the latter half of the 1980s, particularly around the issue of growth in full time employees (FTEs), which was concentrated on AIDS research at the same time FTEs shrunk for cancer research; see National Cancer Advisory Board, "May 19–21, 1986 Summary of Meeting," 6–7 (National Cancer Institute Division of Extramural Activities, NCAB digital archive) [hereafter NCAB digital archive], https://deainfo.nci.nih.gov/advisory/ncab/archive/index.htm; National Cancer Advisory Board, "November 16–17, 1987 Summary of Meeting," 17 (NCAB digital archive); National Cancer Advisory Board, "May 9–11, 1988 Summary of Meeting," 33 (NCAB digital archive).

4. National Cancer Advisory Board, "May 19–21, 1986 Summary of Meeting," 6 (NCAB digital archive).

5. National Cancer Advisory Board, "October 7–8, 1985 Summary of Meeting," 12 (NCAB digital archive).

6. National Cancer Advisory Board, "November 16–17, 1987 Summary of Meeting," 43 (NCAB digital archive).

7. "DCE Board Demands Other Agencies Pay for NCI AIDS Support Contract," *Cancer Letter* 11, no. 21 (May 24, 1985): 4.

8. "DCE Board Demands Other Agencies Pay for NCI AIDS Support Contract," *Cancer Letter*, 4.

9. National Cancer Advisory Board, "February 2–4, 1987 Summary of Meeting," 5–6 (NCAB digital archive).

10. Panem, *The AIDS Bureaucracy*, 93.

11. Victoria Harden, *AIDS at 30: A History* (Washington, D.C.: Potomac Books, 2012), 130.

12. "Annual Report of the Metabolism Branch," *Annual Report of Program Activities, National Cancer Institute, Fiscal Year 1980, Part II-A* (Bethesda, MD: U.S. Department of Health and Human Services, 1980), 843.

13. As political conflicts over the use of fetal tissues emerged in the ensuing years, many of these tools became increasingly scarce and consequential resources for labs studying HIV/AIDS in vitro.

14. Transcript of Samuel Broder oral history, conducted by Victoria Harden and Caroline Hannaway, February 2, 1997, 8 (Oral History Archive, Office of NIH History) [hereafter Broder oral history]. https://history.nih.gov/archives/downloads/broderfeb97.pdf.

15. Broder oral history, 16–17.

16. Broder oral history, 8.

17. Broder oral history, 11.

18. Broder oral history, 8–9.

19. Harden, *AIDS at 30*, 130.

20. Harden, *AIDS at 30*, 131–32.

21. "Summary Report, Associate Director for Clinical Oncology," *National Cancer Institute Division of Cancer Treatment Annual Report, 1985, Volume II* (Bethesda, MD: U.S. Department of Health and Human Services, 1985), 449.

22. Transcript of Robert Yarchoan oral history, conducted by Victoria Harden and Caroline Hannaway, April 30, 1998, 12 (Oral History Archive, Office of NIH History) [hereafter Yarchoan oral history].https://history.nih.gov/display/history/Yarchoan%2C+Robert+1998.

23. Yarchoan oral history, 8.

24. Yarchoan oral history, 4.

25. Yarchoan oral history, 8–10.

26. Yarchoan oral history, 10.

27. Yarchoan oral history, 11.

28. Peter Arno and Karyn Feiden, *Against the Odds: The Story of AIDS Drug Development, Politics, and Profits* (New York: Harper Perennial, 1992), 40.

29. Mitsuya discusses cultivating these cells by injecting himself seven times with tetanus toxoid in an interview for the documentary *I Am Alive Today*. Vincent Detours and Dominique Henry, directors, *I Am Alive Today: History of an AIDS Drug* [film] (Paris: ADR Productions, 2002).

30. Broder oral history, 21.

31. Yarchoan oral history, 13.

32. Yarchoan oral history, 13.

33. For a classic science and technology studies (STS) statement on the role of scientific collaboration in transferring the tacit knowledge required for experimental reproduction, see Harry M. Collins, "Tacit Knowledge, Trust and the Q of Sapphire," *Social Studies of Science* 31, no. 1 (2001): 71–85.

34. Broder oral history, 21.

35. Yarchoan oral history, 14.

36. Yarchoan oral history, 12.

37. "NCI Restructures AIDS Effort; New Research Thrusts Okayed by Advisors," *Cancer Letter* 10, no. 38 (October 5, 1984): 6.

38. At the time, HTLV-3 was still the term in use in Gallo's lab for the viral cause of AIDS; see Samuel Broder and Robert Gallo, "A Pathogenic Retrovirus (HTLV-III) Linked to AIDS," *New England Journal of Medicine* 311, no. 20 (1984): 1292–97. On suramin, see Hiroaki Mitsuya, Mikulas Popovic, Robert Yarchoan, Shuzo Matsushita, et al., "Suramin Protection of T Cells In Vitro Against Infectivity and Cytopathic Effect of HTLV-III," *Science* 226, no. 4671 (1984): 172–74.

39. Yarchoan oral history, 14.

40. Yarchoan oral history, 14.

41. Yarchoan oral history, 14.

42. Jan Balzarini, Hiroaki Mitsuya, Erik De Clercq, and Samuel Broder, "Comparative Inhibitory Effects of Suramin and Other Selected Compounds on the Infectivity and Replication of Human T-cell Lymphotropic Virus (HTLV-III)/Lymphadenopathy-Associated Virus (LAV)," *International Journal of Cancer* 37, no. 3 (1986): 451–57.

43. Yarchoan oral history, 18.

44. For a succinct discussion, see Steven Epstein, *Impure Science: AIDS, Activism, and the Politics of Knowledge* (Berkeley: University of California Press, 1996), 182.

45. Arno and Feiden, *Against the Odds*, 54.

46. Broder oral history, 13–14.

47. "Project CM07200-03," *National Cancer Institute Division of Cancer Treatment Annual Report, 1985, Volume II* (Bethesda, MD: U.S. Department of Health and Human Services, 1985), 478.

48. Yarchoan oral history, 19.

49. Robert Gallo, *Virus Hunting: AIDS, Cancer, and the Human Retrovirus* (New York: Basic Books, 1991), 202–3.

50. Harden, *AIDS at 30*, 132.

51. Arno and Feiden, *Against the Odds*, 39.

52. Harden, *AIDS at 30*, 132.

53. Yarchoan oral history, 19.

54. Broder oral history, 13.

55. Yarchoan oral history, 19.

56. Yarchoan oral history, 19.

57. Arno and Feiden, *Against the Odds*, 39.

58. Arno and Feiden, *Against the Odds*, 39.

59. Yarchoan oral history, 21.

60. Arno and Feiden, *Against the Odds*, 40–41.

61. Yarchoan oral history, 20.

62. Arno and Feiden, *Against the Odds*, 40.

63. Broder oral history, 21.

64. Broder oral history, 22.

65. Arno and Feiden, *Against the Odds*, 41.

66. Arno and Feiden, *Against the Odds*, 269.

67. Royalties for technology transfer in the NIH were not enshrined into law until 1986.

68. Yarchoan oral history, 22.

69. Arno and Feiden, *Against the Odds*, 42.

70. Broder oral history, 26.

71. Broder oral history, 23–24.

72. Yarchoan oral history, 27.

73. Yarchoan oral history, 26.

74. Yarchoan oral history, 28.

75. Yarchoan oral history, 28.

76. "Project CM07181-01," *National Cancer Institute Division of Cancer Treatment Annual Report, 1986* (Bethesda, MD: U.S. Department of Health and Human Services, 1986), 282.

77. "Annual Report of the Laboratory of Medicinal Chemistry, Developmental Therapeutics Program," *National Cancer Institute Division of Cancer Treatment Annual Report, 1986* (Bethesda, MD: U.S. Department of Health and Human Services, 1986), 221.

78. Yarchoan oral history, 29.

79. Yarchoan oral history, 29.

80. Yarchoan oral history, 29.

81. Yarchoan oral history, 30.

82. Broder oral history, 22–23.

83. As Yarchoan put it, the COP's nucleoside experiments were always "moving on to the next drug. There was initially not so much the idea of combining drugs. We just hoped that the next one was going to be better." Yarchoan oral history, 30.

84. "Summary Report, Associate Director for Clinical Oncology Program," *Division of Cancer Treatment Annual Report, 1989, Volume II* (Bethesda, MD: U.S. Department of Health and Human Services, 1986), 717.

85. "Project CM07209-01," *Division of Cancer Treatment Annual Report, 1989, Volume II* (Bethesda, MD: U.S. Department of Health and Human Services, 1986), 747.

86. "Project CM07209-01," *Division of Cancer Treatment Annual Report, 1989, Volume II* (Bethesda, MD: U.S. Department of Health and Human Services, 1986), 753.

87. "Summary Report, Associate Director for Clinical Oncology Program," *Division of Cancer Treatment Annual Report, 1989, Volume II* (Bethesda, MD: U.S. Department of Health and Human Services, 1986), 715 (emphasis in original).

88. "Project CM07209-01," *Division of Cancer Treatment Annual Report, 1989, Volume II* (Bethesda, MD: U.S. Department of Health and Human Services, 1986), 747.

89. Yarchoan oral history, 30.

90. Yarchoan oral history, 32.

91. Yarchoan oral history, 32.

92. Yarchoan oral history, 32.

93. See Epstein, *Impure Science*, 266–69.

94. See Arno and Feiden, *Against the Odds*, 172–85.

95. NIH Office of Technology Transfer, "Videx© Expanding Possibilities: A Case Study" (Bethesda, MD: National Institutes of Health, 2003), 2. See also Epstein, *Impure Science*, 278–80.

96. NIH Office of Technology Transfer, "Videx© Expanding Possibilities," 1.

97. Broder oral history, 26–27.

98. Harden, *AIDS at 30*, 136.

99. Arno and Feiden, *Against the Odds*, 56.

100. Arno and Feiden, *Against the Odds*, 56.

101. Harden, *AIDS at 30*, 136–38. See also Arno and Feiden, *Against the Odds*, 134–37.

102. Arno and Feiden, *Against the Odds*, 135, 138.

103. Arno and Feiden, *Against the Odds*, 138–139.

104. Harden, *AIDS at 30*, 137.

105. Broder oral history, 30–31.

106. See Arno and Feiden, *Against the Odds*, 267–72.

107. Broder Yarchoan oral history, 29

108. Broder Yarchoan oral history, 30.

109. Broder Yarchoan oral history, 32.

110. Arno and Feiden, *Against the Odds*, 177–78.

111. Arno and Feiden, *Against the Odds*, 178.

112. NIH Office of Technology Transfer, "Videx© Expanding Possibilities," 1.

113.   Arno and Feiden, *Against the Odds*, 178.

114.   Arno and Feiden, *Against the Odds*, 223.

115.   Yarchoan oral history, 36.

116.   Victoria Harden, "The NIH and Biomedical Research on AIDS," in *AIDS and the Public Debate: Historical and Contemporary Perspectives*, ed. Caroline Hannaway, Victoria Harden, and John Parascandola (Washington, D.C.: IOS Press, 1995), 35.

117.   Arno and Feiden, *Against the Odds*, 54.

118.   Arno and Feiden, *Against the Odds*, 48.

119.   Arno and Feiden, *Against the Odds*, 18.

120.   Epstein, *Impure Science*, 280–84.

121.   Epstein, *Impure Science*, 283.

122.   As Arno and Feiden note, "between 1987 and 1991 the National Cancer Institute tested 40,000 compounds at facilities in Frederick, Maryland, and Birmingham, Alabama, to see if any could disable the AIDS virus" (Arno and Feiden, *Against the Odds*, 17)—this even after AZT was licensed by the FDA.

123.   Christine Grady, *The Search for an AIDS Vaccine: Ethical Issues in the Development and Testing of a Preventive HIV Vaccine* (Bloomington: Indiana University Press, 1995), 6.

124.   See Epstein, *Impure Science*.

125.   Grady, *The Search for an AIDS Vaccine*, 6.

126.   See Marissa Mika, *Africanizing Oncology: Creativity, Crisis, and Cancer in Uganda* (Athens: Ohio University Press, 2022).

6. LOST IN TRANSLATION, 1990–2001

1.   The historian of medicine Todd Olszewski traces the ascent of "translational research" as a policy paradigm to the efforts of NIH director Donald Frederickson around the Consensus Development Program in the mid to late 1970s; see Todd M. Olszewski, "Lost in Translation: Linking Biomedical Research and Clinical Practice at the National Institutes of Health, 1977 to 2013," *Annals of Internal Medicine* 168, no. 6 (2018): 431–35. Being as it is a somewhat intuitive metaphor, "translation" had been used colloquially for decades to refer to this process. During the War on Cancer, NCI scientist-bureaucrats used it to refer to "efficient and timely translation of research results into techniques and procedures that can be used for the practical control of cancer in man"; see "National Cancer Program: The Strategic Plan" (January 1973), III-6. National Institutes of Health Office of the Director Central Files (National Archives and Records Administration II, College Park, MD [hereafter NARA II], Record Group 443, UD-06D Entry 1, Box 95). References to this interpretation of translational research, which anticipates its contemporary usage, date back to at least 1967, though the language of translation was overpowered in this period by bellicose Cold War metaphors; see Draft of National Cancer Institute Annual Report of Program Activities, 1967. National Institutes of Health Office of the Director Central Files (NARA II, Record Group 443, UD-06D Entry 1, Box 93), 238.

2.   See Jane Maienschein, Mary Sunderland, Rachel A. Ankeny, and Jason Scott Robert, "The Ethos and Ethics Of Translational Research," *American Journal of Bioethics* 8, no. 3 (2008): 43–51; and Kaushik Sunder Rajan and Sabina Leonelli, "Introduction: Biomedical

Trans-actions, Postgenomics, and Knowledge/Value," *Public Culture* 25, no. 3 (2013): 463–75.

3. Elizabeth Popp Berman, *Creating the Market University* (Princeton, NJ: Princeton University Press, 2011); Daniel Lee Kleinman, *Impure Cultures: University Biology and the World of Commerce* (Madison: University of Wisconsin Press, 2003); and Elizabeth Popp Berman, "Not Just Neoliberalism: Economization in US Science and Technology Policy," *Science, Technology, & Human Values* 39, no. 3 (2014): 397–431.

4. Edward J. Hackett, "Science as a Vocation in the 1990s: The Changing Organizational Culture of Academic Science," *Journal of Higher Education* 61, no. 3 (1990): 241–79; and Donald E. Stokes, *Pasteur's Quadrant: Basic Science and Technological Innovation* (Washington, D.C.: Brookings Institution Press, 2011).

5. Maienschein et al., "The Ethos and Ethics of Translational Research"; Mark Dennis Robinson, *The Market in Mind: How Financialization Is Shaping Neuroscience, Translational Medicine, and Innovation in Biotechnology* (Cambridge, MA: MIT Press, 2019).

6. Steven P. Vallas, Daniel Lee Kleinman, and Dina Biscotti, "Political Structures and the Making of U.S. Biotechnology," in *State of Innovation: The U.S. Government's Role in Technology Development*, ed. Fred Block and Matthew R. Keller (Boulder, CO: Paradigm, 2011), 57–76.

7. Philip Mirowski, *Science-Mart: Privatizing American Science* (Cambridge, MA: Harvard University Press, 2011).

8. Peter Keating and Alberto Cambrosio, *Cancer on Trial: Oncology as a New Style of Practice* (Chicago: University of Chicago Press, 2011).

9. Maienschein et al., "The Ethos and Ethics of Translational Research."

10. "NCI Lab and Branch Chiefs' Meeting," November 11, 1994. Videodisc recording. NLM Unique ID: 101594016 (National Library of Medicine, History of Medicine Division, Bethesda, MD) [hereafter NLM].

11. "Project CM06117-13," *National Cancer Institute Division of Cancer Treatment Annual Report, 1985, Volume I* (Bethesda, MD: U.S. Department of Health and Human Services, 1985), 312.

12. "Project CM07200-03," *National Cancer Institute Division of Cancer Treatment Annual Report, 1985, Volume II* (Bethesda, MD: U.S. Department of Health and Human Services, 1985), 478.

13. Transcript of Samuel Broder oral history, conducted by Victoria Harden and Caroline Hannaway, February 2, 1997, 13 (Oral History Archive, Office of NIH History) [hereafter Broder oral history]. https://history.nih.gov/archives/downloads/broderfeb97.pdf.

14. Broder oral history, 5.

15. Raymond S. Greenberg, *Medal Winners: How the Vietnam War Launched Nobel Careers* (Austin: University of Texas Press, 2020), 294–95; and Vincent T. DeVita, Jr., and Elizabeth DeVita-Raeburn, *The Death of Cancer: After Fifty Years on the Front Lines of Medicine, a Pioneering Oncologist Reveals Why the War on Cancer is Winnable—and How We Can Get There* (New York: Sarah Crichton Books, 2015), 233–35.

16. Broder oral history, 6.

17. Broder oral history, 6.

18. Broder oral history, 7–8.

19. "ASCO, AACR Hold Last Joint Annual Meeting, Vow to Encourage Basic-Clinical Interactions," *Cancer Letter* 19, no. 22 (May 28, 1993): 2.

20. Fax from Michael J. Bishop to Barbara Rimer (January 12, 1995), Harold Varmus papers, Box 6, Folder 8 (NLM).

21. Jon Cohen, *Shots in the Dark: The Wayward Search for an AIDS Vaccine* (New York: Norton, 2001), 182 fn. 11–13.

22. Cohen, *Shots in the Dark*, 182 fn. 11–13.

23. "Number of Clinical R01 Applications Doubles, Funding Rate Below 20 Percent; NCI Execs Not Satisfied," *Cancer Letter* 18, no. 29 (July 17, 1992): 3. The calculation is based on statistics from National Cancer Institute, *Fact Book 1993* (Bethesda, MD: U.S. Department of Health and Human Services, 1993), 61.

24. "Budget Difficulties Aside, Centers Important to NCI, Broder Asserts; Warns Against Sabotage," *Cancer Letter* 17, no. 28 (July 12, 1991): 2.

25. "Budget Difficulties Aside, Centers Important to NCI, Broder Asserts," *Cancer Letter*, 7.

26. National Cancer Advisory Board, "May 6–7, 1991 Summary of Meeting," 39 (National Cancer Institute Division of Extramural Activities, NCAB digital archive) [hereafter NCAB digital archive]. https://deainfo.nci.nih.gov/advisory/ncab/archive/index.htm.

27. "Senate Committee Adds $200 Mil. to NCI Request for FY92; Centers, Women's Health, Targeted," *Cancer Letter* 17, no. 29 (July 19, 1991): 2.

28. "Senate Committee Adds $200 Mil. to NCI Request for FY92," *Cancer Letter*, 3.

29. "Report Urges Coordination of National Cancer Program," *Cancer Letter* 20, no. 38 (October 7, 1994): 8.

30. National Cancer Advisory Board, "May 5–6, 1992 Summary of Meeting," 53 (NCAB digital archive).

31. National Cancer Advisory Board, "May 5–6, 1992 Summary of Meeting," 53.

32. Samuel Broder and Judith E. Karp, "Progress Against Cancer," *Journal of Cancer Research and Clinical Oncology* 121, no. 11 (1995): 633–47.

33. National Cancer Advisory Board, "September 21–22, 1992 Summary of Meeting," 5 (NCAB digital archive).

34. "NCI Develops Plan for Specialized Centers, but Funding $67.5M Program Depends on New $$," *Cancer Letter* 17, no. 27 (July 5, 1991): 2.

35. See Steven Epstein, *Inclusion: The Politics of Difference in Medical Research* (Chicago: University of Chicago Press, 2007), 80–81.

36. National Cancer Advisory Board, "September 21–22, 1992 Summary of Meeting," 4.

37. National Cancer Institute, *Fact Book 1992* (Bethesda, MD: U.S. Department of Health and Human Services, 1992), 76.

38. "NCI Develops Plan for Specialized Centers," *Cancer Letter*, 2.

39. "NCI Develops Plan for Specialized Centers," *Cancer Letter*, 2.

40. "NCI Develops Plan for Specialized Centers," *Cancer Letter*, 3.

41. "Report of SPOREs Cut 'Premature,' Broder Says, Wait for Peer Review," *Cancer Letter* 18, no. 11 (March 13, 1992): 6.

42. National Cancer Advisory Board, "January 25–26, 1992 Summary of Meeting," 8 (NCAB digital archive).

43. National Cancer Advisory Board, "January 25–26, 1992 Summary of Meeting," 8.

44.   National Cancer Advisory Board, "January 25–26, 1992 Summary of Meeting," 9.

45.   "Report of SPOREs Cut 'Premature,' Broder Says," *Cancer Letter*, 6.

46.   "NCI SPOREs Seen as Less than Efficacious by Varmus, Director Favors Individual Investigator Grants," *Blue Sheet* (March 2, 1994), Harold Varmus papers, Box 6, Folder 7 (NLM), 2.

47.   "NCI SPOREs Seen as Less than Efficacious by Varmus," *Blue Sheet*, 2.

48.   "NCI SPOREs Seen as Less than Efficacious by Varmus," *Blue Sheet*, 2.

49.   National Cancer Advisory Board, "September 20, 1993 Summary of Meeting," 5 (NCAB digital archive); and National Cancer Advisory Board, "May 4–5, 1993 Summary of Meeting," 3 (NCAB digital archive).

50.   "NCI SPOREs Seen as Less than Efficacious by Varmus," *Blue Sheet*, 2.

51.   "NCI SPOREs Seen as Less than Efficacious by Varmus," *Blue Sheet*, 2.

52.   National Cancer Advisory Board, "February 24–25, 1994 Summary of Meeting," 14 (NCAB digital archive).

53.   "Kripke: Translational Research Is Greatest Opportunity Today," *Cancer Letter* 20, no. 10 (March 11, 1994): 4.

54.   "NCI SPOREs Seen as Less than Efficacious by Varmus," *Blue Sheet*, 3.

55.   "NCI Director Broder's Year in Review: Avoid Politics, Stay Focused on Science," *Cancer Letter* 20, no. 41 (October 28, 1994): 4.

56.   National Cancer Advisory Board, "January 10–11, 1995 Summary of Meeting," 6 (NCAB digital archive).

57.   National Cancer Advisory Board, "January 10–11, 1995 Summary of Meeting," 48.

58.   "NCI SPOREs Seen as Less than Efficacious by Varmus," *Blue Sheet*, 3.

59.   See Natalie B. Aviles, "The Little Death: Rigoni-Stern and the Problem of Sex and Cancer in 20th-Century Biomedical Research," *Social Studies of Science* 45, no. 3 (2015): 394–415.

60.   Oral history interview with John Schiller, conducted by Natalie B. Aviles, April 22, 2015, Bethesda, MD [hereafter Schiller oral history].

61.   For an account of Frazer and Zhou's HPV research, see Gregory J. Morgan, *Cancer Virus Hunters: A History of Tumor Virology* (Baltimore, MD: Johns Hopkins University Press, 2022), 257–63.

62.   Oral history interview with Douglas Lowy, conducted by Natalie B. Aviles, February 23, 2017, Bethesda, MD [hereafter Lowy oral history].

63.   "Project CB09052-03," *National Cancer Institute Division of Cancer Biology, Diagnosis and Centers Annual Report, 1991* (Bethesda, MD: U.S. Department of Health and Human Services, 1991), 208–10.

64.   "Project CB09052-04," *National Cancer Institute Division of Cancer Biology, Diagnosis and Centers Annual Report, 1992* (Bethesda, MD: U.S. Department of Health and Human Services, 1992), 215.

65.   Reinhard Kirnbauer, et al., "Papillomavirus L1 Major Capsid Protein Self-Assembles Into Virus-like Particles That Are Highly Immunogenic," *Proceedings of the National Academy of Sciences USA* 89, no. 24 (1992): 12180–84.

66.   The recombinant subunit hepatitis B vaccine development at Merck was spearheaded by Edward Scolnick, a former intramural researcher at NCI who had collaborated with Lowy in the 1970s and 1980s before leaving for Merck.

67.   Schiller oral history.

68.   Schiller oral history.

69.   Schiller oral history.

70.   Text of Senate bill, in "Senate Bill Matches $2.01 Billion Bush Request for NCI, Sets Bypass Funding for Breast Cancer," *Cancer Letter* 18, no. 36 (September 18, 1992): 5.

71.   National Cancer Advisory Board, "December 14–15, 1992 Summary of Meeting," 29–34 (NCAB digital archive); National Cancer Advisory Board, "May 4–5, 1993 Summary of Meeting," 25–29 (NCAB digital archive).

72.   National Cancer Institute, *Fact Book 1993*, 2.

73.   Schiller oral history; Lowy oral history.

74.   Schiller oral history.

75.   Schiller oral history.

76.   Statement by Bernadine Healy, Director, National Institutes of Health, Department of Health and Human Services. Senate Select Committee on Aging (February 24, 1993). NCI Office of Government and Congressional Relations, Policy Files 1980–1999 (NARA II, Record Group 443, UD-10W Entry 9, Box 1, Folder 9).

77.   Jordan Goodman and Vivien Walsh, *The Story of Taxol: Nature and Politics in the Pursuit of an Anti-Cancer Drug* (New York: Cambridge University Press, 2001), 160.

78.   "MedImmune Begins Clinical Trial with the First Preventative Human Papillomavirus Vaccine Candidate," *PR Newswire* (February 3, 1997).

79.   Letter from Nancy B. Miller, M.D., Center for Biologics Evaluation and Research, US Food and Drug Administration. "Clinical Review of Biologics License Application for Human Papillomavirus 6, 11, 16, 18 L1 Virus Like Particle Vaccine (S. cerevisiae) (STN 125126 GARDASIL), manufactured by Merck, Inc." (June 8, 2006), 19 (FDA digital archive), https://www.fda.gov/about-fda/about-website/fdagov-archive).

80.   John T. Schiller and Douglas R. Lowy, "Papillomavirus-like Particles and HPV Vaccine Development," *Seminars in Cancer Biology* 7, no. 6 (1996): 373–82.

81.   Lowy oral history.

82.   Schiller oral history.

83.   Jon Cohen, "Is NIH's Crown Jewel Losing Luster? *Science* Examines the NIH Intramural Program and Finds Intramural and Extramural Researchers Agreeing That Strenuous Efforts Must Be Made if Excellence Is to Be Sustained," *Science* 261, no. 5125 (1993): 1120–27.

84.   "Klausner Town Hall Meeting (Extramural)," August 2, 1995. Videocassette recording. NLM Unique ID: 101593946 (NLM).

85.   "Report of the Task Force on the Intramural Research Program of the National Institutes of Health" (Klausner Report), April 1992, Donald Frederickson papers, Box 40, Folder 9 (NLM).

86.   Donald Frederickson, "The Klausner Report." Personal diary entry, September 13, 1993, Donald Frederickson papers, Box 40, Folder 9 (NLM)

87.   Cohen, "Is NIH's Crown Jewel Losing Luster," 1125.

88.   "Recommendations of NIH Scientific Directors for Implementation of the Report of the Task Force on the Intramural Program," March 1993, Donald Frederickson papers, Box 40, Folder 9 (NLM)

89.   Cohen, "Is NIH's Crown Jewel Losing Luster," 1125.

90.   "Force Stronger Peer Review, Cut Weaker Intramural Labs, Advisors Urge NIH in Report," *Cancer Letter* 20, no. 19 (May 20, 1994): 4.

91.   "Report of the External Advisory Committee of the Director's Advisory Committee, National Institutes of Health: The Intramural Program," April 11, 1994, Donald Frederickson papers, Box 40, Folder 20 (NLM).

92.   "Report of the External Advisory Committee of the Director's Advisory Committee, National Institutes of Health: The Intramural Program," Donald Frederickson papers, 2, 10.

93.   "Report of the External Advisory Committee of the Director's Advisory Committee, National Institutes of Health: The Intramural Program," Donald Frederickson papers, 15, 17.

94.   "Implementation Plan and Progress Report: External Advisors' Report on the NIH Intramural Programs" (November 17, 1994), Donald Frederickson papers, Box 40, Folder 21 (NLM), 29.

95.   National Cancer Advisory Board, "December 5-6, 1994 Summary of Meeting," 74-75 (NCAB digital archive).

96.   National Cancer Advisory Board, "A Review of the Intramural Program of the National Cancer Institute: A Report by the Ad Hoc Working Group of the National Cancer Advisory Board," June 9, 1995 (NCAB digital archive).

97.   National Cancer Advisory Board, "May 16-17, 1995 Summary of Meeting," 50 (NCAB digital archive).

98.   National Cancer Advisory Board, "May 16-17, 1995 Summary of Meeting," 51 (NCAB digital archive).

99.   National Cancer Advisory Board, "May 16-17, 1995 Summary of Meeting," 47 (NCAB digital archive).

100.   " 'Leadership Vacuum' at NCI Allows NIH to Look at Reorganization, Varmus Says," *Cancer Letter* 20, no. 38 (October 7, 1994): 1-2.

101.   "Bishop No Longer Candidate for NCI Director; HHS Endorses Intramural Scientist Klausner." *Cancer Letter*, 21, no. 16 (April 21, 1995): 1.

102.   "Klausner Town Hall Meeting (Extramural)," August 2, 1995 (NLM)

103.   "Klausner Town Hall Meeting (Extramural)," August 2, 1995 (NLM).

104.   National Cancer Advisory Board, "September 12-13, 1995 Summary of Meeting," 9-10 (NCAB digital archive).

105.   National Cancer Advisory Board, "September 12-13, 1995 Summary of Meeting," 9-10.

106.   "The New NCI: Structure, Procedures, Advisory Boards to Change, Klausner Says," *Cancer Letter* 21, no. 35 (September 15, 1995): 6.

107.   "New NCI Advisory Boards Appointed, Begin Review," *Cancer Letter* 22, no. 13 (March 29, 1996): 4.

108.   "The New NCI," *Cancer Letter*, 4.

109.   "The New NCI," *Cancer Letter*, 6.

110.   "The New NCI," *Cancer Letter*, 6; and National Cancer Advisory Board, "November 19-20, 1996 Summary of Meeting," 10 (NCAB digital archive).

111. National Cancer Advisory Board, "May 7–8, 1996 Summary of Meeting," 10 (NCAB digital archive).

112. "Raising NIH appropriations is high priority, House Subcommittee chairman says," *The Cancer Letter* 23, no. 9 (March 7, 1997), 2. See Rachel Kahn Best, *Common Enemies: Disease Campaigns in America* (New York: Oxford University Press, 2019).

113. "Specter Comes Through with 7.5 Percent Increase for NIH," *Cancer Letter* 23, no. 29 (July 25, 1997): 7.

114. "The New NCI," *Cancer Letter*, 7.

115. National Cancer Advisory Board, "November 28–29, 1995 Summary of Meeting," 24 (NCAB digital archive).

116. "UNC Oncologist Edison Liu to Direct NCI Intramural Clinical Research Programs," *Cancer Letter* 22, no. 26 (June 28, 1996): 3.

117. National Cancer Advisory Board, "June 17, 1997 Summary of Meeting," 7 (NCAB digital archive).

118. President's Cancer Panel, *Fighting the War on Cancer in an Evolving Health Care System* (Bethesda, MD: National Cancer Institute, 1997), 9.

119. National Cancer Advisory Board, "September 24, 1997 Summary of Meeting," 17 (NCAB digital archive).

120. National Cancer Advisory Board, "May 22–23, 1998 Summary of Meeting," 6 (NCAB digital archive).

121. National Cancer Institute, *Fact Book 2000* (Bethesda, MD: U.S. Department of Health and Human Services, 2000), iii.

122. National Cancer Advisory Board, "February 25–26, 1997 Summary of Meeting," 5 (NCAB digital archive).

123. National Cancer Advisory Board, "December 7–8, 1999 Summary of Meeting," 11 (NCAB digital archive).

124. National Cancer Advisory Board, "September 13–14, 2000 Summary of Meeting," 8 (NCAB digital archive).

125. National Cancer Advisory Board, "December 5–6, 2000 Summary of Meeting," 9 (NCAB digital archive); and National Cancer Institute, *Fact Book 2000*, B-4.

126. "NCI to Merge Two Intramural Divisions to form Center for Cancer Research" *Cancer Letter* 27, no. 2 (January 12, 2001): 1–2.

127. National Cancer Advisory Board, "February 13–14, 2001 Summary of Meeting," 5 (NCAB digital archive).

128. National Cancer Institute, *The Nation's Investment in Cancer Research: A Plan and Budget Proposal for Fiscal Year 2003* (Bethesda, MD: U.S. Department of Health and Human Services, 2001), 15.

129. National Cancer Advisory Board, "December 4–5, 2001 Summary of Meeting," 13 (NCAB digital archive).

130. National Cancer Institute, *The Nation's Investment in Cancer Research: A Plan and Budget Proposal for Fiscal Year 2003*, 25.

131. National Cancer Advisory Board, "September 10–11, 1996 Summary of Meeting," 9 (NCAB digital archive).

132. National Cancer Advisory Board, "November 19–20, 1996 Summary of Meeting," 10 (NCAB digital archive).

133. National Cancer Institute, *The Nation's Investment in Cancer Research: A Budget Proposal for Fiscal Year 1999* (Bethesda, MD: U.S. Department of Health and Human Services, 1997), 9.

134. National Cancer Institute, *The Nation's Investment in Cancer Research: A Budget Proposal for Fiscal Years 1997/1998* (Bethesda, MD: U.S. Department of Health and Human Services, 1996).

135. Lowy oral history.

136. Schiller oral history.

137. National Cancer Advisory Board, "December 4–5, 2002 Summary of Meeting," 33–34 (NCAB digital archive).

138. National Cancer Advisory Board, "September 12–13, 1995 Summary of Meeting," 11 (NCAB digital archive).

139. Schiller oral history.

140. Lowy oral history.

141. National Cancer Advisory Board, "December 9–10 1998 Summary of Meeting," 15 (NCAB digital archive).

142. For an analysis of trans-NIH efforts to improve clinical trial diversity, see Epstein, *Inclusion*.

143. National Cancer Advisory Board, "December 9–10 1998 Summary of Meeting," 15.

144. "NCI Health Disparities Center Describes 'Think Tank' Projects for Policy Change," *Cancer Letter* 27, no. 17 (April 27, 2001): 2.

145. National Cancer Institute, *The Nation's Investment in Cancer Research: A Plan and Budget Proposal for Fiscal Year 2003*, 49.

146. National Cancer Institute, "Report of the Gynecological Cancer Progress Review Group" (November 2001), 7. (NCAB digital archive).

147. Schiller and Lowy, "Papillomavirus-like Particles and HPV Vaccine Development," 373.

148. John T. Schiller and Denise Nardelli-Haefliger, "Second Generation HPV Vaccines to Prevent Cervical Cancer," *Vaccine* 24, suppl. 3 (August 2006): S147–S153.

149. National Cancer Advisory Board, "December 9–10 1998 Summary of Meeting," 15.

150. National Cancer Institute, *The Nation's Investment in Cancer Research: A Plan and Budget Proposal for Fiscal Year 2003*, 82.

151. National Cancer Institute, *The Nation's Investment in Cancer Research: A Plan and Budget Proposal for Fiscal Year 2005* (Bethesda, MD: U.S. Department of Health and Human Services, 2003), 27.

152. National Cancer Institute, *Division of Extramural Activities Annual Report 2003* (Bethesda, MD: U.S. Department of Health and Human Services, 2003), 157.

153. National Cancer Advisory Board, "December 4–5 2002 Summary of Meeting," 33–37 (NCAB digital archive); see also Laura A. Koutsky et al., "A Controlled Trial of a Human Papillomavirus Type 16 Vaccine," *New England Journal of Medicine* 347, no. 21 (2002): 1645–51.

154. Senate Appropriations Committee Report, in "Senate Calls Cancer Research a Priority, Cites Research Task Force Funding Goal," *Cancer Letter* 25, no. 38 (October 8, 1999): 5, 7; Senate Appropriations Committee Report, quoted in "Senate Approves 15 Percent

Increase for NIH; House Passes 5.6 Percent Raise, but Favors More," *Cancer Letter* 26, no. 27 (July 7, 2000): 4.

155.   Merck followed one small group of women who violated protocols for two years and found that a single dose of the vaccine was 97 percent effective at preventing cervical cancer surrogate end points. See "Vaccine Prevented Cervical Pre-Cancers, Non-Invasive Cancers in Phase III Trial." *Clinical Cancer Letter* 28, no. 10 (October 2005), 2.

156.   Schiller oral history.

157.   Schiller oral history; and Lowy oral history.

158.   For a discussion of unsuccessful attempts by Schiller and Lowy's lab to manufacture generics in India after TRIPS, see Natalie B. Aviles, "Situated Practice and the Emergence of Ethical Research: HPV Vaccine Development and Organizational Cultures of Translation at the National Cancer Institute," *Science, Technology, & Human Values* 43, no. 5 (2018): 810–33.

159.   See, for example, Niederhuber's testimony before the Board of Scientific Advisors on June 29, 2006, which substantially echoes the testimony Schiller gave before NCAB in December 2005. NCI Board of Scientific Advisors, "Meeting Minutes, June 29–30 2006," 7 (National Cancer Institute Division of Extramural Activities, Board of Scientific Advisors digital archive) [hereafter BSA digital archive]. https://deainfo.nci.nih.gov/advisory /bsa/bsameetings.htm.

160.   National Cancer Advisory Board, "November 27 2007 Summary of Meeting," 12 (NCAB digital archive).

161.   "Remarks on HPV Vaccines, SPORE Funds Create Controversy for NCI's Niederhuber," *Cancer Letter* 32, no. 14 (April 14 2006): 4–5.

162.   Director, National Cancer Institute, *The Nation's Investment in Cancer Research: A Plan and Budget Proposal for Fiscal Year 2008* (Bethesda, MD: U.S. Department of Health and Human Services, 2006), 7.

163.   Monica J. Casper and Laura M. Carpenter, "Sex, Drugs, and Politics: The HPV Vaccine for Cervical Cancer," *Sociology of Health & Illness* 30, no. 6 (2008): 886–99; Ilana Löwy, *A Woman's Disease: The History of Cervical Cancer* (New York: Oxford University Press, 2011); Laura Mamo and Steven Epstein, "The Pharmaceuticalization of Sexual Risk: Vaccine Development and the New Politics of Cancer Prevention," *Social Science & Medicine* 101 (January 2014): 155–65; and Keith Wailoo, Julie Livingston, Steven Epstein, and Robert Aronowitz, *Three Shots at Prevention: The HPV Vaccine and the Politics of Medicine's Simple Solutions* (Baltimore, MD: Johns Hopkins University Press, 2010).

164.   Kristen Intemann and Inmaculada de Melo-Martín, "Social Values and Scientific Evidence: The Case of the HPV Vaccines," *Biology & Philosophy* 25, no. 2 (2010): 203–13.

165.   The NIH established the Vaccine Clinical Materials Program, an FDA-compliant GMP facility for vaccine manufacture overseen by NIAID, at the Frederick National Laboratory for Cancer Research in 2006. However, the facility's production capacity is only large enough to accommodate intramural projects and small pilot programs.

166.   Kendall Hoyt, *Long Shot: Vaccines for National Defense* (Cambridge, MA: Harvard University Press, 2012).

167.   Hoyt, *Long Shot*, 32–33.

168.   Institute of Medicine and National Research Council, *Vaccine Supply and Innovation* (Washington, D.C.: The National Academies Press, 1985). See also Louis Galambos and Jane Eliot Sewell, *Networks of Innovation: Vaccine Development at Merck, Sharp and Dohme, and Mulford, 1895–1995* (New York: Cambridge University Press, 1997), 244; and Hoyt, *Long Shot*, 33.

169.   Institute of Medicine and National Research Council, *Vaccine Supply and Innovation*, v.

170.   Hoyt, *Long Shot*, 47.

7. FROM ROADMAP TO MOONSHOT, 2002–2016

1.   Stephen Hilgartner, *Reordering Life: Knowledge and Control in the Genomics Revolution* (Cambridge, MA: MIT Press, 2017); and James Mittra, *The New Health Bioeconomy: R&D Policy and Innovation for the Twenty-First Century* (New York: Palgrave MacMillan, 2016).

2.   Notable case studies include Christine Ogilvie Hendren and Sharon Tsai-hsuan Ku, "The Interdisciplinary Executive Scientist: Connecting Scientific Ideas, Resources and People," in *Strategies for Team Science Success*, ed. Kara L. Hall, Amanda L. Vogel, and Robert T. Croyle (Cham, Switzerland: Springer, 2019), 363–73; Steven Shapin, *The Scientific Life: A Moral History of a Late Modern Vocation* (Chicago: University of Chicago Press, 2009); Steven Shapin and Simon Schaffer, *Leviathan and the Air-Pump: Hobbes, Boyle, and the Experimental Life*, vol. 32 (Princeton, NJ: Princeton University Press, 1985); Charles Thorpe and Steven Shapin, "Who Was J. Robert Oppenheimer? Charisma and Complex Organization," *Social Studies of Science* 30, no. 4 (2000): 545–90; and Janet Vertesi, *Seeing Like a Rover: How Robots, Teams, and Images Craft Knowledge of Mars* (Chicago: University of Chicago Press, 2015). For a more general overview, see Edward J. Hackett, John N. Parker, Niki Vermeulen, and Bart Penders, "The Social and Epistemic Organization of Scientific Work," in *The Handbook of Science and Technology Studies*, ed. Ulrike Felt, Rayvon Fouché, Clark A. Miller, and Laurel Smith-Doerr (Cambridge, MA: MIT Press, 2017), 733–64.

3.   Pierre Azoulay, Wesley H. Greenblatt, and Misty L. Heggeness, "Long-Term Effects from Early Exposure to Research: Evidence from the NIH 'Yellow Berets,' " *Research Policy* 50, no. 9 (2021): 104332; Sandeep Khot, Buhm Soon Park, and W.T. Longstreth, Jr., "The Vietnam War and Medical Research: Untold Legacy of the U.S. Doctor Draft and the NIH 'Yellow Berets,' " *Academic Medicine* 86, no. 4 (April 2011): 502–8; and Raymond S. Greenberg, *Medal Winners: How the Vietnam War Launched Nobel Careers* (Austin: University of Texas Press, 2020).

4.   See especially Greenberg, *Medal Winners*.

5.   McDonnell uses the concept of "influence effect" to describe how socialization into the subcultures of distinctively effective niches in the Ghanian civil service instills a bureaucratic ethos in new government employees that allows these units to remain both effective and committed to the public good. See Erin Metz McDonnell, *Patchwork Leviathan: Pockets of Bureaucratic Effectiveness in Developing States* (Princeton, NJ: Princeton University Press, 2020), 55.

6.   David E. Lewis, *The Politics of Presidential Appointments: Political Control and Bureaucratic Performance* (Princeton, NJ: Princeton University Press, 2010).

7. Sean Gailmard and John W. Patty, *Learning While Governing: Expertise and Accountability in the Executive Branch* (Chicago: University of Chicago Press, 2012), 231.

8. National Cancer Advisory Board, "May 22–23, 1998 Summary of Meeting," 5 (National Cancer Institute Division of Extramural Activities, NCAB digital archive) [hereafter NCAB digital archive]. https://deainfo.nci.nih.gov/advisory/ncab/archive/index.htm.

9. National Cancer Advisory Board, "May 22–23, 1998 Summary of Meeting," 5.

10. Rachel Kahn Best, *Common Enemies: Disease Campaigns in America* (New York: Oxford University Press, 2019), 119–26; and "Senate Committee Approves 15 Percent Increase for NCI," *Cancer Letter* 24, no. 34 (September 11, 1998): 6.

11. "Bush Budget Stresses Research Now, Public Health Interventions Later," *Cancer Letter* 27, no. 15 (April 13, 2001): 1–2.

12. "Bush Budget Stresses Research Now, Public Health Interventions Later," *Cancer Letter*, 3.

13. "With NIH 'Accountability' as Background, Advocates Support Budget Increases," *Cancer Letter* 27, no. 13 (March 30, 2001): 1.

14. National Cancer Advisory Board, "September 11, 2001 Summary of Meeting," 6 (NCAB digital archive).

15. "Swearing In Ceremony for the New NCI Director Andrew C. von Eschenbach M.D" (February 4, 2002). NIH Videocast archive. https://videocast.nih.gov/summary .asp?Live=1454.

16. "Swearing In Ceremony for the New NCI Director Andrew C. von Eschenbach M.D.," comments by Bert Vogelstein (February 4, 2002).

17. "New NCI Director Plans Greater Support for Translational Research, Collaboration," *Cancer Letter* 28, no. 9 (March 1, 2002): 1, 3.

18. "Von Eschenbach's Goal: Speed the Development of Products to Benefit Patients," *Cancer Letter* 28, no. 13 (March 29, 2002): 2.

19. "Barker Named NCI Deputy for Strategic Initiatives," *Cancer Letter* 28, no. 45 (December 6, 2002): 5.

20. "National Cancer Advisory Board (NCAB) Day 1." 125th Regular Meeting of the National Cancer Advisory Board (February 11, 2003). NIH Videocast archive. https://videocast .nih.gov/watch=2202.

21. "National Cancer Advisory Board (NCAB) Day 1." 125th Regular Meeting of the National Cancer Advisory Board (February 11, 2003).

22. "NCI Director Sets a Goal: Eliminate Suffering, Death from Cancer by 2015," *Cancer Letter* 29, no. 7 (February 14, 2003): 2.

23. "NCI Director Sets a Goal: Eliminate Suffering, Death from Cancer by 2015," *Cancer Letter*, 2. Subsequent announcements of the 2015 Challenge Goal, such as to the Board of Scientific Advisors, were met with visible headshakes. See "NCI—Board of Scientific Advisors (Day 1)—Morning Session." 23rd Regular Meeting of the National Cancer Institute Board of Scientific Advisors (February 11, 2003). NIH Videocast archive. https:// videocast.nih.gov/watch=8774 (time stamp 38:21).

24. "June 2003 National Cancer Advisory Board." 24th Regular Meeting of the National Cancer Institute Board of Scientific Advisors (June 10, 2003). NIH Videocast archive. https://videocast.nih.gov/watch=8769.

25. "NCI Director Sets a Goal: Eliminate Suffering, Death from Cancer by 2015," *Cancer Letter*, 4.

26. "NCI Director Sets a Goal: Eliminate Suffering, Death from Cancer by 2015," *Cancer Letter*, 4.

27. "The 2015 Goal: Science or Science Fiction?" *Cancer Letter*, Special Report: The NCI 2015 Goal (August 12, 2003): 1.

28. See, e.g., "NCI's Use of Dialogue for NBN Blueprint Raises Legal, Procedural Questions," *Cancer Letter* 29, no. 46 (December 12, 2003).

29. "NCI—Board of Scientific Advisors (Day 1)—Morning Session." 23rd Regular Meeting of the National Cancer Institute Board of Scientific Advisors (March 3, 2003). NIH Videocast archive. https://videocast.nih.gov/watch=8774.

30. "NCI Deputy Barker Hits FDA, Calls for New Incentives for Pharmaceutical Industry," *Cancer Letter* 29, no. 22 (May 30, 2003).

31. "NCI—Board of Scientific Advisors (Day 1)—Afternoon Session." 23rd Regular Meeting of the National Cancer Institute Board of Scientific Advisors (March 3, 2003). NIH Videocast archive. https://videocast.nih.gov/watch=8772.

32. "New Grant Program to Fund Partnerships Between Academia, Industry, Non-profits," *Cancer Letter* 29, no. 11 (March 14, 2003): 2.

33. "New Grant Program to Fund Partnerships Between Academia, Industry, Non-profits," *Cancer Letter*, 2.

34. "NCI—Board of Scientific Advisors (Day 1)—Afternoon Session." 23rd Regular Meeting of the National Cancer Institute Board of Scientific Advisors (March 3, 2003). NIH Videocast archive. https://videocast.nih.gov/watch=8772.

35. "New Grant Program to Fund Partnerships Between Academia, Industry, Non-profits," *Cancer Letter*, 3.

36. "Von Eschenbach Presents His '2015 Goal' As Logical Progression of Cancer Program," *Cancer Letter* 29, no. 20 (May 16, 2003): 6.

37. "Von Eschenbach Presents His '2015 Goal' As Logical Progression of Cancer Program," *Cancer Letter*, 6.

38. "Von Eschenbach Presents His '2015 Goal' As Logical Progression of Cancer Program," *Cancer Letter*, 8.

39. "Von Eschenbach Presents His '2015 Goal' As Logical Progression of Cancer Program," *Cancer Letter*, 8–9.

40. "Von Eschenbach Presents His '2015 Goal' As Logical Progression of Cancer Program," *Cancer Letter*, 9.

41. "The Emergence of The National Dialogue On Cancer, 2000–2002: Special Report," *Cancer Letter*, Special Report: The Emergence of The National Dialogue on Cancer, 2000–2002 (August 8, 2003): 1.

42. "The Emergence of The National Dialogue On Cancer, 2000–2002: Special Report," *Cancer Letter*, 1.

43. In addition to formulating policy strategies such as the 2015 Challenge Goal without extensive input, von Eschenbach also distributed a $2 million subsidy to the American Association for Cancer Research without consultation from other NCI managers or

advisors. See "AACR Thanks NCI for Funds, Provides Platform for Von Eschenbach's 2015 Goal," *Cancer Letter* 29, no. 29 (July 18, 2003): 2.

44. See, e.g., "Karen Antman to Work at NCI on Centers, SPORE Programs," *Cancer Letter* 29, no. 40 (October 31, 2003): 2.

45. "National Cancer Advisory Board (NCAB) February 2004—Day 1." 129th Regular Meeting of the National Cancer Advisory Board (February 18, 2004). NIH Videocast archive. https://videocast.nih.gov/watch=3059.

46. "NCI Exceeds Employment Ceilings, Must Cut Personnel in FY 2004, NIH Says," *Cancer Letter* 30, no. 5 (January 30, 2004): 5.

47. "Starting Year 3, Director Plans New Management Structure," *Cancer Letter* 30, no. 8 (February 20, 2004): 10.

48. "National Cancer Advisory Board (NCAB) February 2004—Day 1." 129th Regular Meeting of the National Cancer Advisory Board (February 18, 2004). NIH Videocast archive. https://videocast.nih.gov/watch=3059.

49. In addition to those conflicts of interest pertaining to his role in the National Dialogue on Cancer, von Eschenbach at various points in his tenure as director used inappropriate communication channels and violated policies barring federal employees from giving gifts to organizations such as the FDA that had supervisory authority over their conduct; on this and skepticism toward the Challenge Goal, see "FDA Commissioner Says Science Is Far from Eliminating Cancer as a Threat," *Cancer Letter* 30, no. 6 (February 6, 2004): 2, 4.

50. Von Eschenbach in fact anticipated that in the near future, cancer-oriented public health would soon yield to personalized medicine, a move that would entirely obviate this prong of the NCI's mission; see Kirsten Boyd Goldberg, "Johnson to ASCO Members: Reconnect to Patients, Recommit to Profession," *Cancer Letter* 31, no. 20 (May 20, 2005): 3.

51. "In Odd Aftermath of McClellan's Lecture, NCI Director Forwards Note to 3,000 Staff," *Cancer Letter* 30, no. 11 (March 12, 2004): 2.

52. Kristen Boyd Goldberg, "A 2.7 Percent Increase in FY 2005 Insufficient to Cover Commitments, NCI Director Says," *Cancer Letter* 30, no. 45 (December 3, 2004): 2.

53. "The Cancer Letter Wins Journalism Awards for 'Authoritative Examination' of NCI," *Cancer Letter* 30, no. 24 (June 11, 2004): 1.

54. "NCI Board of Scientific Advisors—March 2005 (Day 2)," 30th Regular Meeting of the National Cancer Institute Board of Scientific Advisors (March 8, 2005). NIH Videocast archive. https://videocast.nih.gov/watch=3955.

55. "NCI Board of Scientific Advisors—March 2005 (Day 2)." 30th Regular Meeting of the National Cancer Institute Board of Scientific Advisors (March 8, 2005).

56. Kristen Boyd Goldberg, "Advisors Reject NCI's $89 Million Plan for Proteomics as Too Much, Too Soon," *Cancer Letter* 31, no. 10 (March 11, 2005): 10. This plan was eventually approved after major revisions, which among other things shifted funding timelines to ones deemed more reasonable to advisors (and, not coincidentally, thus ruled out promising results ahead of a 2015 Challenge Goal framework). See Kristen Boyd Goldberg, "Advisors Approve NCI's Revised Plan for $104M Proteomics Research Program," *Cancer Letter* 31, no. 27 (July 8, 2005).

57. "Onward to 2010? NCI Pledges Faster Result for More Money," *Cancer Letter* 31, no. 20 (May 20, 2005): 6.

58. Kristen Boyd Goldberg, "Senate Appropriators Endorse NCI's 'Bold Goal' for 2015," *Cancer Letter* 31, no. 29 (July 22, 2005).

59. Kristen Boyd Goldberg. "Money Would Speed Progress, NCI Says, but Backs Off Meeting 2015 Goal by 2010," *Cancer Letter* 31, no. 30 (July 29, 2005).

60. Kristen Boyd Goldberg, "Von Eschenbach's NCI: From 'Humility' to Grandiose Plans," *Cancer Letter* 31, no. 35 (September 30, 2005): 6.

61. Goldberg, "Von Eschenbach's NCI: From 'Humility' to Grandiose Plans," 7–8.

62. Goldberg, "Von Eschenbach's NCI: From 'Humility' to Grandiose Plans," 8.

63. Kristen Boyd Goldberg and Paul Goldberg, " 'Excitement' Building Toward 2015 Goal, NCI Director Says in FY07 Budget Request," *Cancer Letter* 31, no. 44 (December 2, 2005): 1.

64. Most infamous among these was Bush's patronage appointment of Michael Brown as director of the Federal Emergency Management Agency (FEMA), whose incompetence led to a botched federal response to Hurricane Katrina in 2005; see Lewis, *The Politics of Presidential Appointments.*

65. "NCI Board of Scientific Advisors—November 2005." 32nd Regular Meeting of the National Cancer Institute Board of Scientific Advisors (November 14, 2005). NIH Videocast archive. https://videocast.nih.gov/watch=4562.

66. Kristen Boyd Goldberg, "Scientists, Advocates Voice Objections to Von Eschenbach's Conflicts, 2015 Goal," *Cancer Letter* 31, no. 43 (November 23, 2005).

67. Goldberg and Goldberg, " 'Excitement' Building Toward 2015 Goal, NCI Director Says in FY07 Budget Request," 2.

68. Paul Goldberg, "DeVita: 50 Years of Stories on Cancer Wars and Skirmishes," *Cancer Letter* 41, no. 41 (November 6, 2015): 6.

69. NCI Board of Scientific Advisors, "Meeting Minutes, June 26–7 2003," 5 (National Cancer Institute Division of Extramural Activities, Board of Scientific Advisors digital archive) [hereafter BSA digital archive]. https://deainfo.nci.nih.gov/advisory/bsa/bsameetings .htm.

70. "April 17 1996 Minutes of the NIH Extramural Program Management Committee." Extramural Program Management Committee Minutes, 1986–1998 (National Archives and Records Administration II, College Park, MD [hereafter NARA II], Record Group 443, UD-12W Entry 7, Box 2), 2; and National Cancer Advisory Board, "December 4–5 2002 Summary of Meeting," 3 (NCAB digital archive).

71. National Cancer Institute, "Congressional Justification, FY 2003," 22. https://www.cancer .gov/about-nci/budget/congressional-justification.

72. National Cancer Institute, "Congressional Justification, FY 2003," 22.

73. National Cancer Advisory Board, "February 11–12 2003 Summary of Meeting," 10 (NCAB digital archive).

74. "Managing Biomedical Research to Prevent and Cure Disease in the 21st Century: Matching NIH Policy with Science." Joint Hearing Before the Committee on Energy and Commerce, U.S. House of Representatives, and the Committee on Health, Education, Labor, and Pensions (October 2, 2003), 3.

75. "NCI Exceeds Employment Ceilings, Must Cut Personnel in FY 2004, NIH says," *Cancer Letter* 30, no. 5 (January 30, 2004): 2.

76. National Cancer Advisory Board, "February 18–19 2004 Summary of Meeting," 1–2. (NCAB digital archive).

77. National Cancer Advisory Board, "February 18–19 2004 Summary of Meeting," 1 (NCAB digital archive).

78. "Von Eschenbach Presents His '2015 Goal' As Logical Progression of Cancer Program," *Cancer Letter*, 6.

79. National Cancer Advisory Board, "September 13–14, 2000 Summary of Meeting," 5. (NCAB digital archive).

80. National Cancer Advisory Board, "December 2–3 2003 Summary of Meeting," 24 (NCAB digital archive).

81. National Cancer Advisory Board, "December 2–3 2003 Summary of Meeting," 24–25 (NCAB digital archive).

82. "National Cancer Advisory Board (NCAB) December 2003—Day 2." 128th Regular Meeting of the National Cancer Advisory Board (December 3, 2003). NIH Videocast archive. https://videocast.nih.gov/watch=2913.

83. National Cancer Advisory Board, "December 2–3 2003 Summary of Meeting," 25 (NCAB digital archive).

84. "National Cancer Advisory Board (NCAB) December 2003—Day 2." 128th Regular Meeting of the National Cancer Advisory Board (December 3, 2003).

85. J. Carl Barrett, "NCI Director Dr. Andrew von Eschenbach Visits the CCR," *CCR Frontiers in Science* 3 (July 2004): 5.

86. "NCI Board of Scientific Advisors (Day 1) November 2003." 25th Regular Meeting of the National Cancer Institute Board of Scientific Advisors (November 13, 2003). NIH Videocast archive. https://videocast.nih.gov/watch=2856

87. National Cancer Advisory Board, "November 30-December 1 2004 Summary of Meeting," 2 (NCAB digital archive).

88. National Cancer Advisory Board, "November 30-December 1 2004 Summary of Meeting," 3 (NCAB digital archive).

89. President's Cancer Panel, "Translating Research to Reduce the Burden of Cancer Meeting Summary" (August 30, 2004), 6. President's Cancer Panel digital archives. https://deainfo.nci.nih.gov/advisory/pcp/pcpmeetings.htm.

90. "National Cancer Advisory Board (NCAB) September 2004—Day 1." 131st Regular Meeting of the National Cancer Advisory Board (September 14, 2004). NIH Videocast archive. https://videocast.nih.gov/watch=3380.

91. "National Cancer Advisory Board (NCAB) September 2004—Day 1." 131st Regular Meeting of the National Cancer Advisory Board (September 14, 2004).

92. National Cancer Institute, "Congressional Justification, FY 2005," 15. https://www.cancer.gov/about-nci/budget/congressional-justification.

93. "National Cancer Advisory Board (NCAB) September 2004—Day 1." 131st Regular Meeting of the National Cancer Advisory Board (September 14, 2004).

94. Robert H. Wiltrout, "NCI Director Dr. Andrew von Eschenbach Visits the CCR." *CCR Frontiers in Science* 4 (May 2005): 9.

95. "National Cancer Advisory Board (NCAB) June 2005—Day 1." 134th Regular Meeting of the National Cancer Advisory Board (June 7, 2005). NIH Videocast archive. https://videocast.nih.gov/watch=4093.

96. "National Cancer Advisory Board (NCAB) November 2006—Day 1." 140th Regular Meeting of the National Cancer Advisory Board (November 30, 2006). NIH Videocast archive. https://videocast.nih.gov/watch=5545.

97. National Cancer Advisory Board, "September 6–7 2006 Summary of Meeting," 25 (NCAB digital archive); see also "National Cancer Advisory Board (NCAB) June 2005—Day 1." 134th Regular Meeting of the National Cancer Advisory Board (June 7, 2005).

98. Translational Research Working Group, "Transforming Translation: Harnessing Discovery for Patient and Public Benefit (Executive Summary)" (June 2007), 3 (NCAB digital archive); and National Cancer Institute, *Advancing Basic, Clinical, and Translational Research: A Strategic Plan for the Center for Cancer Research* (Bethesda, MD: U.S. Department of Health and Human Services, 2007).

99. National Cancer Advisory Board, "November 30-December 1 2006 Summary of Meeting," 12 (NCAB digital archive).

100. National Cancer Advisory Board, "November 30-December 1 2006 Summary of Meeting," 12 (NCAB digital archive).

101. National Cancer Advisory Board, "December 4–5 2002 Summary of Meeting," 6 (NCAB digital archive).

102. National Cancer Advisory Board, "December 4–5 2002 Summary of Meeting," 6–7 (NCAB digital archive).

103. National Cancer Institute Board of Scientific Counselors, June 26–7 2003 Meeting minutes, 23 (FAC25160AR; Newspaper, Periodical, and Government Publication Collection, Library of Congress, Washington, D.C.).

104. National Cancer Advisory Board, "December 4–5 2002 Summary of Meeting," 3 (NCAB digital archive).

105. "National Cancer Advisory Board (NCAB) February 2004—Day 1." 129th Regular Meeting of the National Cancer Advisory Board (February 18, 2004). NIH Videocast archive. https://videocast.nih.gov/watch=3059.

106. National Cancer Advisory Board, "February 11–12, 2003 Summary of Meeting," 3 (NCAB digital archive).

107. National Cancer Advisory Board, "February 11–12, 2003 Summary of Meeting," 2 (NCAB digital archive).

108. National Cancer Institute Board of Scientific Advisors, "Meeting Minutes, June 26–7 2003," 5 (BSA digital archive).

109. National Cancer Advisory Board, "December 2–3 2003 Summary of Meeting," 24 (NCAB digital archive).

110. "NIH Roadmap Overview" (September 2003), Harold Varmus papers, Box 9, Folder 20 (Bethesda, MD: National Library of Medicine, 2003), 4.

111. "NCI—Board of Scientific Advisors—June 2004 (Day 1)." 27th Regular Meeting of the NCI Board of Scientific Advisors (June 24, 2004). NIH Videocast archive. https://videocast.nih.gov/watch=3176.

112. "NCI—Board of Scientific Advisors—June 2004 (Day 1)." 27th Regular Meeting of the NCI Board of Scientific Advisors (June 24, 2004).

113. National Cancer Advisory Board, "June 2–3 2004 Summary of Meeting," 17 (NCAB digital archive).

114. National Cancer Advisory Board, "June 2–3 2004 Summary of Meeting," 17.

115. Annie Nguyen, "Re-engineering the Clinical Research Enterprise: A Look at the Roadmap's RAID for Translational Research Core Services," *NIH Catalyst* 13, no. 1 (January-February 2005): 2.

116. "National Cancer Advisory Board." 116th Regular Meeting of the National Cancer Advisory Board (December 5, 2000). NIH Videocast archive. https://videocast.nih.gov/watch=503.

117. Mark Dennis Robinson, *The Market in Mind: How Financialization Is Shaping Neuroscience, Translational Medicine, and Innovation in Biotechnology* (Cambridge, MA: MIT Press, 2019); see also James Mittra, *The New Health Bioeconomy: R&D Policy and Innovation for the Twenty-First Century* (New York: Palgrave MacMillan, 2016), 66–71.

118. "NCI—Board of Scientific Advisors (Day 1)." 21st Regular Meeting of the NCI Board of Scientific Advisors, June 24, 2002. NIH Videocast archive. https://videocast.nih.gov/watch=1205.

119. "NCI—Board of Scientific Advisors (Day 1)." 21st Regular Meeting of the NCI Board of Scientific Advisors (June 24, 2002). NIH Videocast archive.

120. "NCI—Board of Scientific Advisors (Day 1)." 21st Regular Meeting of the NCI Board of Scientific Advisors (June 24, 2002).

121. "NCI—Board of Scientific Advisors (Day 1)." 21st Regular Meeting of the NCI Board of Scientific Advisors (June 24, 2002).

122. See NCI Board of Scientific Advisors, "Meeting Minutes, March 13, 2006" (BSA digital archive); NCI Board of Scientific Advisors, "Meeting Minutes, June 29–30, 2006" (BSA digital archive); and NCI Board of Scientific Advisors, "Meeting Minutes, November 2–3, 2006" (BSA digital archive).

123. "NCI Board of Scientific Advisors—June 2006 (Day 1)." 34th Regular Meeting of the NCI Board of Scientific Advisors (June 29, 2006). NIH Videocast archive. https://videocast.nih.gov/watch=5071.

124. "NCI Board of Scientific Advisors—March 2006." 33rd Regular Meeting of the NCI Board of Scientific Advisors (March 13, 2006). NIH Videocast archive. https://videocast.nih.gov/watch=4832.

125. "NCI—Board of Scientific Advisors (Day 1)." 21st Regular Meeting of the NCI Board of Scientific Advisors (June 24, 2002).

126. "NCI—Board of Scientific Advisors (Day 1)." 21st Regular Meeting of the NCI Board of Scientific Advisors (June 24, 2002).

127. Quoted in "Varmus: Expect Another CR for Funding Through December," *Cancer Letter* 40, no. 35 (September 19, 2014): 11.

128. National Cancer Advisory Board, "June 14 2006 Summary of Meeting," 12–14 (NCAB digital archive).

129. "Introduction: Strategic Planning and Roadmap 1.5," in National Institutes of Health, *Biennial Report of the Director, Fiscal Years 2006 & 2007* (Bethesda, MD: U.S. Department of Health and Human Services, 2008).

130. "Introduction: Strategic Planning and Roadmap 1.5," in National Institutes of Health, *Biennial Report of the Director, Fiscal Years 2006 & 2007.*

131. National Cancer Advisory Board, "June 2–3 2004 Summary of Meeting," 17 (NCAB digital archive).

132. National Cancer Institute Board of Scientific Advisors, "Meeting Minutes, June 29–30 2006," 16 (BSA digital archive).

133. National Cancer Advisory Board, "November 27 2007 Summary of Meeting," 10 (NCAB digital archive).

134. "NCI Hits Grant Targets, but Labs Feel the Pain of Budget Cuts, Director Says," *Cancer Letter* 34, no. 43 (November 23, 2007): 2–3.

135. Goldberg and Goldberg, " 'Excitement' Building Toward 2015 Goal, NCI Director Says in FY07 Budget Request," 1.

136. "Remarks on HPV Vaccines, SPORE Funds Create Controversy for NCI's Niederhuber," *Cancer Letter* 32, no. 14 (April 14, 2006): 2.

137. Kristen Boyd Goldberg, "2015 Goal Not Mentioned as NCI Faces Life After Andy," *Cancer Letter* 32, no. 23 (June 16, 2006): 5.

138. Kristen Boyd Goldberg, "NCI 'Garbage Can'—The Director's Office—Gets Makeover in Reorganization Plan," *Cancer Letter* 32, no. 44 (December 8, 2006).

139. Paul Goldberg. "Stimulus Bill Gives NIH A $10 Billion Boost Over Two Years, and $1.1 Billion for AHRQ," *Cancer Letter* 35, no. 6 (February 13, 2009): 2.

140. Goldberg, "Stimulus Bill Gives NIH A $10 Billion Boost Over Two Years, and $1.1 Billion for AHRQ," 2.

141. Fran Visco, President of the National Breast Cancer Coalition, quoted in "Funds Put Pressure on NIH to Make Rapid Decisions," *Cancer Letter* 35, no. 6 (February 13, 2009): 4.

142. Kirsten Boyd Goldberg, "New NCI Director Varmus 'Glad to Be Back,' Says Goal Is to Control Cancer Through Science," *Cancer Letter* 36, no. 27 (July 16, 2010): 7.

143. Goldberg, "New NCI Director Varmus 'Glad to Be Back,' Says Goal Is to Control Cancer Through Science," 7.

144. "NCI Town Hall Meeting—July 2010" (July 12, 2010). NIH Videocast archive. https://videocast.nih.gov/watch=9433.

145. "NCI Town Hall Meeting—July 2010" (July 12, 2010). NIH Videocast archive.

146. "NCI Town Hall Meeting—July 2010" (July 12, 2010). NIH Videocast archive.

147. Paul Goldberg. "How NCI Will Spend New Money (if It Comes)," *Cancer Letter* 41, no. 26 (July 3, 2015): 2.

148. Barack Obama, "Presidential Memorandum—White House Cancer Moonshot Task Force" (January 28, 2016). https://obamawhitehouse.archives.gov/the-press-office/2016/01/28/memorandum-white-house-cancer-moonshot-task-force.

149. "NCI Board of Scientific Advisors Meeting—March 2016." 57th Regular Meeting of the NCI Board of Scientific Advisors (March 29, 2016). NIH Videocast archive. https://videocast.nih.gov/watch=18674.

150. Matthew Bin Han Ong, "Biden's Moonshot Goals Are Flexible Enough to Be Realistic," *Cancer Letter* 42, no. 26 (July 1, 2016).

151. "NCI Board of Scientific Advisors Meeting—September 2010." 155th Regular Meeting of the National Cancer Advisory Board (September 7, 2010). NIH Videocast archive. permalink: https://videocast.nih.gov/watch=9493.

152. The NCI team had been attempting to manufacture generics and create second-generation HPV vaccines with several biotechnology and pharmaceutical companies in India; see Natalie B. Aviles, "Situated Practice and the Emergence of Ethical Research: HPV Vaccine Development and Organizational Cultures of Translation at the National Cancer Institute," *Science, Technology, & Human Values* 43, no. 5 (2018): 810–33.

153. National Cancer Advisory Board, "September 7–8, 2010 Summary of Meeting," 3 (NCAB digital archive).

154. "NCI Board of Scientific Advisors Meeting—March 2016." 57th Regular Meeting of the NCI Board of Scientific Advisors (March 29, 2016).

155. Douglas R. Lowy and Francis S. Collins, "Aiming High—Changing the Trajectory for Cancer," *New England Journal of Medicine* 374, no. 20 (2016): 1901–4.

156. Lowy and Collins, "Aiming High—Changing the Trajectory for Cancer," 1903. Lowy also discussed the importance of these vaccines in initial moonshot planning meetings with the NCI's Board of Scientific Advisors; "NCI Board of Scientific Advisors Meeting—March 2016." 57th Regular Meeting of the NCI Board of Scientific Advisors (March 29, 2016).

157. Tyler Jacks, Elizabeth Jaffee, and Dinah Singer, "Cancer Moonshot Blue Ribbon Panel Report 2016" (October 17, 2016) (NCAB digital archive). Per the timeline presented by Dinah Singer in the March 2016 BSA meeting, the panel (which had not yet been staffed) was required to submit its final report to the NCAB in August 2016; "NCI Board of Scientific Advisors Meeting—March 2016." 57th Regular Meeting of the NCI Board of Scientific Advisors (March 29, 2016).

158. "Lowy: Implementation Will Depend on NCI Funding in Fiscal Year 2017 and 2018," *Cancer Letter* 42, no. 33 (September 9, 2016).

159. "The Moonshot's Metric for Success: Avoiding a Single, Tangible Endpoint," *Cancer Letter* 42, no. 25 (June 24, 2016).

160. "The Moonshot's Metric for Success: Avoiding a Single, Tangible Endpoint," *Cancer Letter*.

161. "The Moonshot's Metric for Success: Avoiding a Single, Tangible Endpoint," *Cancer Letter*.

162. Ong, "Biden's Moonshot Goals Are Flexible Enough to Be Realistic."

163. "White House's Danielle Carnival: I'm Moving the Cancer Moonshot Forward with an All-of-Government Approach," *Cancer Letter* 48, no. 7 (February 18, 2022).

164. "CDC Contribution to National Dialogue Raises Questions About Ties with ACS," *Cancer Letter*, Special Report: The Emergence of The National Dialogue on Cancer, 2000–2002 (August 8, 2003), 20.

165. Gailmard and Patty, *Learning While Governing*; and Lewis, *The Politics of Presidential Appointments*.

166. Conor Hale, "Rising Costs at NCI Threaten to Overtake Slim Increases in Budget Appropriations," *Cancer Letter* 40, no. 13 (March 28, 2014): 8.

167. "Varmus: 'We Are Shrinking Everything' to Keep Grant Numbers Level During Cuts," *Cancer Letter* 39, no. 43 (November 15, 2013): 7.

168. For a discussion of the broad political economy of biomedicine under neoliberalism, see Kaushik Sunder Rajan, *Biocapital: The Constitution of Postgenomic Life* (Durham, NC: Duke University Press, 2006).

CONCLUSION

1. Joan Fujimura, *Crafting Science: A Sociohistory of the Quest for the Genetics of Cancer* (Cambridge, MA: Harvard University Press, 1996).

2. Robin Wolfe Scheffler and Natalie B. Aviles, "State Planning, Cancer Vaccine Infrastructure, and the Origins of the Oncogene Theory," *Social Studies of Science* 52, no. 2 (2022): 174–98.

3. To the extent it analyzes the productive capacity of the NCI, this study complements and expands upon work done by Peter Keating and Alberto Cambrosio, *Cancer on Trial: Oncology as a New Style of Practice* (Chicago: University of Chicago Press, 2011); Fujimura, *Crafting Science*; Robin Wolfe Scheffler, *A Contagious Cause: The American Hunt for Cancer Viruses and the Rise of Molecular Medicine* (Chicago: University of Chicago Press, 2019); and Scheffler and Aviles, "State Planning, Cancer Vaccine Infrastructure, and the Origins of the Oncogene Theory."

4. Donald P. Moynihan and Joe Soss, "Policy Feedback and the Politics of Administration," *Public Administration Review* 74, no. 3 (2014): 320–32.

5. Edgar Kiser, "Comparing Varieties of Agency Theory in Economics, Political Science, and Sociology: An Illustration from State Policy Implementation," *Sociological Theory* 17, no. 2 (1999): 146–70.

6. For examples of sociologists who examine principal-agent theory from such a perspective, see Julia Adams, "Principals and Agents, Colonialists and Company Men: The Decay of Colonial Control in the Dutch East Indies," *American Sociological Review* 61, no. 1 (1996): 12–28; and Isaac Ariail Reed, *Power in Modernity: Agency Relations and the Creative Destruction of the King's Two Bodies* (Chicago: University of Chicago Press, 2020).

7. Erin Metz McDonnell, *Patchwork Leviathan: Pockets of Bureaucratic Effectiveness in Developing States* (Princeton, NJ: Princeton University Press, 2020).

8. Mariana Mazzucato, *The Entrepreneurial State: Debunking Public vs. Private Sector Myths* (New York: Public Affairs, 2015).

9. For a collection of essays on the agencies that support the hidden industrial policies of the United States, see Fred Block and Matthew R. Keller, eds., *State of Innovation: The U.S. Government's Role in Technology Development* (Boulder, CO: Paradigm, 2011).

10. Fred Block, "Innovation and the Invisible Hand of Government," in *State of Innovation: The U.S. Government's Role in Technology Development*, ed. Fred Block and Matthew R. Keller (Boulder, CO: Paradigm, 2011), 20–24.

11. Karen Orren and Stephen Skowronek, *The Policy State: An American Predicament* (Cambridge, MA: Harvard University Press, 2017); and Rachel Augustine Potter, *Bending the Rules: Procedural Politicking in the Bureaucracy* (Chicago: University of Chicago Press, 2019).

12. For a discussion of these failed attempts to innovate low-cost HPV vaccine alternatives, see Natalie B. Aviles, "Situated Practice and the Emergence of Ethical Research: HPV Vaccine Development and Organizational Cultures of Translation at the National Cancer Institute," *Science, Technology, & Human Values* 43, no. 5 (2018): 810–33.

13. Josh Whitford and Andrew Schrank, "The Paradox of the Weak State Revisited: Industrial Policy, Network Governance, and Political Decentralization," in *State of Innovation:*

The U.S. Government's Role in Technology Development, ed. Fred Block and Matthew R. Keller (Boulder, CO: Paradigm, 2011), 261–81.

14. A cognate concept of "system failure" exists in economics to describe this phenomenon; see Mazzucato, *The Entrepreneurial State*, 46.

15. Daniel Carpenter and David A. Moss, "Introduction," in *Preventing Regulatory Capture: Special Interest Influence and How to Limit It*, ed. Daniel Carpenter and David A. Moss (New York: Cambridge University Press, 2013), 3.

16. Deepak Hegde and Bhaven Sampat, "Can Private Money Buy Public Science? Disease Group Lobbying and Federal Funding for Biomedical Research," *Management Science* 61, no. 10 (2015): 2281–98.

17. Etienne Billette de Villemeur, Jack W. Scannell, and Bruno Versaevel, "Biopharmaceutical R&D Outsourcing: Short-Term Gain for Long-Term Pain?" *Drug Discovery Today* 27, no. 11 (2022): 1–9.

18. Mazzucato, *The Entrepreneurial State*; Fred Block and Margaret Somers, *The Power of Market Fundamentalism: Karl Polanyi's Critique* (Cambridge, MA: Harvard University Press, 2014); and Karl Polanyi, *The Great Transformation: The Political and Economic Origins of Our Time* (Boston: Beacon Press, 1944).

19. Aviles, "Situated Practice and the Emergence of Ethical Research."

20. Steven Epstein, *Inclusion: The Politics of Difference in Medical Research* (Chicago: University of Chicago Press, 2007).

21. Jane Maienschein, Mary Sunderland, Rachel A. Ankeny, and Jason Scott Robert, "The Ethos and Ethics of Translational Research," *American Journal of Bioethics* 8, no. 3 (2008): 43–51; and Caragh Brosnan and Mike Michael, "Enacting the 'Neuro' in Practice: Translational Research, Adhesion and the Promise of Porosity," *Social Studies of Science* 44, no. 5 (2014): 680–700.

22. Scheffler, *A Contagious Cause*, 4.

23. See James Mahoney and Kathleen Thelen, "A Theory of Gradual Institutional Change," in *Explaining Institutional Change: Ambiguity, Agency, and Power*, ed. James Mahoney and Kathleen Thelen (New York: Cambridge University Press, 2010), 1–37.

24. Walter W. Powell and Paul J. DiMaggio, eds., *The New Institutionalism in Organizational Analysis* (Chicago: University of Chicago Press, 2012); and Neil Fligstein and Doug McAdam, *A Theory of Fields* (New York: Oxford University Press, 2012).

25. Donald Moynihan, "Delegitimization, Deconstruction and Control: Undermining the Administrative State," *Annals of the American Academy of Political and Social Science* 699, no. 1 (2022): 36–49.

26. Gordon Gauchat, "Politicization of Science in the Public Sphere: A Study of Public Trust in the United States, 1974 to 2010," *American Sociological Review* 77, no. 2 (2012): 167–87.

27. Raymond S. Greenberg, *Medal Winners: How the Vietnam War Launched Nobel Careers* (Austin: University of Texas Press, 2020), 294.

28. Vincent T. DeVita, Jr., and Elizabeth DeVita-Raeburn, *The Death of Cancer: After Fifty Years on the Front Lines of Medicine, a Pioneering Oncologist Reveals Why the War on Cancer Is Winnable—and How We Can Get There* (New York: Sarah Crichton Books, 2015), 233; and Greenberg, *Medal Winners*, 295.

29. Transcript of Samuel Broder oral history, conducted by Victoria Harden and Caroline Hannaway, February 2, 1997, 7–8 (Oral History Archive, Office of NIH History). https://history.nih.gov/archives/downloads/broderfeb97.pdf.

30. Kendall Hoyt, *Long Shot: Vaccines for National Defense* (Cambridge, MA: Harvard University Press, 2012).

31. Selam Gebrekidan and Matt Apuzzo, "Rich Countries Signed Away a Chance to Vaccinate the World," *New York Times*, March 25, 2021, https://www.nytimes.com/2021/03/21/world/vaccine-patents-us-eu.html?smid=tw-share.

32. For a discussion of the shifting conceptions of the social contract of science as they pertain to NIH policy, see David H. Guston, *Between Politics and Science: Assuring the Integrity and Productivity of Research* (Cambridge: Cambridge University Press, 2000).

BIBLIOGRAPHY

Abbott, Andrew. *Processual Sociology*. Chicago: University of Chicago Press, 2016.

Adams, Julia. "Principals and Agents, Colonialists and Company Men: The Decay of Colonial Control in the Dutch East Indies." *American Sociological Review* 61, no. 1 (1996): 12–28.

Argyris, Chris, and Donald A. Schön. *Organizational Learning: A Theory of Action Perspective*. Reading, MA: Addison-Wesley, 1978.

Arno, Peter, and Karyn Feiden. *Against the Odds: The Story of AIDS Drug Development, Politics, and Profits*. New York: Harper Perennial, 1992.

Aviles, Natalie B. "The Little Death: Rigoni-Stern and the Problem of Sex and Cancer in 20th-Century Biomedical Research." *Social Studies of Science* 45, no. 3 (2015): 394–415.

——. "Scientific Innovation as Environed Social Learning." In *Inquiry, Agency, and Democracy: The New Pragmatist Sociology*, ed. Neil Gross, Isaac Ariail Reed, and Christopher Winship, 231–55. New York: Columbia University Press, 2022.

——. "Situated Practice and the Emergence of Ethical Research: HPV Vaccine Development and Organizational Cultures of Translation at the National Cancer Institute." *Science, Technology, & Human Values* 43, no. 5 (2018): 810–33.

Azoulay, Pierre, Wesley H. Greenblatt, and Misty L. Heggeness. "Long-Term Effects from Early Exposure to Research: Evidence from the NIH 'Yellow Berets.'" *Research Policy* 50, no. 9 (2021): 104332.

Berman, Elizabeth Popp. *Creating the Market University: How Academic Science Became an Economic Engine*. Princeton, NJ: Princeton University Press, 2011.

——. "Not Just Neoliberalism: Economization in US Science and Technology Policy." *Science, Technology, & Human Values* 39, no. 3 (2014): 397–431.

Besley, Timothy, and Maitreesh Ghatak. "Competition and Incentives with Motivated Agents." *American Economic Review* 95, no. 3 (2005): 616–36.

Best, Rachel Kahn. *Common Enemies: Disease Campaigns in America*. New York: Oxford University Press, 2019.

Block, Fred. "Innovation and the Invisible Hand of Government." In *State of Innovation: The U.S. Government's Role in Technology Development*, ed. Fred Block and Matthew R. Keller, 1–26. Boulder, CO: Paradigm, 2011.

Block, Fred, and Matthew R. Keller, eds. *State of Innovation: The U.S. Government's Role in Technology Development*. Boulder, CO: Paradigm, 2011.

Block, Fred, and Margaret Somers. *The Power of Market Fundamentalism: Karl Polanyi's Critique.* Cambridge, MA: Harvard University Press, 2014.

Blume, Stuart. "Towards a History of 'the Vaccine Innovation System,' 1950–2000." In *Biomedicine in the Twentieth Century: Practices, Policies, and Politics*, ed. Caroline Hannaway, 255–86. Washington, D.C.: IOS, 2008.

Braun, Dietmar. "Who Governs Intermediary Agencies? Principal-Agent Relations in Research Policy-Making." *Journal of Public Policy* 13, no. 2 (1993): 135–62.

Brosnan, Caragh, and Mike Michael. "Enacting the 'Neuro' in Practice: Translational Research, Adhesion and the Promise of Porosity." *Social Studies of Science* 44, no. 5 (2014): 680–700.

Calvert, Jane. "The Idea of 'Basic Research' in Language and Practice." *Minerva* 42, no. 3 (2004): 251–68.

Cantor, David. "Radium and the Origins of the National Cancer Institute." In *Biomedicine in the Twentieth Century: Practices, Policies, and Politics*, ed. Caroline Hannaway, 95–146. Amsterdam: IOS Press, 2008.

Carpenter, Daniel. *The Forging of Bureaucratic Autonomy.* Princeton, NJ: Princeton University Press, 2001.

——. *Reputation and Power.* Princeton, NJ: Princeton University Press, 2014.

Carpenter, Daniel, and David A. Moss. "Introduction." In *Preventing Regulatory Capture: Special Interest Influence and How to Limit It*, ed. Daniel Carpenter and David A. Moss, 1–22. New York: Cambridge University Press, 2013.

Carrese, Louis M., and Carl G. Baker. "The Convergence Technique: A Method for the Planning and Programming of Research Efforts." *Management Science* 13, no. 8 (1967): B420–B438.

Carroll, Patrick. *Science, Culture, and Modern State Formation.* Berkeley: University of California Press, 2006.

Casper, Monica J., and Laura M. Carpenter. "Sex, Drugs, and Politics: The HPV Vaccine for Cervical Cancer." *Sociology of Health & Illness* 30, no. 6 (2008): 886–99.

Casper, Monica J., and Adele E. Clarke. "Making the Pap Smear Into the 'Right Tool' for the Job: Cervical Cancer Screening in the USA, Circa 1940–95." *Social Studies of Science* 28, no. 2 (1998): 255–90.

Caswill, Chris. "Principals, Agents and Contracts." *Science and Public Policy* 30, no. 5 (2003): 337–46.

Chubin, Daryl E., and Kenneth E. Studer. "The Politics of Cancer." *Theory and Society* 6, no. 1 (1978): 55–74.

Clarke, Adele, and Susan Leigh Star. "The Social Worlds Framework: A Theory/Methods Package." In *The Handbook of Science and Technology Studies*, 3rd ed., ed. Edward J. Hackett et al., 113–37. Cambridge, MA: MIT Press, 2008.

Clemens, Elisabeth, and James M. Cook. "Politics and Institutionalism: Explaining Durability and Change." *Annual Review of Sociology* 25, no. 1 (1999): 441–66.

Cohen, Jon. *Shots in the Dark: The Wayward Search for an AIDS Vaccine.* New York: Norton, 2001.

Coleman, James S. *Foundations of Social Theory.* Cambridge, MA: Harvard University Press, 1990.

Collins, Harry M. "Tacit Knowledge, Trust and the Q of Sapphire." *Social Studies of Science* 31, no. 1 (2001): 71–85.

Collins, Harry M., and Robert Evans. *Rethinking Expertise.* Chicago: University of Chicago Press, 2008.

Creager, Angela N. H. "Mobilizing Biomedicine: Virus Research Between Lay Health Organizations and the U.S. Federal Government, 1935–1955." In *Biomedicine in the Twentieth Century: Practices, Policies, and Politics*, ed. Caroline Hannaway, 171–201. Amsterdam: IOS Press, 2008.

Crewdson, John. *Science Fictions: A Scientific Mystery, a Massive Cover-up, and the Dark Legacy of Robert Gallo*. New York: Little, Brown, 2002.

Daipha, Phaedra. *Masters of Uncertainty: Weather Forecasters and the Quest for Ground Truth*. Chicago: University of Chicago Press, 2015.

DeVita, Vincent T., Jr., and Elizabeth DeVita-Raeburn. *The Death of Cancer: After Fifty Years on the Front Lines of Medicine, a Pioneering Oncologist Reveals Why the War on Cancer Is Winnable—and How We Can Get There*. New York: Sarah Crichton Books, 2015.

de Villemeur, Etienne Billette, Jack W. Scannell, and Bruno Versaevel. "Biopharmaceutical R&D Outsourcing: Short-Term Gain for Long-Term Pain?" *Drug Discovery Today* 27, no. 11 (2022): 1–9.

Easterby-Smith, Mark, Mary Crossan, and Davide Nicolini. "Organizational Learning: Debates Past, Present and Future." *Journal of Management Studies* 37, no. 6 (September 1, 2000): 783–96.

Epstein, Steven. *Impure Science: AIDS, Activism, and the Politics of Knowledge*. Berkeley: University of California Press, 1996.

——. *Inclusion: The Politics of Difference in Medical Research*. Chicago: University of Chicago Press, 2007.

Ezrahi, Yaron. *The Descent of Icarus: Science and the Transformation of Contemporary Democracy*. Cambridge, MA: Harvard University Press, 1990.

Feldman, Martha S., and Wanda J. Orlikowski. "Theorizing Practice and Practicing Theory." *Organization Science* 22, no. 5 (2011): 1240–53.

Finkielsztein, Mariusz, and Izabela Wagner. "The Sense of Meaninglessness in Bureaucratized Science." *Social Studies of Science* 53, no. 2 (2022): 271–86.

Fligstein, Neil, and Doug McAdam. *A Theory of Fields*. New York: Oxford University Press, 2012.

Frickel, Scott, and Kelly Moore, eds. *The New Political Sociology of Science: Institutions, Networks, and Power*. Madison: University of Wisconsin Press, 2006.

Fujimura, Joan. *Crafting Science: A Sociohistory of the Quest for the Genetics of Cancer*. Cambridge, MA: Harvard University Press, 1996.

Gailmard, Sean. "Multiple Principals and Oversight of Bureaucratic Policy-Making." *Journal of Theoretical Politics* 21, no. 2 (2009): 161–86.

Gailmard, Sean, and John W. Patty. *Learning While Governing: Expertise and Accountability in the Executive Branch*. Chicago: University of Chicago Press, 2012.

Galambos, Louis, and Jane Eliot Sewell. *Networks of Innovation: Vaccine Development at Merck, Sharp and Dohme, and Mulford, 1895–1995*. New York: Cambridge University Press, 1997.

Gallo, Robert. *Virus Hunting: AIDS, Cancer, and the Human Retrovirus*. New York: Basic Books, 1991.

Gauchat, Gordon. "Politicization of Science in the Public Sphere: A Study of Public Trust in the United States, 1974 to 2010." *American Sociological Review* 77, no. 2 (2012): 167–87.

Gaudillière, Jean-Paul, and Ilana Löwy, eds. *Heredity and Infection: The History of Disease Transmission*. New York: Routledge, 2012.

Goodman, Jordan, and Vivien Walsh. *The Story of Taxol: Nature and Politics in the Pursuit of an Anti-Cancer Drug*. New York: Cambridge University Press, 2001.

Grady, Christine. *The Search for an AIDS Vaccine: Ethical Issues in the Development and Testing of a Preventive HIV Vaccine.* Bloomington: Indiana University Press, 1995.

Greenberg, Raymond S. *Medal Winners: How the Vietnam War Launched Nobel Careers.* Austin: University of Texas Press, 2020.

Guston, David H. *Between Politics and Science: Assuring the Integrity and Productivity of Research.* Cambridge: Cambridge University Press, 2000.

——. "Stabilizing the Boundary Between US Politics and Science: The Role of the Office of Technology Transfer as a Boundary Organization." *Social Studies of Science* 29, no. 1 (1999): 87–111.

Hackett, Edward J. "Science as a Vocation in the 1990s: The Changing Organizational Culture of Academic Science." *Journal of Higher Education* 61, no. 3 (1990): 241–79.

Hackett, Edward J., John N. Parker, Niki Vermeulen, and Bart Penders. "The Social and Epistemic Organization of Scientific Work." In *The Handbook of Science and Technology Studies,* ed. Ulrike Felt, Rayvon Fouché, Clark A. Miller, and Laurel Smith-Doerr, 733–64. Cambridge, MA: MIT Press, 2017.

Hammond, Thomas H., and Jack H. Knott. "Who Controls the Bureaucracy? Presidential Power, Congressional Dominance, Legal Constraints, and Bureaucratic Autonomy in a Model of Multi-institutional Policy-Making." *Journal of Law, Economics, and Organization* 12, no. 1 (1996): 119–66.

Harden, Victoria A. *AIDS at 30: A History.* Washington, D.C.: Potomac Books, 2012.

——. *Inventing the NIH: Federal Biomedical Research Policy, 1887–1937.* Baltimore, MD: Johns Hopkins University Press, 1986.

——. "The NIH and Biomedical Research on AIDS." In *AIDS and the Public Debate: Historical and Contemporary Perspectives,* ed. Caroline Hannaway, Victoria Harden, and John Parascandola, 30–46. Washington, D.C.: IOS Press, 1995.

Haydu, Jeffrey. "Making Use of the Past: Time Periods as Cases to Compare and as Sequences of Problem Solving." *American Journal of Sociology* 104, no. 2 (1998): 339–71.

Hegde, Deepak, and Bhaven Sampat. "Can Private Money Buy Public Science? Disease Group Lobbying and Federal Funding for Biomedical Research." *Management Science* 61, no. 10 (2015): 2281–98.

Hendren, Christine Ogilvie, and Sharon Tsai-hsuan Ku. "The Interdisciplinary Executive Scientist: Connecting Scientific Ideas, Resources and People." In *Strategies for Team Science Success,* ed. Kara L. Hall, Amanda L. Vogel, and Robert T. Croyle, 363–73. Cham, Switzerland: Springer, 2019.

Hilgartner, Stephen. *Reordering Life: Knowledge and Control in the Genomics Revolution.* Cambridge, MA: MIT Press, 2017.

Hoffman, Beatrix. *Health Care for Some: Rights and Rationing in the United States Since 1930.* Chicago: University of Chicago Press, 2012.

Hoyt, Kendall. *Long Shot: Vaccines for National Defense.* Cambridge, MA: Harvard University Press, 2012.

Huzair, Farah, and Steve Sturdy. "Biotechnology and the Transformation of Vaccine Innovation: The Case of the Hepatitis B Vaccines 1968–2000." *Studies in History and Philosophy of Science Part C: Studies in History and Philosophy of Biological and Biomedical Sciences* 64 (2017): 11–21.

Intemann, Kristen, and Inmaculada de Melo-Martín. "Social Values and Scientific Evidence: The Case of the HPV Vaccines." *Biology and Philosophy* 25, no. 2 (2010): 203–13.

Jain, S. Lochlann. *Malignant: How Cancer Becomes Us*. Berkeley: University of California Press, 2013.

Jasanoff, Sheila. *Designs on Nature: Science and Democracy in Europe and the United States*. Princeton, NJ: Princeton University Press, 2011.

——. *The Fifth Branch: Science Advisers as Policymakers*. Cambridge, MA: Harvard University Press, 1998.

Kalyanaraman, V. S., M. G. Sarngadharan, Marjorie Robert-Guroff, Isao Miyoshi, Douglas Blayney, David Golde, and Robert C. Gallo. "A New Subtype of Human T-cell Leukemia Virus (HTLV-II) Associated with a T-cell Variant of Hairy Cell Leukemia." *Science* 218, no. 4572 (1982): 571–73.

Keating, Peter, and Alberto Cambrosio. *Cancer on Trial: Oncology as a New Style of Practice*. Chicago: University of Chicago Press, 2011.

Khot, Sandeep, Buhm Soon Park, and W. T. Longstreth, Jr. "The Vietnam War and Medical Research: Untold Legacy of the U.S. Doctor Draft and the NIH 'Yellow Berets.' " *Academic Medicine* 86, no. 4 (April 2011): 502–8.

Kirnbauer, Reinhard, F. Booy, N. Cheng, Douglas R. Lowy, and John. T. Schiller. "Papillomavirus L1 Major Capsid Protein Self-Assembles Into Virus-like Particles That Are Highly Immunogenic." *Proceedings of the National Academy of Sciences USA* 89, no. 24 (1992): 12180–84.

Kiser, Edgar. "Comparing Varieties of Agency Theory in Economics, Political Science, and Sociology: An Illustration from State Policy Implementation." *Sociological Theory* 17, no. 2 (1999): 146–70.

Kleinman, Daniel Lee. *Impure Cultures: University Biology and the World of Commerce*. Madison: University of Wisconsin Press, 2003.

——. *Politics on the Endless Frontier: Postwar Research Policy in the United States*. Durham, NC: Duke University Press, 1995.

Koopman, Colin. *Pragmatism as Transition: Historicity and Hope in James, Dewey, and Rorty*. New York: Columbia University Press, 2009.

Koutsky, Laura A., Kevin A. Ault, Cosette M. Wheeler, Darron R. Brown, Eliav Barr, Frances B. Alvarez, Lisa M. Chiacchierini, and Kathrin U. Jansen. "A Controlled Trial of a Human Papillomavirus Type 16 Vaccine." *New England Journal of Medicine* 347, no. 21 (2002): 1645–51.

Levitt, Barbara, and James G. March. "Organizational Learning." *Annual Review of Sociology* 14 (1988): 319–40.

Lewis, David E. *The Politics of Presidential Appointments: Political Control and Bureaucratic Performance*. Princeton, NJ: Princeton University Press, 2010.

Löwy, Ilana. *A Woman's Disease: The History of Cervical Cancer*. New York: Oxford University Press, 2011.

Mahoney, James, and Kathleen Thelen. "A Theory of Gradual Institutional Change." In *Explaining Institutional Change: Ambiguity, Agency, and Power*, ed. James Mahoney and Kathleen Thelen, 1–37. New York: Cambridge University Press, 2010.

Maienschein, Jane, Mary Sunderland, Rachel A. Ankeny, and Jason Scott Robert. "The Ethos and Ethics of Translational Research." *American Journal of Bioethics* 8, no. 3 (2008): 43–51.

Mamo, Laura, and Steven Epstein. "The Pharmaceuticalization of Sexual Risk: Vaccine Development and the New Politics of Cancer Prevention." *Social Science & Medicine* 101 (January 2014): 155–65.

Mandel, Richard. *A Half-Century of Peer Review: 1946–1996*. Bethesda, MD: Division of Research Grants, National Institutes of Health, 1996.

Mazzucato, Mariana. *The Entrepreneurial State: Debunking Public vs. Private Sector Myths*. New York: Public Affairs, 2015.

McCubbins, Matthew D., and Thomas Schwartz. "Congressional Oversight Overlooked: Police Patrols versus Fire Alarms." *American Journal of Political Science* 28, no. 1 (1984): 165–79.

McDonnell, Erin Metz. *Patchwork Leviathan: Pockets of Bureaucratic Effectiveness in Developing States*. Princeton, NJ: Princeton University Press, 2020.

Mettler, Suzanne. *The Submerged State: How Invisible Government Policies Undermine American Democracy*. Chicago: University of Chicago Press, 2011.

Mika, Marissa. *Africanizing Oncology: Creativity, Crisis, and Cancer in Uganda*. Athens: Ohio University Press, 2022.

Miller, Gary J. "The Political Evolution of Principal-Agent Models." *Annual Review of Political Science* 8, no. 1 (2005): 203–25.

Mirowski, Philip. *Science-Mart: Privatizing American Science*. Cambridge, MA: Harvard University Press, 2011.

Mitsuya, Hiroaki, Mikulas Popovic, Robert Yarchoan, Shuzo Matsushita, Robert Gallo, and Samuel Broder. "Suramin Protection of T Cells In Vitro Against Infectivity and Cytopathic Effect of HTLV-III." *Science* 226, no. 4671 (1984): 172–74.

Mittra, James. *The New Health Bioeconomy: R&D Policy and Innovation for the Twenty-First Century*. New York: Palgrave MacMillan, 2016.

Montagnier, Luc. *Virus: The Co-Discoverer of HIV Tracks Its Rampage and Charts the Future*. New York: Norton, 2000.

Morange, Michel. *A History of Molecular Biology*. Trans. Matthew Cobb. Cambridge, MA: Harvard University Press, 1998.

Morgan, Gregory J. *Cancer Virus Hunters: A History of Tumor Virology*. Baltimore, MD: Johns Hopkins University Press, 2022.

——. "Ludwik Gross, Sarah Stewart, and the 1950s Discoveries of Gross Murine Leukemia Virus and Polyoma Virus." *Studies in History and Philosophy of Science Part C: Studies in History and Philosophy of Biological and Biomedical Sciences* 48, part B (December 2014): 200–209.

Morgan, Kimberly J., and Ann Shola Orloff, eds. *The Many Hands of the State: Theorizing Political Authority and Social Control*. New York: Cambridge University Press, 2017.

Moynihan, Donald. "Delegitimization, Deconstruction and Control: Undermining the Administrative State." *Annals of the American Academy of Political and Social Science* 699, no. 1 (2022): 36–49.

Moynihan, Donald P., and Joe Soss. "Policy Feedback and the Politics of Administration." *Public Administration Review* 74, no. 3 (2014): 320–32.

Mukerji, Chandra. *A Fragile Power: Scientists and the State*. Princeton, NJ: Princeton University Press, 1989.

——. *Territorial Ambitions and the Gardens of Versailles*. New York: Cambridge University Press, 1997.

Mukherjee, Siddhartha. *The Emperor of All Maladies: A Biography of Cancer*. New York: Scribner, 2010.

Olszewski, Todd M. "Lost in Translation: Linking Biomedical Research and Clinical Practice at the National Institutes of Health, 1977 to 2013." *Annals of Internal Medicine* 168, no. 6 (2018): 431–35.

Orlikowski, Wanda J. "Material Knowing: The Scaffolding of Human Knowledgeability." *European Journal of Information Systems* 15, no. 5 (2006): 460–66.

Orren, Karen, and Stephen Skowronek. *The Policy State: An American Predicament.* Cambridge, MA: Harvard University Press, 2017.

Padgett, John F., and Walter W. Powell. *The Emergence of Organizations and Markets.* Princeton, NJ: Princeton University Press, 2012.

Panem, Sandra. *The AIDS Bureaucracy: Why Society Failed to Meet the AIDS Crisis and How We Might Improve Our Response.* Cambridge, MA: Harvard University Press, 1988.

Park, Buhm Soon. "Disease Categories and Scientific Disciplines: Reorganizing the NIH Intramural Program, 1945–1960." In *Biomedicine in the Twentieth Century: Practices, Policies, and Politics,* ed. Caroline Hannaway, 27–58. Amsterdam: IOS Press, 2008.

Polanyi, Karl. *The Great Transformation: The Political and Economic Origins of our Time.* Boston: Beacon Press, 1944.

Porter, Theodore M. *Trust in Numbers: The Pursuit of Objectivity in Science and Public Life.* Princeton, NJ: Princeton University Press, 1996.

Potter, Rachel Augustine. *Bending the Rules: Procedural Politicking in the Bureaucracy.* Chicago: University of Chicago Press, 2019.

Powell, Walter W., and Paul J. DiMaggio, eds. *The New Institutionalism in Organizational Analysis.* Chicago: University of Chicago Press, 2012.

Rajan, Kaushik Sunder. *Biocapital: The Constitution of Postgenomic Life.* Durham, NC: Duke University Press, 2006.

Rajan, Kaushik Sunder, and Sabina Leonelli. "Introduction: Biomedical Trans-Actions, Postgenomics, and Knowledge/Value." *Public Culture* 25, no. 3 (2013): 463–75.

Rauscher, Frank J., Jr., and Michael B. Shimkin. "Viral Oncology." In *NIH: An Account of Research in Its Laboratories and Clinics,* ed. DeWitt Stetten and W. T. Carrigan, 350–67. Orlando, FL: Academic Press, 1984.

Reed, Isaac Ariail. *Power in Modernity: Agency Relations and the Creative Destruction of the King's Two Bodies.* Chicago: University of Chicago Press, 2020.

Rettig, Richard. *Cancer Crusade: The Story of the National Cancer Act of 1971.* Lincoln, NE: iUniverse, 2005.

Rheinberger, Hans-Jörg. *Toward a History of Epistemic Things: Synthesizing Proteins in the Test Tube.* Stanford, CA: Stanford University Press, 1997.

Robinson, Mark Dennis. *The Market in Mind: How Financialization Is Shaping Neuroscience, Translational Medicine, and Innovation in Biotechnology.* Cambridge, MA: MIT Press, 2019.

Rose, Nikolas. *The Politics of Life Itself: Biomedicine, Power, and Subjectivity in the Twenty-First Century.* Princeton, NJ: Princeton University Press, 2007.

Rouse, Joseph. *Articulating the World.* Chicago: University of Chicago Press, 2015.

Sampat, Bhaven N. "Mission-Oriented Biomedical Research at the NIH." *Research Policy* 41, no. 10 (2012): 1729–41.

Sawyer, R. Keith. *Explaining Creativity: The Science of Human Innovation.* Oxford: Oxford University Press, 2011.

Schatzki, Theodore R. "On Organizations as They Happen." *Organization Studies* 27, no. 12 (2006): 1863–73.

Scheffler, Robin Wolfe. *A Contagious Cause: The American Hunt for Cancer Viruses and the Rise of Molecular Medicine.* Chicago: University of Chicago Press, 2019.

Scheffler, Robin Wolfe, and Natalie B. Aviles. "State Planning, Cancer Vaccine Infrastructure, and the Origins of the Oncogene Theory." *Social Studies of Science* 52, no. 2 (2022): 174–98.

Shapin, Steven. *The Scientific Life: A Moral History of a Late Modern Vocation*. Chicago: University of Chicago Press, 2009.

Shapin, Steven, and Simon Schaffer. *Leviathan and the Air-Pump: Hobbes, Boyle, and the Experimental Life*, vol. 32. Princeton, NJ: Princeton University Press, 1985.

Shorter, Edward. *The Health Century*. New York: Doubleday, 1987.

Sledge, Daniel. *Health Divided: Public Health and Individual Medicine in the Making of the Modern American State*. Lawrence: University Press of Kansas, 2017.

Sontag, Susan. *Illness as Metaphor*. New York: Farrar, Straus and Giroux, 1978.

Star, Susan Leigh, and James R. Griesemer. "Institutional Ecology, 'Translations' and Boundary Objects: Amateurs and Professionals in Berkeley's Museum of Vertebrate Zoology, 1907–39." *Social Studies of Science* 19, no. 3 (August 1, 1989): 387–420.

Starr, Paul. *The Social Transformation of American Medicine: The Rise of a Sovereign Profession and the Making of a Vast Industry*. New York: Basic Books, 1982.

Steinmetz, George, ed. *State/Culture: State Formation After the Cultural Turn*. Ithaca, NY: Cornell University Press, 1999.

Stokes, Donald E. *Pasteur's Quadrant: Basic Science and Technological Innovation*. Washington, D.C.: Brookings Institution Press, 2011.

Strickland, Stephen P. *Politics, Science, and Dread Disease: A Short History of United States Medical Research Policy*. Cambridge, MA: Harvard University Press, 1972.

Studer, Kenneth E. and Daryl E. Chubin. *The Cancer Mission: Social Contexts of Biomedical Research*. Beverly Hills, CA: Sage, 1980.

Swedberg, Richard. "Colligation." In *Concepts in Action: Conceptual Constructionism*, ed. Håkon Leiulfsrud and Peter Sohlberg, 63–78. Leiden: Brill, 2017.

Thorpe, Charles, and Steven Shapin. "Who Was J. Robert Oppenheimer? Charisma and Complex Organization." *Social Studies of Science* 30, no. 4 (2000): 545–90.

Tilly, Charles. *Coercion, Capital, and European States, AD 990–1992*. Cambridge, MA: Blackwell, 1992.

Turner, Stephen P. "Forms of Patronage." In *Theories of Science in Society*, ed. Susan E. Cozzens and Thomas F. Gieryn, 185–211. Bloomington: Indiana University Press, 1990.

Vallas, Steven P., Daniel Lee Kleinman, and Dina Biscotti. "Political Structures and the Making of U.S. Biotechnology." In *State of Innovation: The U.S. Government's Role in Technology Development*, ed. Fred Block and Matthew R. Keller, 57–76. Boulder, CO: Paradigm, 2011.

van Helvoort, Ton. "A Century of Research Into the Cause of Cancer: Is the New Oncogene Paradigm Revolutionary?" *History and Philosophy of the Life Sciences* 21, no. 3 (1999): 293–330.

Varmus, Harold. *The Art and Politics of Science*. New York: Norton, 2009.

Vaughan, Diane. *The Challenger Launch Decision: Risky Technology, Culture, and Deviance at NASA*. Chicago: University of Chicago Press, 1996.

——. "The Role of the Organization in the Production of Techno-Scientific Knowledge." *Social Studies of Science* 29, no. 6 (1999): 913–43.

Vertesi, Janet. *Seeing Like a Rover: How Robots, Teams, and Images Craft Knowledge of Mars*. Chicago: University of Chicago Press, 2015.

——. *Shaping Science: Organizations, Decisions, and Culture on NASA's Teams*. Chicago: University of Chicago Press, 2020.

Viergever, Roderik F., and Thom C. C. Hendriks. "The 10 Largest Public and Philanthropic Funders of Health Research in the World." *Health Research Policy and Systems* 14, no. 12 (2016): 1–15.

Voorn, Bart, Marieke van Genugten, and Sandra van Thiel. "Multiple Principals, Multiple Problems: Implications for Effective Governance and a Research Agenda for Joint Service Delivery." *Public Administration* 97, no. 3 (2019): 671–85.

Wailoo, Keith, Julie Livingston, Steven Epstein, and Robert Aronowitz. *Three Shots at Prevention: The HPV Vaccine and the Politics of Medicine's Simple Solutions.* Baltimore, MD: Johns Hopkins University Press, 2010.

Weber, Max. "Bureaucracy." In *From Max Weber: Essays in Sociology*, ed. H. H. Girth and C. Wright Mills, 196–244. Oxford: Oxford University Press, 1958.

Whitford, Josh. "Pragmatism and the Untenable Dualism of Means and Ends: Why Rational Choice Theory Does Not Deserve Paradigmatic Privilege." *Theory and Society* 31, no. 3 (2002): 325–63.

Whitford, Josh, and Andrew Schrank. "The Paradox of the Weak State Revisited: Industrial Policy, Network Governance, and Political Decentralization." In *State of Innovation: The U.S. Government's Role in Technology Development*, ed. Fred Block and Matthew R. Keller, 261–81. Boulder, CO: Paradigm, 2011.

Yi, Doogab. "Governing, Financing, and Planning Cancer Virus Research: The Emergence of Organized Science at the U.S. National Cancer Institute in the 1950s and 1960s." *Korean Journal for the History of Science* 38, no. 2 (2016): 321–49.

INDEX

GPSR Authorized Representative: Easy Access System Europe, Mustamäe tee
50, 10621 Tallinn, Estonia, gpsr.requests@easproject.com

www.ingramcontent.com/pod-product-compliance
Lightning Source LLC
Chambersburg PA
CBHW021848020426
42334CB00013B/230